CODEX ALTERNUS™

A RESEARCH COLLECTION OF
Alternative and Complementary Treatments for
Schizophrenia, Bipolar Disorder and
Associated Drug-induced Side Effects

Revised Edition

On The Cover
Rauwolfia Serpentina "Herb Against Insanity"

Photograph ©2015 Michael Balick, Steven Foster Group, Inc.

Cover design done by Julie Lundy http://www.juliekaren.com

LEGAL NOTICE

ISBN: Softcover 978-0692532430

Printed by CreateSpace, An Amazon.com Company
Available from Amazon.com and other retail outlets

CODEX ALTERNUS™

SAFE HARBOR CONTRIBUTORS

DION ZESSIN
Researcher and Writer

DAN STRADFORD
Contributor and Writer

CRAIG WAGNER
EditorAssistance

JARROD GUTMAN
Media Coordinator

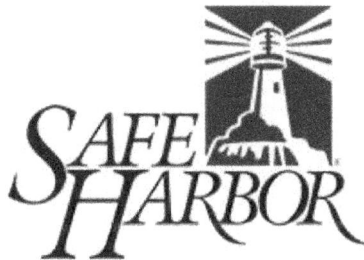

SAFE HARBOR

2333 Lincoln Avenue, Altadena, CA. 91001
Phone: (626)-791-7858   Fax: (626)-791-7867

www.AlernativeMentalHealth.com
mail@altenativementalhealth.com

This book is dedicated to all those in support of natural alternative and complementary therapies for the treatment of serious mental illness and their medication-induced side effects.

> *Behold, I will bring health and cure, and I will cure them, and will reveal unto them the abundance of peace and truth. (Jeremiah 33:6)*

Table of Contents

Foreword

It is not often that I am invited to write the introduction for a landmark publication. But that is what Dion Zessin has created, an exhaustive compendium of psychiatric research that has never been seen before as a single collection of data.

What Dion has assembled here – for the first time – are many of the pieces of one of man's greatest puzzles: "How does one fix a broken mind?"

Those in the mental health professions are only too familiar with how daunting this healing effort has been since the dawn of time.

A century ago, Emil Kraeplin, known as "The Father of Psychiatry," wrote in his classic essay *One Hundred Years of Psychiatry*, "The magnitude of the efforts to be expended on our task, the impenetrable darkness that hides the innermost workings of the brain and their relation to psychic manifestations, and finally the inadequacy of our instruments for dealing with extremely complicated issues, must cause even the most confident investigator to doubt whether it is possible to make any appreciable progress toward psychiatric knowledge and understanding."

By 1985, three decades after pharmaceuticals became the mental health treatment of choice, the "impenetrable darkness" continued to confound the efforts of psychiatrists. "What do you do when you don't know what to do?" wrote British psychiatrist R.D. Laing at the time in his book *Wisdom, Madness, and Folly*. "No wonder there are more suicides among psychiatrists than in any other profession."

In the year 2000, King County, Washington, became the first American county required by law to report on the effectiveness of its mental health department. Their first report in 2001 showed that, of 9302 patients treated, only five could be classified as "recovered." The report for 2002 showed similar results. As a result of making this information public, King County was ridiculed by mental health advocates across the country as the poster child for psychiatry's inability to effectively treat mental illness. King County no longer reports the recovery rates of its patients.

Clearly much of the "impenetrable darkness" remains.

Psychiatric jargon has changed. Patients are treated humanely, by and large. The mentally ill receive disability payments. The general public has a much better understanding of bipolar disorder, depression, autism. Modern meds control symptoms for some though the side effects are debilitating for many.

But the impenetrable darkness that hides the innermost workings... the causes and remedies of these terrible warpings of the mind and behavior...ah, that remains as elusive as ever.

Or does it?

Since the advent of the germ theory of disease, medical specialties, including psychiatry, have hunted their own magic bullets for the causes of the ills they encounter. If bacterial diseases can be wiped out in one fell swoop, why not schizophrenia and depression? When Freudian theory failed to deliver for psychiatry in the first half of the twentieth century, pharmaceuticals became (and remain) the carrot just out of reach, promising some relief now and a cure in some distant tomorrow.

However, as Dion's work in this volume clearly shows, there is no magic bullet. If there were, it would not be necessary for researchers to investigate such a broad variety of treatments to reduce symptomology in the mentally unwell. And remarkably, so many modalities, even those from primitive times, work to some degree!

What this research shows is that the human mind has numerous components – physical, psychological, spiritual, energy flows, and, no doubt, others. Understanding this, we can see that the mind can be deranged through one or more of these components. Conversely, we can see that the healing of the mind would have to occur by addressing these same components.

And each component has a cornucopia of avenues through which it can be addressed! Just look at the list of physical treatments that Dion has compiled. And this does not include the massive collection of medical issues that can cause mental disorders (another subject where Dion has created historic research compilations and published them). Seeing this vast array of physical treatments – herbs, nutrients, exercise, yoga, treating medical issues, etc., etc. – this alone tells us that MANY factors derange the mind and there are MANY avenues to fixing it.

We can also see that no single treatment works for everyone so each person needs a tailor-made treatment program for his/her particular needs and individuality – a program that will likely need to be readjusted as the person works his/her path to healing.

We also see that the health of the mind is the result of the net sum of the influences upon it. Certainly one issue – such as celiac disease (gluten intolerance) – can cause a mental disorder. But sometimes it may be many issues. Or that person with celiac can be made to feel better or worse by many other influences. That person's ability or willingness to stick to a gluten-free diet can be improved or weakened by many factors.

Thus, it is worth looking for the cause of the disorder, since many causes have been identified. And even if we cannot find the cause of the disorder, *we may be able to raise the person's wellness level through many other means until the individual can rise above the disorder or the disorder simply heals on its own through the person's improved general health.*

This multitudinous approach, this giant tool box, this awareness that our mind is not a single-piece puzzle – THIS is what Dion's work brings to the psychiatric profession – in minute detail. It is, in my experience, the keys to the kingdom of healing.

When I first met Dion Zessin, our nonprofit Safe Harbor was one of the only mental health organizations educating the public and medical field on the many medical problems that can cause mental disorders. This has been one of the topics we have monitored and specialized in since our inception in 1998. At the time Dion contacted us, the best compilations in the world listed perhaps 300 medical problems that could cause mental issues.

Dion, working on his own, had compiled a list double that size and sent it to me. I was shocked. I am an expert in this field and I've worked with many of America's other experts and I'd never seen such a collection. Working as a Safe Harbor volunteer, Dion has since built that list to 1500 through his research – with full journal citations – and promises he has more coming.

This man has put in thousands of hours doing what no medical researcher in the world has done. He has gathered up, in a few documents, a sizable and never-before-seen share of humanity's hard-won knowledge of what harms – and importantly, what heals – the mind. I thank him every time he stuns me with yet another of these astounding gifts to mankind and the medical field.

I don't think it is overstating the matter to say that, used wisely and intelligently by practitioners and researchers alike, this single volume in front of you could significantly impact our civilization by opening the door to a true renaissance in mental health treatment.

I will say it once more: Thank you, Dion.

Dan Stradford
President and Founder
Safe Harbor
Altadena, California

Preface

Codex Alternus is a research collection of citations and summaries of articles on alternative and complementary therapies for schizophrenia, bipolar disorders, and associated drug-induced side effects. It represents both old and new, novel and experimental therapies that researchers and clinicians may want to utilize in their practice, laboratory, or clinical trial. The Codex citations and summaries are organized by therapy class, disease category, or medical condition.

Codex Alternus is about the plethora of research and therapies that is available for persons suffering from psychotic or affective disorders. It offers approximately 900 citations and summaries on CAM therapies for treatment of schizophrenia, bipolar disorder, and medication-induced side effects. From this the reader will gain insight into the number of therapies available for treatment of psychotic, affective disorders and/or related conditions and will learn of the therapeutic efficacy of some of these therapies from case reports and clinical trials. This book best serves clinicians and researchers. However, patients and their care givers can benefit from therapies listed in the Codex if caution is taken and proper research is conducted before utilizing chosen therapy.

In 1995, after my first visit to a psychiatrist, being prescribed Depakote for Bipolar Disorder and gaining 30 pounds in a couple short months, was the first time I considered using natural medicine for mental health related conditions. Years later, after a serious mental breakdown and being hospitalized for a considerable amount of time, it was time to give natural medicine and lifestyle changes another consideration. Having research skill from past life experiences in forestry, law, and general psychiatritry; I started researching holistic medicine for mental health in the state hospital. When I returned to society, I continued my research, bought many books on alternative medicine for mental health and used the Safe Harbor database to learn more. I also became interested in somatopsychic disorders, the consumer/survivor/ex-patient movement, and iatrogenic injury from psychotropic drugs. These things furthered my interest in CAM therapies for the treatment of psychotic disorders and other mental illnesses.

Though I have no medical background, and little college education, I have extensive life experience as a psychiatric patient who has been surrounded by both allopathic and holistic mental health professionals. I have learned a lot from them and have learned much on my own. As an avid bookworm, I have been researching PubMed, EBSCO host, Web of Science, Google Scholar and Cochrane databases for 10 years. I have sorted through an estimated 1.0 million articles in the past 10 years. I have compiled exhaustive lists and research on somatopsychic disorders, environmental disorders (toxins), as well as alternative and complementary medicine for all types of psychiatric conditions. I correspond with a small network of like-minded researchers, doctors, social workers, lawyers, and friends, with whom I share these unconventional therapeutic ideas and theories. Even though I lack a formal college education in mental health or medicine, researchers and integrative clinicians have learned from and used the ideas and information I share in the laboratory and in academic research. Moreover, some authors have used my research to further their own publications.

I chose to research and compile the Codex Alternus directory because I needed to research therapies for my own healing and also wanted to help others. I find researching new and novel mental health therapies exhilarating because I feel I have found something few conventional doctors have explored and may be helpful in my own pursuits. I feel others may feel the same way when new information is presented providing them with more treatment options. This directory may also help researchers for clinical trials, integrative physicians, psychologists, social workers, holistic psychiatrists, as well as patients, and their care givers. For me, researching Codex Alternus is a therapy in itself; it keeps me busy, it keeps my mind off my problems and it helps condition my brain muscles.

Most of my research for Codex Alternus was carried out using a home laptop computer. PubMed was the primary database used for most of the research; however some research did come from Google Scholar. Initially, while conducting an extensive search for medical disorders that cause psychiatric symptoms on PubMed, I searched over approximately 355,000 citations and abstracts and retrieved some of these CAM medicine citations. However, you can't retrieve all these CAM medicine references with a general query. PubMed does not link all related citations together, or neither can they be found in a general search. Moreover, if you don't know what you're looking for it's hard to find that "unknown" therapy. So, the searching was exhaustive at times.

Research for Codex Alternus included additional queries and broad searches to gather information. It took hundreds of hours and putting the research into a directory; tedious work which is not complete. I hope you will find this Revised Edition useful despite the lack of resources on the usage and negative side effects of the therapies listed.

My hopes for the book of Codex Alternus: Revised Edition are to be massively circulated and known as a comprehensive research collection for CAM and non-drug therapies for psychotic and bipolar affective disorders, and medication-induced side effects. I believe there are a lack of authors in this area of concern that write about CAM treatments and other forms of unconventional medicine. My hope is that this issues will be used to help those suffering with psychotic and bipolar affective disorders.

Acknowledgments

The making of Codex Alternus and the discovery of new therapies which were unfamiliar to me before this reseach, has been exhausting and exhilarating. In the beginning, Codex Alternus started as a 20 page document in the fall of 2011. By 2012, the document grew to 40 pages, then 88 pages by 2014. In February 2015, Codex Alternus grew to over 300 pages of condensed citations and summaries. We now have nearly 500 pages of citation and summaries that are in this edition.

As the document grew, along the way the people who helped were Safe Harbor's CEO, Dan Stradford—who helped name the document Codex Alternus. He has also published several of my documents prior to the official Codex Alternus book.

I would like to thank Safe Harbor for having so much information on alternatives for mental illness available to the public. It has been a blessing having an outlet to publish and post my work. I would also like to thank members of the Safe Harbor list serve for helping with questions I had while researching this book.

Safe Harbor volunteer, Craig Wagner was a great help. He helped edit, structure and produce Codex Alternus: Depression and Anxiety Spectrum Disorders. He also worked very hard on restructuring Codex Alternus: A Research Collection of Alternative and Complementary Treatments for Schizophrenia, Bipolar Disorder and Associated Medication-induced Side Effects. He has done some minor writing and editing to the first introduction that was written, plus edited the summaries in the main document. He also provides technical assistance for Word documents in production of the book.

Further gratitude goes to David Moyer, LCSW for his assistance in technical advice for a few of the articles that were out of the ordinary. Also, for his help promoting Codex Alternus in his books and seminars. Thanks also goes to Safe Harbor volunteer Jarrod Gutman for promotion of Codex Alternus through Safe Harbor. Thanks to Robert Whitaker of Mad in America for the publication of Codex Alternus and special thanks to their supporters for taking time to review the manuscript. Sincerest thanks to Robyn Sederstrom from informing me of errors I had in the book. That was very important.

Appreciation goes to Martha Grenzeback and the Interlibrary loan staff at the Omaha Public Library for filling so many ILL requests of journals and books in a timely manner. Thanks also goes to library staff at University Nebraska Medical Center, McGoogan Library, Creighton Health Sciences Library for procurement of journal articles, and the University of Nebraska—Omaha (UNO) Criss Library for filling journal requests.

Many thanks goes to Shawn Woodman Esq. for copyright consulting and social support during the research and writing process. I would also like to thank Kara Goddard for information about technical writing and editing syntax in the book. Thank you to my mother

Diane King for support while I was researching these therapies and writing Codex Alternus. Also, I would like to thank Community Alliance in Omaha, Nebraska for their work receiving an enrichment grant, which was used for a new laptop computer and laser printer for research purposes.

Though all the information provided by these people did not make into this issue—I am very grateful for their assistance. Gratitude goes out to Dr. Chanel Heermann for providing advice on mal-practice insurance and liability for integrative psychiatrists, and providing information on how to evaluate clinical trials. I am grateful for Dr. Garry Vickar, who also provided information about orthomolecular treatments of inpatients. Hopefully my next book will provide the information these people provided.

Rosemary Reiss, Technical Library Assistant from David D. Palmer Health Sciences Library, was of great help finding articles on chiropractic sanitariums. Anna Mullen from the Museum of Osteopathic Medicine was of great help finding articles on osteopathic sanitariums. Leslie Ching D.O. was of great assistance in helping find information on osteopathic sanitariums. I would also like to also thank Dr. James Whorton and psychotherapist Will Hall, MA, DiplPW for granting permission to use their articles in the book.

Would like to thank Julie Lundy of http://www.juliekaren.com for her work on the cover art and Safe Harbor contributor's page and inner art work. She doses great work.

I would like to thank God for the blessings often forgotten, and the fact I am not hospitalized and able to do this research and write this book.

Best wishes to all those consumers/survivors/ex-patients that are either using CAM therapies or thinking about using CAM therapies, and becoming psychotropic drug-free. The combination may be your best alternative.

Thanks to all the readers who make this worthwhile.

Be Well,

Dion Zessin
- *Safe Harbor*
  Volunteer Researcher

Introduction

Definition of CAM Medicine

Complementary and alternative medicine (CAM) is the popular term for health and wellness therapies that have typically not been part of conventional Western medicine. Complementary means treatments that are used along with conventional medicine. Alternative means treatments used in place of conventional medicine. CAM focuses on the whole person and includes physical, emotional, mental and spiritual health. For example, CAM includes mind-body medicine (such as meditation, acupuncture and yoga), manipulative and body-based practices (such as massage therapy and spinal manipulation), and natural products (such as herbs and dietary supplements).

Definition of Non-Pharmaceutical Therapies

In this book—the Codex Alternus defines non-pharmaceutical therapies as primary non-psychological. However, included are a limited number of psychological non-drug therapies such as mindfulness, imagery, hypnosis, meditation, and several others. These items are typically considered CAM therapies. Codex Alternus focus is primarily on CAM therapies but other non-pharmaceutical allopathic and alternative therapies have been included. Some include oxygen therapy, hyperbaric oxygen therapy, hemodialysis, and transcranial direct current stimulation, among others.

Scope of Inclusion

Codex Alternus citations and summaries are procured from PubMed and Google Scholar databases. PubMed is a database of more than 23 million citations for biomedical literature from MEDLINE, life science journals, and online books. This document is a compilation of PubMed citations and other citations that meet the following criteria:

> **Time.** Citations occur between January 1850 to July 2015

> **Non-drug psychiatric therapy focus.** Citations are for studies that demonstrate or suggest the efficacy of alternative and complementary, or primarily non-psychological, non-drug psychiatric treatments—those treatments that fall outside the domains of pharmaceuticals, counseling, and other mainstream psychiatric therapies.

> **Psychiatric and EPS diagnoses.** The studies associated with the citations address one or more of the following psychiatric diagnoses: schizophrenia, schizoaffective disorder, typical psychosis and tardive psychosis, bipolar I

disorder, bipolar II disorder, and extrapyramidal symptoms including tardive dyskinesia, orofacial dyskinesia, tardive dystonia, akathisia, parkinsonian-- tremors, motor tics, and tremors.

> **Drug-induced Side Effects.** The studies include citations on alternative treatments for neuroleptic-malignant syndrome, metabolic syndrome, insulin resistance, cardiac disease prevention, sexual dysfunction prevention, weight gain prevention, polydipsia treatment, dyslipidemia treatment, homocysteine treatment, hypersalvation treatments, hyperprolactinemia treatments, and amenorrhea treatments, drug-induced constipation, GI upset, nausea and vomiting treatments, lithium side effect treatments and valproic acid toxicity prevention.

Methods

Articles were located by doing a computerized literature search of PubMed from 1950 up to January 2015 using the search terms "schizophrenia" OR "psychotic disorder" OR "psychosis" OR "bipolar disorder" OR "mania" OR "manic-depression" OR "tardive dyskenisia" OR "tardive dystonia "OR "neuroleptic-induced parkinsons" OR "akathisia" OR "extrapyramidal symptoms" OR any "psychiatric diagnostic terminology that was relevant for this research" in combination with a range of alternative and complementary therapies and other unconventional therapies. There were also broad searches done with these terms using generic terms as queries (e.g. alternative, natural, herbal, complementary, etc.). The clinical trial studies included in Codex Alternus: Revised Edition was not evaluated for insufficient data, small samples sizes, and or adequate control size. The author felt this compilation of research, as such, summarize relevant findings in respect to possible therapeutic outcomes despite variations in clinical trial designs. The case reports included were based on novelty and each one was not securitized for its methodology. The search did have language limits, but English abstracts of articles written in foreign languages were included. Some documents are written in Chinese, German, Russian, French, Dutch, Spanish, etc., but most are English.

This book, even though it contains 900 citations on alternative and complementary treatments, has several weak areas in research. There are few citations on CAM therapies for schizophrenia on anxiety, insomnia, depression and substance abuse. These topics have to be researched separately. This document does not include family therapy, occupational therapy, nicotine therapies, CBT, web support based programs, psychoeducation, group therapy, or peer support citations. Left out were documents from Chinese and Japanese medical databases, which contain more information on traditional Chinese medicine and Kampo medicine for schizophrenia and bipolar disorder.

More about the Codex Alternus:

This book is primarily intended for use by clinicians and researchers due to its complex language and lack of detail on therapy usage. It can be useful to those with psychiatric diagnosis and their supporters if further individual study is undertaken. It is a valuable resource for those seeking clinical efficacy of alternative treatments for schizophrenia and bipolar disorder that choose to not use psychiatric drugs. This resource is also useful for those who are forced used psychiatric drugs, and are aware of iatrogenic harm, and are interested in methods in reducing harm, or treating dyskinesia's, dystonia, akathisia, atypical antipsychotic-induced weight gain, treating dopaminergic supersensitivity. However, some of these therapies have only been utilized in research settings—clinical outcome may vary, and clinical use may be limited for some therapies. Further, there are several therapies which can only be obtained by doctors' prescription and made in a compound pharmacy. Others may have to be ordered through special pharmacies or chemical suppliers. It is mostly advisable for many patients seeking use of natural health products and other herbal forms of therapy to consult the advice of an experienced clinician before attempting to use these therapies. Further, some of these therapies have had negative clinical trials that have shown them insufficient in the majority of patients tested; however they have demonstrated positive results in some clinical trials, and case reports, so they have been included in this book. Some may even exacerbate certain psychiatric conditions. Please do your homework before utilizing some of these therapies.

> ➤ **Intent of this document for clinicians and researchers:** this document was designed to inform clinicians and researchers on as many possible alternative and complementary options available to the professional as possible. It may further enhance the clinicians' therapeutic toolbox. Further research may be needed to evaluate each therapy and its safety and therapeutic efficacy. It may also aid a reference tool for researchers doing clinical trials and clinical research.

This book contains references to Ayurvedic medicine, Kampo medicine, and Chinese traditional medicine as well as alternative medicine used in the Western world such as orthomolecular medicine. Other non-invasive therapies such as neurofeedback, biofeedback, dark therapy, and sound therapy, and many, many more are included. There are also neuroprotective treatments that can be found in current psychiatric and medical scientific literature, including treatment to reverse structural atrophy of the brain, and help reduce the oxidative damages of neuroleptic drugs. There is a very long section on natural herbal and peptide antipsychotics in the book. These are some of the many alternative and natural treatments that improve the outcome of schizophrenia and bipolar disorder that have been validated by scientific literature. All these and more are included in this book.

How to Use This book

On each citation there is a PMID number. This is a PubMed identification number. Go to http://www.ncbi.nlm.nih.gov/pubmed and in the search box enter the PMID number of the citation you are reviewing. This will take you directly to that citation and abstract (if there is an abstract). From the PubMed citation or abstract you may be able to directly access the publishers of your document. Then you may be able to order the article for a fee. However, there are free methods of obtaining documents. See next paragraph for details.

On almost each citation there is a digital object identifier number (DOI number). You can search http://www.crossref.org/ and enter your DOI number. CrossRef's database has 74 million records for authors, titles, DOIs, ORCIDs, ISSNs, FundRefs, license URIs, etc. You can even paste entire references into the search box and discover their DOIs. Using crossref.org you can access your article directly from the journal publishing the article through the DOI number.

From Google, Bing, or Yahoo you may be able to find your document by entering the long DOI number into the search box. But this method may bring up unrelated results of articles using your DOI as a reference. It is much easier to use the PMID numbers or Crossref.org.

Some citations have ISSN numbers and they can be found at http://www.crossref.org/. There are also several citations with web addresses and you will have to either Google the citation or put the address in the browser to find the article.

To make best use of this book search Google Scholar for your document. It may be located on Google Scholar for free. If that doesn't work, or if you have numerous documents to procure use your local public library, college library, or university medical school library to order the document you are interested in by interlibrary loan. Often this can be done from your home via the internet from the libraries home page via WorldCat https://www.worldcat.org/ and a library card ID number. If you have a medical school, or nursing school near your residence or place of business, it would be recommended if you are acquiring numerous articles to use their databases for free. If you are a student, or medical student your local college, nursing school, or medical library will provide articles either for free or at a drastically reduced price. They often only charge for copies and print outs.

These journal articles and case reports contain more information than what is listed in this document— dosages, contact names, e-mail addresses, supplier information, etc., etc. Hope you find this book useful.

Countercultural Healing: A Brief History of Alternative Medicine in America

By James Whorton M.D. Reprinted with permission by James Whorton M.D.

So explosive has been the growth of interest in complementary and alternative medicine (CAM) over the last decade, one could easily draw the conclusion that unconventional approaches to healing must be a new phenomenon in American society. In fact, the current surge of enthusiasm for unorthodox treatments is merely the latest of three waves of popularity in the past century-and-a-half (the first was the mid-1800s, the second the early 1900s). And although it is true that the present environment differs in certain critical respects from previous cycles, there are still more ways in which historical patterns are mirrored by the interest in CAM today. It is therefore vital to have some familiarity with the historical background of unconventional medicine in order to understand our contemporary situation.

Unorthodox systems of medical treatment were first developed in Europe and the United States in the late 1700s; by 1850, Americans dissatisfied with conventional medicine could choose from among Thomsonianism (which employed botanical drugs and steam baths), hydropathy (which used various applications of cold water), magnetic healing (which relied on hypnotism and suggestion), and a number of other schemes. Most popular of all—comparable in scale to chiropractic today--was homeopathy, which prescribed drugs that were supposed to cure by duplicating the symptoms experienced by the patient, a form of "like cures like" ("homeopathy" is derived from the Greek roots omeos, or "similar," and pathos, or suffering; homeopathy thus means using treatments that are "like the disease"). Following the Civil War, a second generation of unorthodox systems emerged: osteopathy in the 1870s, and chiropractic and naturopathy in the 1890s. Many more alternative methods would establish a foothold in the twentieth century, most notably massage therapy and, since the 1970s, acupuncture.

From the beginning, doctors utilizing unconventional methods were dismissed by orthodox medicine as unscientific pretenders, and were collectively branded "irregular practitioners" ("alternative practitioners" would not become the common designator until the 1970s). Not surprisingly, through the entire nineteenth century and all but the last quarter or so of the twentieth, relations between MDs and irregulars were hostile. Venom flowed through all their exchanges with one another. In the mid-1800s, for example, a regular physician addressed the question of what should be the attitude of true medicine toward homeopathy. "It should be that of abomination, loathing and hate," he declared; "It should be considered the unclean thing--foul to the touch, wicked and treacherous to the soul...the death of every upright principle." In reply, a homeopath voiced his profession's feelings about regulars: "Spurn them beneath your feet as foul and slimy reptiles," he urged. "Dogs may return to their vomit, and sows to their wallowing in the mire," but homeopathy must never return to orthodox methods, "the chaos from whence it came forth."

(It was the founder of homeopathy, Samuel Hahnemann, who coined the term allopathy, from Greek words meaning "different from the disease," as a label for conventional medicine. "Allopathic medicine" has been revived and come into common use in recent years as a synonym for mainstream medicine, and many MDs today accept the designation uncomplainingly; in the nineteenth and early twentieth centuries, however, regular practitioners bitterly resented the name, as it implied their medicine was just one more "pathy," no more valid than homeopathy or naturopathy).

Conflict between regulars and irregulars has been a war not just of words, but of action too. Establishment medicine has striven all along to suppress alternative practitioners by pressing legal authorities to arrest, fine, and jail them as threats to public safety for practicing medicine without a license; as a result, many irregular doctors have indeed paid hefty fines and/or spent time in jail. In return, they have struck back forcefully. On one hand, they have successfully campaigned for legislation granting them legal standing in states throughout the union. On the other, they have refined a public image of being superior care givers that has proved very attractive to American consumers. It is an image drawn from a distinctive medical philosophy crafted in the early nineteenth century, and held in common by alternative practitioners of all stripes ever since. In considering the tenets of that philosophy, one can see several telling parallels between the irregular medicine of the past and the alternative medicine of today.

The emergence of irregular medicine in the late 1700s was encouraged first of all by the perceived ineffectiveness, even danger, of conventional allopathic therapies. Standard treatment up to the middle of the 1800s was centered on evacuation of morbid matter from the body through blood-letting, vomiting, purging of the bowels, blistering of the skin, and similar depletive measures. There were theoretical justifications for such therapies, physicians believed, but to observers guided only by common sense, they appeared useless if not murderous. The most frequently prescribed drug of all, for instance, was the purgative calomel, a mercury compound that caused ulceration of the gums, loss of teeth, and, in some cases, destruction of the jawbone. Even MDs acknowledged that "the mercurial treatment" left the sick "maimed and disfigured," objects "of pity and horror" not unlike cancer patients who a century and more later would be subjected to chemotherapy. Similarly, today a significant factor in the appeal of alternative medicine is public fear of the side effects of not just cancer drugs, but pharmaceuticals in general.

People are also drawn to alternative medicine today in hope of assistance for conditions that often are not curable by conventional medicine. Cancer, diabetes, AIDS, and other afflictions are the modern equivalents of the lethal infectious diseases that ravaged the country in the 1800s and early 1900s. Particularly important for encouraging nineteenth-century Americans to look to irregulars for help was Asiatic cholera, an acute intestinal infection that invaded the United States in epidemic waves in the early 1830s and late 1840s. Cholera killed through dehydration, so absolutely the worst thing to do to a cholera patient was to administer bleeding, vomiting, and purging. Standard treatment reinforced the effects of the disease, no doubt sometimes killing people who otherwise would have survived, and allopaths' obvious impotence when faced with cholera—or yellow fever or typhus or other epidemic infections—drove patients to irregulars. They, at least, did not make the situation worse.

They did not make it worse, irregular doctors believed, partly because their treatments were gentle and non-toxic, but fundamentally because they acted in concert with nature. Alternative doctors throughout the past two centuries have identified themselves as practitioners of "natural healing," by which they have meant they use remedies and procedures that support and stimulate the healing power of nature, the innate tendency of the body to react to illness and work to restore itself to equilibrium and wholeness. As the botanic healer Samuel Thomson announced in the 1820s, his approach had "always been...to learn the course pointed out by nature," then to provide "those things best calculated to aid her in restoring health." Compare that position to the first principle of naturopathic medicine as stated in 1999: "Naturopathic physicians believe that the body has considerable power to heal itself. It is the physician's role to facilitate and enhance this process with the aid of natural, nontoxic therapies." These are sentiments that have been expressed as bedrock philosophy by the proponents of every alternative approach to healing from the 1700s through to the present.

There has also been a consistent response from regular physicians throughout the history of alternative medicine, that the cures attributed to natural remedies are in truth nothing more than demonstrations of the power of a patient's belief in his doctor and the ability of the body to heal itself. As a mid-1800s regular said of homeopaths, they would be every bit as successful if they replaced their symptom-duplicating drugs with "atoms of taffy or sawdust [providing they] give their patients room to exercise their faith, and nature time and opportunity to do the work." The power of the placebo effect continues to be the explanation offered by many mainstream physicians today to account for patients who recover under alternative medical care.

To the extent that patient faith contributes to recovery, irregular practitioners have had an advantage from the outset by virtue of cultivating a more intimate and empathic doctor-patient relationship, by in truth offering what in present times we are calling holistic medicine. The word "holistic" was not introduced into medical circles until the 1970s, when it gained vogue as a catchphrase for providing personalized, humane treatment of the whole patient, psyche and soul as well as body. Nineteenth-century alternative doctors thus didn't know they were practicing "holistic medicine," yet they repeatedly cited their engagement with patients as complicated individual human beings, and not mere organ containers, as one of the chief marks of their superiority to allopathic medicine (it was during the first half of the nineteenth century that mainstream medicine began to focus diagnostic attention on physical pathology seated in specific organs or tissues, and to lose touch with the sick person whose life was being disrupted by that pathology). The words of homeopathy's Samuel Hahnemann in 1810 could have come from the leaders of any of the irregular systems in his day or after: "all parts of the organism are so intimately connected as to form an indivisible whole in feelings and functions." One sees this repeated in another of the basic principles of naturopathic medicine today, that naturopaths "view an individual as a whole entity composed of a complex interaction of physical, mental-emotional, spiritual, social, and other factors."

Nevertheless, the appeal of gentle, natural therapies delivered holistically has waxed and waned over time. The first stage of popular excitement for unconventional medicine, the period from roughly 1830 to 1870, was fueled by distaste for calomel and other harsh allopathic drugs, the more detached bedside manner of regular physicians, and not least by the seeming determination of MDs to understand the human body as a purely mechanical construct, ignoring or denying the operation of forces or agencies that could not be quantified or accounted for by chemistry and physics. Lay people, after all, were inclined to see life as a more mysterious process, and so found satisfaction in homeopaths' declarations of faith in a vital spirit roused to activity by their drugs, and in magnetic healers' claims to manipulate a cosmic vital energy. Similarly, the current period of excitement over alternative medicine was stimulated in part by the reaction in the 1960s and 1970s against biomedical reductionism, the explanation of all vital phenomena in biochemical terms. Recent decades have witnessed a revival of faith that life is more complicated than the biochemists acknowledge, and many patients have opted for healing methods that presume the existence of a vital force (naturopathy) or some form of life energy (the human energy field of Therapeutic Touch, the qi of acupuncture, the prana of Ayurveda).

The initial phase of popular enthusiasm for irregular medicine wound down in the 1870s and 1880s as the germ theory of disease was developed and applied to drug therapy, surgery, and public health. By 1900, allopathic medicine had undergone a revolutionary transformation into an enterprise based on a far more solid scientific foundation and capable of treating, and preventing, disease with a degree of effectiveness not previously approached. Deeply impressed by this new medicine, the public shifted allegiance in great measure back to regular practice. Adding to the decline of medical alternatives was the internal professional dissension that weakened many irregular groups.

But during the decade from 1892 through 1901, three new alternative systems opened schools and began to send graduates out into practice. Osteopaths, chiropractors, and naturopaths all sensed that people actually felt a fair amount of ambivalence about the recent advances in allopathic medicine, realizing that the new surgical operations, vaccines, and drugs could not only do more for them—they could also do more to them. Campaigning under the banner of "drugless healing," all three systems grew rapidly in support, as measured both in patient visits and enactment of state licensing provisions. Surveys conducted in the 1920s indicated that anywhere from one-quarter to three-quarters of the American population received treatment from a drugless healer at least occasionally (surveys published in the 1990s showed that 30% to 40% of Americans used some form of alternative medicine, though usually in conjunction with conventional treatment).

This second stage of prominence for non-allopathic medicine ended in the 1940s, with the introduction of antibiotics and other so-called "wonder drugs." A honeymoon with regular medicine ensued, but it turned out to be brief. By the 1960s patients were once again growing restless, unsettled by news of the untoward effects of many of the new drugs (the thalidomide tragedy having an especially profound impact) and disaffected with the clinical style of allopathic physicians who were more than ever directed toward an objective diagnosis of pathology at the expense of relating to the patient's subjective experience of the illness. Further, doctors trained to intervene decisively to cure infections with antibiotics were poorly equipped to deal with the emotional needs of patients suffering from cancer, heart disease, diabetes, and the other chronic degenerative diseases that came to the fore as infectious disease was brought under control. It was this lack of attention to the whole person that generated the holistic health backlash of the 1970s, and alternative medicine, whose practitioners had always preached a holistic philosophy, benefited from the popular demand for more personal care. Over time, "holistic" would be expanded in meaning to include all the principles of alternative medical philosophy, until by the 1990s "holistic medicine" had become virtually synonymous with alternative medicine.

Unconventional doctors profited as well from the counter-culture movements of the 1960s, particularly the call to return to a more natural way of life (and more natural ways of healing) and rebellion against authority and the establishment; alternative practitioners had been rebelling against the authority of the medical establishment for more than a century. Renewed awareness of alternative medicine snowballed through the 1970s and 1980s, culminating in 1992 in the establishment by the United States Congress of an Office of Alternative Medicine (OAM) at the National Institutes of Health. Given the charge of promoting and funding research into the efficacy of alternative therapies, OAM saw its budget increase forty-five-fold during its first decade.

In 1998, the status of OAM was upgraded by Congress to the National Center for Complementary and Alternative Medicine, in recognition of the strengthening conviction that many alternative methods could actually serve as complements to standard therapy. This idea of complementariness is what is most distinctive about the current era of unconventional medicine. Prior to the last quarter of the twentieth century, cooperation between the two sides was unthinkable, and as much so for irregular as for regular physicians. Historically, alternative systems operated on the assumption they were capable of treating all disease, and anticipated they would one day drive allopathic medicine (as well as all other irregular groups) into extinction. "Hydropathy aims not at a reform," a water-cure doctor proclaimed in the 1840s, "but a total annihilation of the present system." As alternative medicine matured through the twentieth century, however, practitioners came to accept both their own limitations and the strengths of allopathic medicine. Alternative doctors today accept that for the treatment of trauma and acute infections, conventional medicine is unsurpassed. For other problems, however, they feel their medicine is often superior and almost always useful. "If I get into a serious accident," a naturopath has recently written, "take me directly to the hospital emergency department. Do not take me to a naturopathic physician." But, she continues, "once they stop the hemorrhaging, I want the hospital to call my naturopathic doctor, because then I want to integrate. I want the best of both medicines."

Integrating the best of all medical systems into a single grand program of healing is the new goal of advocates of CAM from both the alternative and the allopathic camps. But integration will not be achieved easily, for wounds from past conflicts have not fully healed and are easily reopened. Distrust and wariness remain on both sides. It will take time, coupled with continuing demonstrations of the efficacy of alternative therapies, to put the turbulent past of irregular medicine to rest (FRONTLINE | PBS, 2015).

Prevalence and Common CAM Therapies used for Treatment of Serious Mental Illness

Introduction

Conventional treatments for psychotic and affective disorders commonly include the use of antipsychotics, lithium and other AED mood stabilizers, and antidepressants. These psychotropic drugs may not eliminate all the symptoms and they have serious and life threating adverse effects. Research has suggested that patients with psychotic disorders may turn to complementary and alternative medicine (CAM) to treat their mental and physical problems and improve their quality of life. Previous studies suggest that CAM is primary used in addition to conventional therapy. It helps reduce side effects of the psychotropics, and reduces readmission rates to the psychiatric hospital by reducing symptom severity. High prevalence of CAM has been reported in North Americans and Europeans, with recent trends toward increasing use. The literature suggests that patients suffering from psychotic and affective symptoms may be especially high users of CAM. Studies cited in this book report CAM use in psychotic patients to be an estimated 88% and 63% for natural health products.

Statistics on Complementary and Alternative Methods
Used in the Treatment of Bipolar Affective Disorders

According to a study done by Dr. Amy M. Kilbourne that was published the 2007 *Psychopharmacology Bulletin* the most common types of CAM therapies used by schizoaffective and bipolar patients were; prayer/spiritual healing (54%), relaxation/breathing exercises (41%), meditation (34%), vitamins and minerals (47.3%). Massage represented (12.8%) and special diets represented (17.9%), see Table 1 for full description of therapies and percentages (Kilbourne et al. 2007).

Table 1—Complementary and Alternative Medicine (CAM) Use By Patients With Bipolar Disorder	
N=435	**N(%)**
Any Physical CAM	
Acupuncture/Acupressure	80 (18.6)
Chiropractic	3 (0.7)
Massage	55 (12.8)
Any Oral CAM	
Herbs/Herbal Medication	48 (11.1)
Homeopathy	11 (2.6)
St. John's Wort	15 (3.5)

Vitamins/Minerals	204 (47.3)
Any Cognitive CAM	
Imagery	36 (8.4)
Meditation	146 (33.9)
Relaxation/Breathing Exercises	178 (41.2)
Any Diet-Based CAM	
Dietary or Weight Loss Supplement	37 (8.6)
Special Diet	77 (17.9)
Self-Help/Support Groups	143 (33.2)
Prayer/Spiritual Healing	230 (53.5)

A study in done in 2010 in the journal of *Complementary and Integrative Medicine* by Monica Hazra showed the life-time prevalence of the most commonly used natural health products by patients with psychotic disorders were: chamomile (34.3%), cod liver oil (30.8%), ginseng (27.3%), Echinacea (16.9%), and garlic (15.7%). Multivitamin (36%), Vitamin C (32%) and calcium (22.1%) were the most used vitamins and minerals. Furthermore from this study, Yoga (23.3%), Tai Chi (11.6%) and meditation or relaxation techniques (39.5%) were the most commonly used in their study for alternative therapies. Use of a chiropractor (20.9%) and massage therapist were the most popular CAM therapists, with acupuncturist/Traditional Chinese Medicine therapist third (9.9%). See Table 2 for more details (Hazra et al. 2010).

CAM Dimensions	Type of Therapy	Lifetime Prevalence (%)	Past Year Prevalence (%)
Table 2—Lifetime and past year prevalence of complementary and alternative medicine (CAM) dimensions			
Alternative Therapies	Biofeedback	2.3	1.7
	Homeotherapy	4.7	3.5
	Hypnosis	5.8	0.6
	Meditation or relaxation techniques	39.5	25
	Tai Chi	11.6	4.1
	Traditional Chinese Medicine	3.5	2.9
	Yoga	23.3	11.6
Vitamin and Mineral Supplements	Vitamin A or Beta carotene	8.7	7.5
	Vitamin B	14.5	8.9
	Vitamin C	32.0	20.3
	Vitamin E	15.7	11.0
	Calcium	22.1	18.0
	Magnesium	9.3	8.3
	Multivitamin	54.1	36.0

Other Natural	Chamomile	34.3	16.9
Health Products	Cod liver oil	30.8	5.2
	Echinacea	16.9	9.3
	Evening Primrose Oil	5.2	2.3
	Garlic	15.7	8.7
	Ginkgo	7.6	3.5
	Ginseng	27.3	11.0
	Glucosamine Sulphate	5.2	3.5
	Kava Kava	1.2	0.0
	Valerian	4.7	1.2
	St. John's Wort	8.7	1.7
	Saw Palmentto	1.7	0.6

A study was done by Dr. Ziatka Russinova (2002) published in the *American Journal of Public Health* on the use of alternative health care practices by persons with serious mental illness. The article states the following; "First, some individuals with SMI seem to benefit from a variety of alternative practices, including body-manipulation modalities such as massage and chiropractic. More frequently used practices include meditation, massage, yoga, and guided imagery. Second, religious or spiritual activities, such as prayer, worship attendance, and religious or spiritual reading, appear to be commonly practiced and experienced as beneficial by individuals with SMI. Third, alternative practices seem to promote a recovery process beyond the management of emotional and cognitive impairments by also enhancing social, spiritual, general, and self-functioning. Fourth, alternative practices appear to benefit not only individuals diagnosed with the predominantly studied conditions of anxiety and depression but also persons with the most severe psychiatric disorders. Fifth, psychiatric diagnosis may influence the choice of alternative health care practices. For example, meditation and guided imagery seem to be used less frequently by individuals with schizophrenia spectrum disorder (Russinova et al. 2002)." See Table 3 for details on distribution of diagnosis and use of CAM.

Table 3—Distribution of Use of Alternative Health Care Practices, by Psychiatric Diagnosis		
Practices	**Schizophrenia (n=40), No.(%)**	**Bipolar (n=70) No. (%)**
Religious/spiritual activities	23 (57.5)	29 (41.4)
Meditation	11(27.5)	38 (54.3)
Massage	8 (20.0)	25 (35.7)
Yoga	9 (22.5)	12 (17.1)
Guided Imagery	2 (5.0)	16 (22.9)
Herbs	6 (15.0)	14 (20.0)
Chiropractic	6 (15.0)	8 (11.4)

Nutritional Supplements	6 (15.0)	10 (14.3)

A study was conducted by Clayton Brown, Karen Wohlheiter, and Lisa Dixon from the University of Maryland at Baltimore where 100 participants with schizophrenia and 100 participants with affective disorder were interviewed. Participants were asked whether they had visited a provider of any of 12 categories of alternative treatment during the previous 12 months and the reason for their visit. The categories included chiropractic; acupuncture; nutritional advice of lifestyle diets; massage therapy; herbal remedies; biofeedback training; training of practice of meditation; imagery, or relaxation techniques; homeopathic treatment; spiritual healing or prayer; hypnosis; traditional medicine (Chinese, Ayurvedic); and other treatments.

37% and 68% of the schizophrenia and affective disorder samples were women. 73% and 72% of the schizophrenia and affective disorders group had high school diplomas. 11% of the patients with schizophrenia and 30% of the patients with an affective disorder had consulted an alternative care practitioner for either physical or psychiatric symptoms. The highest consultation rate among the schizophrenia patients were for spiritual healing or prayer (4%), nutritional advice or lifestyle diets (3%). The highest consultation rates in the affective disorder group were for herbal remedies (10%), spiritual healing or prayer (9%), and acupuncture (8%). Only 16% of patients with affective disorder reported seeking alternative care specifically for mental illness or emotional problems, compared to 36% of those patients with schizophrenia.

An analysis of 1996 MEPS sample found national rates of use of practitioner-based alternative care by persons in the general population across self-reported mental conditions of between 9% among 40 participants who reported a psychotic disorder. A rate of 10% was reported among 846 participants with affective disorder. These rates are comparable to those in the outpatient schizophrenia sample (11%) but not to the rates reported for affective disorders in their study of 30%

Table 4--Highest Consultation Rates for CAM Practitioners		
CAM Therapy	**Schizophrenia (%)**	**Affective Disorder (%)**
Spiritual Healing/Prayer	4%	9%
Nutritional advice/lifestyle diets	3%	N/A
Herbal remedies	N/A	10%
Acupuncture	N/A	8%

Common Types of Complementary and Alternative Methods
Used in the Treatment of Psychotic and Bipolar Affective Disorders

The most popular supplements used in the traditional mental health system in America are: multivitamins, fish oil, thiamine and vitamin D_3. These are primary used in the government and public inpatient psychiatric hospitals because of the rising popularity of these supplements and their increasing exposure in psychiatric literature. Thiamine is used primarily for treatment of alcohol related nutritional deficiencies. However, the use of herbs, acupuncture, Chinese Traditional Medicine, or Ayurveda is mostly disregarded as viable treatment in most US psychiatric hospitals. Other alternatives such as music therapy, art therapy, poetry, exercise, aerobic exercise, animal therapy, weight lifting, breathing exercises, imagery, progressive muscle relaxation, and mindfulness are used in government and public psychiatric inpatient hospitals, community day rehabilitation centers, and out-patient services.

Today, there are many new forms of natural therapies due to the development of vitamins, minerals and other dietary supplements synthesized from natural plant and animal products. Since the development of vitamins, and minerals we have many new dietary supplements that are popularized through psychiatric research for the treatment of psychotic and affective disorders (i.e. schizophrenia and bipolar disorder). They include; omega-3 fatty acids (DHA and EPA), glycine, ginkgo biloba, N-acetylcysteine, L-tryptophan, melatonin, and lecithin. Multivitamins and gluten-free/casein free diets are also popular alternative choices for treatments. Nearly all vitamins and some minerals have therapeutic value in the treatment of psychotic and bipolar affective disorders. They have now been popularized by orthomolecular practitioners and will only cover niacin, vitamin D, vitamin B6, cobalamin, and folate, for vitamins, and for minerals; magnesium.

These are some of the most common supplements and dietary methods researched in psychiatric literature;

> **Cobalamin (Vitamin B12):** In cases of cobalamin deficiency mental disturbances such as dementia (especially in elderly subjects), fatigue, mood disorders and even psychoses have been described. In some instances, the psychiatric disturbances may occur as the main or sole symptom, in the absence of any neurological or hematological abnormalities. Although the presentation of psychosis alone is considered a rare condition, determination of serum vitamin B12 levels is still recommended as an essential test in the workup of mental status changes (Masalha, 2001). In one case report, chronic psychosis improves dramatically with short-term antipsychotic medication and intramuscular cobalamin injections in a 31 year old male, who presented to a tertiary care psychiatric facility (Rajkumar , 2008). In another article, three patients recovered only on a combination of B12 supplementation and psychiatric medication (Bhat , 2007). This case report states: a patient recovers from schizophrenia-like psychotic episode with oral cobalamin supplementation and short course antipsychotic treatment and remained asymptomatic and functionally independent at 1 year of follow-up (Kuo, 2009).

➤ **Folate, Folic Acid, L-methylfolate:** Folate is a general term for a group of water soluble b-vitamins, and is also known as B9. Folic acid refers to the oxidized synthetic compound used in dietary supplements and food fortification, whereas folate refers to the various tetrahydrofolate derivatives naturally found in food. The body converts dietary folate or folic acid to l-methylfolate through a series of enzymatic processes. The final stage is done with the enzyme methyltetrahydrofolate reductase (MTHFR). In a study published in the *Lancet* (1990), 33% of both depressed and schizophrenic patients with either borderline methylfolate levels or deficiency significantly improved clinically and had social recovery (Godfrey, 1990). Some schizophrenia patients with high serum homocysteine levels may have the genetic defect of having low folate serum levels. In such cases, folate ingestion may be a good management modality for clinical improvement according to a 2011 study in *Psychiatry Investigation* (Kim, 2011). Based on findings published in *Acta Psychiatrica Scandinavica* (2009) folic acid seems to be an effective adjunctive to sodium valproate in the treatment of the acute phase of mania in patients with bipolar disorder (Behzahi, 2009).

➤ **Ginkgo Biloba:** Native to China, the tree is widely cultivated and it has various uses in traditional medicine and as a source of food. It is also used in the treatment of schizophrenia, dementia, depression, dizziness, migraine and impotence with vascular types. In a combination with standard antipsychotics it is recommended for schizophrenia. Ginkgo biloba may also enhance the effectiveness of antipsychotic drugs and reduce their extrapyramidal side effects (Zhang, 2001). Ginkgo biloba is also effective for reducing positive symptoms in refractory schizophrenia (Knable, 2002; Atmaca, 2005). Ginkgo biloba is also an effective add-on therapy for treatment of negative symptoms in chronic schizophrenia (Singh, 2010). Further, it is effective for enhancing Clozapine's treatment of negative symptoms in schizophrenic patients (Doruk 2008). The usual dose is 360 mg / day (Babic, 2009).

➤ **Gluten free/Casein free diet:** Diet that has no gluten (from wheat) and casein (from milk) improves schizophrenic symptoms. Dr. Fredrick Curtis Dohan and his associates in the two studies examined the relationship between diet and schizophrenia. From 65,000 respondents in Papua, the Solomon Islands and Micronesia there were only two recorded cases of schizophrenia, while the expected number in the same sample in Europe would be 130. This prompted Dr. Dohan to conduct a thorough research that showed that these people do not eat wheat. In 1969, and 1973 Dohan conducted clinical trials in which showed those schizophrenics assigned to a cereal-free milk-free diet were discharged more than twice as fast as those on a high cereal diet (Dohan, 1969, 1973). Robert Cade the inventor of the sports drink Gatorade did a study on autistic children and schizophrenics. He found that seven schizophrenics assigned to a gluten free/casein free diet showed significant improvement in 4 months on the diet (Cade, 2000). Jackson et al (2012) found that people with schizophrenia on a gluten free diet often leads to improvement in extrapyramidal side effects and akathisia (Jackson., 2012). Rice et al. 1978 had a case study in which a woman that was in a psychiatric hospital for 13 years was discharged due to her improvement on a gluten free diet (Rice et al., 1978). Some researchers believe that schizophrenic symptoms can significantly improve by the removal of bread, rice paste, starch and refined sugar from their diets (Potkin, 1981, Ross-Smith Nero 1980).

- **Glycine:** There are numerous studies that show that amino acid glycine increases the activity of neurotransmitters and reduces the negative symptoms of schizophrenia when used with an antipsychotic therapy, especially with haloperidol, thioridazine and perphenazine (Waziri 1996, Heresco, 1999, Javitt, 1994). Glycine augmentation may ameliorate depressive and extrapyramidal symptoms in schizophrenics (Strzelecki et al., 2013). Adjunctive glycine induces a significant reduction in negative symptoms, depression, and improves cognitive functions in schizophrenics (Heresco-Levy, 1996). Glycine has been shown to reduce muscle stiffness and extrapyramidal dysfunction in schizophrenics on conventional neuroleptics (Rosse, 1989). Glycine has also been shown to reduce positive symptoms in schizophrenic patients (Strzelecki, 2011). In the treatment of schizophrenia, the recommended dose is 40-90 grams per day (Babic, 2009).

- **Lecithin:** Lecithin is a fundamental substance in cell membranes. When there is shortage, the membrane becomes weak, especially the brain system. Therefore, it can be used when there is a reduction in concentration and memory. It has a much broader function in protecting other cells in our body and a soothing effect on the nervous system. It also reduces the amount of cholesterol, cleanses the walls of blood vessels, and increases the work of the heart muscle. Lecithin may also be used in the treatment of schizophrenia. According to a study in the *American Journal of Clinical Nutrition* (1982), six schizophrenics receiving Choline were reported to experience modest improvement in their symptoms, and neuroleptics were clearly more efficacious (Rosenburg, 1982; Davis, 1978). However, there is more literature on the use of lecithin in mania. Lecithin's effect on four manic patients has been investigated. When lecithin was administered in the 90% pure form, all patients rapidly improved. Three of the four patients then worsened after withdrawal of lecithin (Cohen, 1980). A double-blind, placebo controlled trial of pure lecithin for the treatment of mania was conducted and improvement was significantly greater than placebo in five of six patients studied (Cohen, 1982). Another case was of a bipolar, 13 year old girl on lithium was not responding to her mood stabilizer and was placed on lecithin and she appeared to respond well to lecithin alone (Schreier, 1982) The recommended dose is 1-2 capsules of 1250 mg a day.

- **L-tryptophan:** Tryptophan, the natural amino acid precursor in 5-HT biosynthesis, increases 5-HT synthesis in the brain and, therefore, may stimulate 5-HT release and function. Since it is a natural constituent of the diet, tryptophan should have low toxicity and produce few side effects. Based on these advantages, dietary tryptophan supplementation has been used in the management of schizophrenia and bipolar disorder with some success. In one study, tryptophan has been useful in the treatment of aggressive schizophrenics (Morand, 1983). Tryptophan has also been shown to enhance memory in schizophrenic patients (Levoritz, 2003). Combined with lithium, tryptophan results in significantly greater improvement in bipolar and schizoaffective symptoms (Brewerton, 1983). In the treatment of mania, tryptophan has been found effective (Chouinard, 1985). Tryptophan may be considered an alternative maintenance treatment in bipolar patients unresponsive or unable to take lithium (Beitman, 1982). Tryptophan has also been found effective for the treatment of depressive symptoms and normalizes sleep patterns in a patient with bipolar disorder (Cooke et al. 2010).

- **Magnesium:** Magnesium is a calming mineral that nourishes the nervous system and helps prevent anxiety, fear, nervousness, restlessness and irritability. A study on magnesium deficiency in schizophrenic and manic-depressive patients suggests that oral Mg supplementation should be considered as an adjunct to the treatment in psychiatric patients (Kirov 1990). Though according to one journal article published in *Magnesium Research* (2008) after 3 weeks of antipsychotic treatment, in both haloperidol and risperidone treated patients, the magnesium erythrocyte concentrations expressed a significant increase. In the same article it was said that increasing intracellular brain levels of magnesium determines a decreasing glutamate-induced activation of NMDA receptors and consequently alleviates manic psychomotor hyperactivity. They considered the increase in magnesium an important element in the mechanism of action of mood stabilizers for bipolar disorder (Nechifor, 2008).

➤ **Melatonin:** Melatonin is a hormone made by the pineal gland. The hormone can be used as a sleep aid and in the treatment of sleep disorders. It can be taken orally as capsules, tablets, or liquid. It is also available in a form to be used sublingually, and there are transdermal patches. In a study of schizophrenic outpatients done by Suresh et al. (2007), "melatonin significantly improved the quality and depth of sleep of nighttime sleep, reduced the number of nighttime awaking's, and increased the duration of sleep without producing a morning hangover. Subjectively, melatonin also reduced sleep-onset latency, heightened freshness on awaking, improved mood, and improved daytime functioning. (Suresh , 2007)" In another study, it was found that melatonin improves sleep efficiency in patients with schizophrenia whose sleep quality is low (Shamir, 2000). Lastly, there is one case where melatonin treatment leads to rapid relief of insomnia and aborts manic episode in boy with bipolar disorder (Robertson, 1997). Dosages of melatonin can range from 1mg a night to as much as 45mg a night depending on doctors recommendations. Common average dose is 5 mg per night.

➤ **Multivitamins:** For the majority of patients suffering from schizophrenia it is recommended to use multivitamin products due to their poor diet. However, in scientific literature there are no studies on the use of multivitamins in schizophrenic patients. Orthomolecular practitioners often do not recommend multivitamins to undermethylated schizophrenic and bipolar patients due to the folate, and folic acid content of the multivitamin. However, this may only represent up to 20% of the bipolar/schizophrenia group spectrum. There are a few case reports with patients with bipolar disorder that describe positive effects of multivitamins. One case study with a bipolar II patient with comorbid ADHD showed significant improvement in mood, anxiety, and hyperactivity/impulsivity after 8 weeks on multivitamin (Rucklidge, 2010). Another study showed multivitamin Empower Plus resulted in outcome superior to conventional treatment (Frazier, 2009). Dermot et al. (2009) demonstrated in a study that a mean symptom score could be lowered by 41% than baseline after 3 months, and 45% lower after 6 months with a multivitamin. In his study 50% experienced improvement in 6 months (Dermot et al. 2009).

➤ **N-acetylcysteine:** N-acetylcysteine comes from the amino acid L-cysteine. N-acetylcysteine has been used for a wide variety of uses in medicine including treatment of bipolar disorder and schizophrenia. By augmenting production of glutathione (GSH), N-acetyl cysteine (NAC) treatment may be of clinical benefit in the treatment of schizophrenia and bipolar disorder. Cysteine is the rate-limiting precursor for GSH synthesis, but oral supplementation with pure cysteine is not efficiently bioavailable However, oral NAC rapidly increases plasma cysteine levels, replenishing depleted

GSH systemically. Systemic administration of NAC prevents brain GSH depletion , with neuroprotective benefits (Berk, 2008). In one case study a treatment-resistant schizophrenic patient improves considerably with add-on NAC (Bulut,2009). NAC has been shown to be a potential therapeutic agent for hallucinations and psychosis associated with hallucinogen use and schizophrenia (Lee, 2014). NAC has been found effective for alleviating negative symptoms of schizophrenia (Farokhnia, 2013). Add-on treatment with NAC for bipolar II achieves full remission of both depressive and manic symptoms (Magalhaes, 2011). NAC demonstrates robust depression scores in bipolar disorder (Berk , 2011). As an ad-on to antipsychotics, 2 g daily (1 g twice daily [b.i.d.]) of NAC is suggested dosage.

➤ **Niacin (Vitamin B3):** Insufficient niacin in the diet can cause nausea, skin and mouth lesions, anemia, headaches, and tiredness. Chronic niacin deficiency leads to a disease called pellagra .In the journal *European Review for Medical and Pharmacological Sciences* (2015) the author concluded "Niacin deficiency seems to be an important contributor in the development of the clinical picture of schizophrenia. Studies and sparse case reports indicate that niacin augmentation could help a subset of patients suffering from schizophrenia." In the *Canadian Medical Association Journal* (1973), Abram Hoffer described a young woman who first showed manifestations of schizophrenia in childhood. Improvement commenced shortly after the institution of megavitamin therapy, notably nicotinic acid 3 grams daily. No medication other than nicotinic acid was required." Another article on hospital readmission rates was published by Abram Hoffer in 1964 in *Acta Psychiatrica Scandinavica*. It showed that "The group which received nicotinic acid had the best record which showed most clearly in the total days of rehospitalization, i.e. about 11 days per patient per year. The comparison group required about 19 days per patient per year." Hoffer had several articles reporting the reduction of hospital readmission rates. A case report in *General Hospital Psychiatry* (2008) by Ravi Prakash detailed a case of pellagra causing delusional parasitosis which responded rapidly to niacin therapy.

➤ **Omega-3 Fatty Acids (DHA & EPA):** This is recommended as a complementary therapy to a standard psycho pharmacotherapy with various forms of depression, and in the treatment of a bipolar affective disorder and schizophrenia. Psychiatrists often will prescribe omega-3 fatty acids for elevated triglycerides also. According to these studies; Omega-3 fatty acids may be effective for treatment of bipolar depression (Montgomery, 2008; Sarris, 2012). Omega-3 fatty acids have been shown to reduce irritability of persons with bipolar disorder (Sagduyu, 2005). Omega-3's DHA and EPA are helpful adjunct treatments for bipolar disorder and demonstrate significant improvements (Turnbull, 2008). Research shows that people with schizophrenia can have up to 25% reduction in symptoms when taking Omega-3 (Emsley, 2003). Ethyl eicosapentaenoic acid has procognitive effects and improves positive symptoms in patients with schizophrenia (Reddy, 2011). Following clinical improvement, ethyl eicosapentaenoic acid has been shown to change the hemispheric balance symmetry between right and left hand at 3-month follow-up in schizophrenic patients (Richardson, 1999). Omega-3's may also increase the efficacy of atypical antipsychotics (Jamilain, 2014). The recommended dose is 1-2 grams for the prevention and 4-6 grams a day for the treatment.

- ➢ **Pyridoxine (Vitamin B6):** Pyridoxine 5'-phosphate, vitamin B-6, is an essential cofactor in various transamination, decarboxylation, glycogen hydrolysis, and synthesis pathways involving carbohydrate, sphingolipid, amino acid, heme, and neurotransmitter metabolism. Pyridoxine deficiency causes blood, skin, and nerve changes (Medscape, 2015). In schizophrenics that have pyridoxine deficiency a pilot study in September 1970 had shown that supplementation of 50 mg of pyridoxine showed significant improvement within 8 to 10 weeks. The study claimed the schizophrenic patients were more alert, responsive; more active had lost their blunted effects, nor were indifferent to personal habits or their environment (Bucci, 1973). Another study researching the antidepressant effects of pyridoxine in schizophrenic patients results were as follows: "Two of nine patients (22%), characterized by higher initial HAM-D and SANS scores, and by older age and longer duration of illness, experienced marked improvements in depressive symptoms (23% and 28% decrease in HAM-D scores) following 4 weeks of pyridoxine administration"(Shiloh , 2001). This report describes the treatment of an 18-year-old male diagnosed (DSM II) as having an acute schizophrenic reaction, catatonic type (APA, 1968) in association with multiplex psychological findings which were partially congruous with several neuropsychobehavioral disorders. The complex findings and clinical success with pyridoxine HCI in this case parallel a previously unreported case of an 11 year-old female with schizophrenia, catatonic type and minimal brain dysfunction who demonstrated initial trifluperazine and thiothixene intolerance but sequent responsiveness to pyridoxine HCI at 500 mg daily. Experience with both cases estimated the effective dosage of pyridoxine HCI (vitamin B6) at 500 mg daily was therapeutically effective in eliminating the major schizophrenic reaction (Brooks, 1983).

- ➢ **Vitamin D3:** Cholecalciferol (toxiferol, vitamin D3) is one of the five forms of vitamin D. A 2014 study in the journal of *Therapeutic Advances in Psychopharmacology* recommend that, "serum vitamin D levels should be measured in patients with schizophrenia especially in long term care. Appropriate further treatment with add-on vitamin D supplements and diets that are rich in vitamin D should be considered." Another study in *Schizophrenia Research* (2014) done by James Clelland states; "these findings strongly support vitamin D supplementation in patients, particularly for those with elevated proline." Another study done in *Schizophrenia Research* (2014) by Kristina Cieslak came to the conclusion that "vitamin D may be considered as a potential therapy in women who present with aggressive manifestations of schizophrenia."

Conclusion

While there is a plethora of treatments available for the treatment of psychotic and bipolar affective disorder, we are only covered the most common supplements in this section. CAM use in this population is high with one study finding CAM use in psychotic patients to be an estimated 88% and 63% for natural health products. The traditional mental health system uses some of these CAM therapies, but however limits the use to cognitive and mind-body CAM therapies mostly. Many patients using CAM medicine are using it for purposes other than for mental health purposes. Patient satisfaction on the efficacy is considerably high with CAM therapies for bipolar disorder. A survey of 200 bipolar patients in Colombia and Argentina published in the *Journal of Affective Disorders* (2013) found that 52% of patients found CAM-usage as "useful" and "very useful" (Strejielevich, 2013).

Evaluating Evidence-based Medicine: How to Appraise a Journal Article

Introduction

In Codex Alternus there is nearly 900 citations and summaries and quotations that are from case reports, case series reports, cohort studies, case-controlled studies, controlled trials, editorials, opinions, and meta-analysis. Many are from peer reviewed journals however all are scholarly articles and some may be included based on factors of novelty to the treatment of psychotic disorders, bipolar affective disorders, or medication-induced side effects. Codex Alternus was not designed to criticize and evaluate each therapy published in the journals, nor was it designed to criticize or evaluate each journals and authors claims. Codex Alternus was designed to provide as many new, novel, and traditional therapies as could be data mined from medical databases that contained positive results. It is intended to be used as a research reference tool and clinician guide for therapies with positive outcomes. Its weaknesses is that it does not review negative reports and criticisms. Though, the books positive side it allows the reader to evaluate the quality of the journal reporting and authorship.

Below we will show the hierarchy of medical research and show you a way to evaluate the literature of the therapies you are reviewing. The chart below helps you sort out the volume of research that is sometimes available for some therapies.

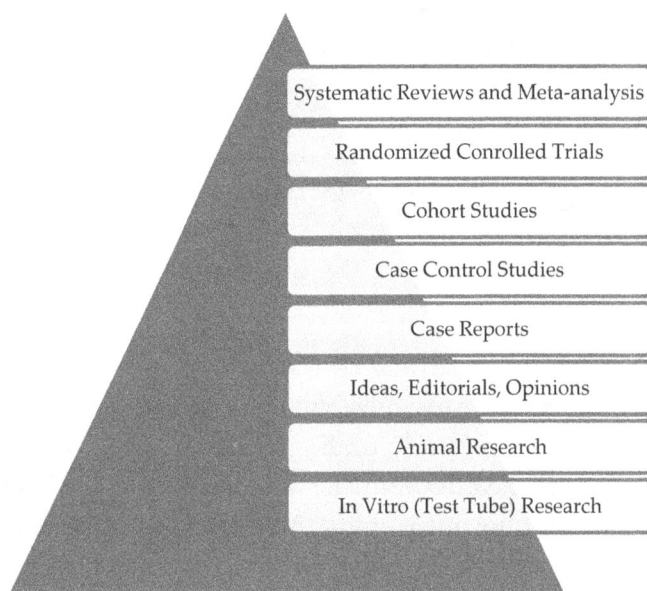

Systematic Reviews and Meta-analysis

Randomized Conrolled Trials

Cohort Studies

Case Control Studies

Case Reports

Ideas, Editorials, Opinions

Animal Research

In Vitro (Test Tube) Research

1.1 Table of Hierarchy of Evidence in Health Care

In this chapter we will examine evidence based medicine and how to appraise a journal article. It is in this chapter the reader will gain insight on how to evaluate the references, summaries, and journal articles cited in Codex Alternus. This is the best way for an evaluation to be performed; by the reader.

The Basics of Appraising a Journal Article

Appraising journal articles

The best way to find high quality information is to carry out a literature search on one or more databases and to download, copy or request relevant current publications. Once you have obtained the papers most relevant to your question you should consider a number of things before using the results. This applies even when the publications are from peer reviewed journals:

- ➢ Authorship
- ➢ Publication bias

- ➢ Journal ranking and impact factors
- ➢ Abstract quality

Publication bias

1. Negative results don't (often) get published – If you want to carry out a detailed or systematic review of a subject area, you might consider trying to get hold of unpublished studies.

2. Reviewers may be biased against unconventional versus conventional techniques (e.g. orthodox drug versus alternative therapy).

Authorship

Are the authors based at a well-established Centre of Excellence? Are there any issues of sponsorship or competing interests?

Journal ranking and impact factors

Although the impact factor of a journal is clearly going to be linked to its popularity and accessibility, the journals with higher impact factors in a subject area are generally well respected for good reason.

Abstract quality

Read the paper carefully and don't rely on the abstract alone. Around 24%-60% of abstracts in peer reviewed journals have deficiencies. Three common types of inaccuracies are: 1) data inconsistent in abstract and body of the paper, tables, and figures; 2) data or information in the abstract do not appear elsewhere; and 3) conclusions in the abstract not substantiated in the paper itself. [see Ward LG et al. Annals of Pharmacotherapy 2004; 38(7-8): 1173-7].

Critical Appraisal of an Individual Journal Article Describing a Piece of Research

---

Review of Structured Abstract

An abstract should summarize the research concisely and include the objectives, study design, important results, and the authors' conclusions. When starting to appraise an article reviewing a structured abstract is particularly helpful because the different constituents of the research can readily be identified. Serious flaws may be detected at this stage (Huth, 1987; Lock, 1988).

What are the Objectives of the Research?

The next step is to identify the precise objectives of the research. These should be stated in the introduction to the paper or may be given in the abstract. A principal goal of appraisal is to establish whether research objectives have been met, and the most precise form of the objectives should be sought. For example, the specific objective "To determine the effect of EDTA chelation therapy on bipolar manic depressives symptoms of depression in patients with high vanadium, compared to manic patients", one objective would be to have to compare vanadium levels in relation to symptomology in both bipolar depressive patients, compared to manic patients.

What is the Overall Study Design?

Before dissecting the methods in detail the overall design of the study should be clarified, as this helps to determine those aspects of the appraisal on which to concentrate. The design should be stated in the abstract and at the beginning of the methods section. Most studies comprise one of six designs: case report, case series, cross sectional, cohort, case-control, and controlled trial. Many others are simply combinations and nuances of these six. The formats are as follows (figure).

Case report: A case report is a description of one interesting and unusual case.

Case series: A case series is a description of several cases in which no attempt is made to answer specific hypotheses or to compare the results with another group of cases.

Example: Mental health and medical records were reviewed to study the clinical features of HIV diagnosed in one depressed incarcerated inmate, and one inmate with serve mental illness. Discussion focused upon recommended treatment of mental illness and HIV. No other cases were studied (Watts, 2006).

Cross sectional study: A cross sectional study is a survey of the frequency of disease, risk factors, or other characteristics in a defined population at one particular time.

Example: A survey of self-reported quality of sleep in a population of psychiatric in-patients on the acute ward of a psychiatric hospital. Subject's quality of sleep was assessed by the administration of the Pittsburg Sleep Quality Index (PSQI). The aim was to compare clinical, demographic, and PSQI data between poor sleepers and good sleepers (Donaldson et al., 2009).

Cohort study: A cohort study is an observational study of a group of people with a specified characteristic or disease who are followed up over a period of time to detect new events. Comparisons may be made with a control group. No interventions are normally applied to the groups.

Example: Between August 1992 and December 1998, seven wave cohort study of adolescent health in the Australian state of Victoria was conducted. The study involved 1601 students and was conducted over seven years. The study was to determine whether cannabis use in adolescence predisposes to higher rates of depression and anxiety in young adulthood. Some 60% of participants had used cannabis by the age of 20;7% were daily users at that point. Daily use in young women was associated with an over fivefold increase in the odds of reporting a state of depression and anxiety after adjustment for intercurrent use of other substances (odds ratio 5.6, 95% confidence interval 2.6 to 12), (Patton, et al., 2002).

Case-control study: A case-control study is an observational study in which characteristics of people with a disease (cases) are compared with those of selected people without the disease (controls).

Example: A study was undertaken to evaluate the association between mood and anxiety disorders in Hashimoto disease and Euthyroid Goitre in a case control study. Cases included 19 subjects with Hashimoto disease in euthyroid phase, 19 subjects with euthyroid goiter, 2 control groups of each 76 subjects matched (4/1) according to age and sex drawn from data base of community sample (Carta, 2005).

Controlled trial: A controlled trial is an experimental study in which an intervention is applied to one group of people and the outcome compared with that in a similar group (controls) not receiving the intervention.

Example: A total of 519 adults with severe and persistent mental illness were recruited from outpatient community mental health settings in 6 Ohio communities and randomly assigned to the 8-week intervention or a wait-list control condition. The purpose of the study was to determine the efficacy of a peer-led illness self-management intervention called Wellness Recovery Action Planning (WRAP) by comparing it with usual care (Cook, 2011).

Guidelines

The following six guidelines (labeled A-F), each in the form of a question about the research and including a checklist of criteria, are summarized below:

A. Study Design Appropriate To Objectives?

Deciding if the overall study design is appropriate may require more common sense than a detailed knowledge of epidemiological methods. If, for example, the purpose of a study is to evaluate a new treatment a controlled trial is almost vital, as a trial without a control group would be troubled with difficulties in knowing whether improvement in patients was due to the treatment. Similarly, a project examining prognosis would normally require follow up by means of a cohort study. On the other hand, research investigating the cause of ADHD might adopt any of the designs shown in the figure.

B. Study Sample Representative?

Source of sample: If research is to be applicable and relevant to other populations the study sample (group selected to participate) must be representative of the group from which it is drawn (study population), which in turn should be typical of the wider population to whom the research might apply (target population). Appropriateness of the target and study populations is usually a subjective assessment based on our knowledge of the topic under investigation. For example, research concerned with the pathogenesis of schizophrenia might be of limited value if restricted to a target population of men over 50 years of age.

Sampling method: In population based studies random sampling is the ideal method of avoiding selection bias and producing a sample typical of the study population. In other studies non-random sampling may be adequate; for example, consecutive patients attending a mental health clinic may be included in a controlled trial, or every ninth person may be selected from a register. In studies based in hospital, however, beware that referral bias may lead to an atypical study sample.

Sample size: A statement in the methods section that a sample size was chosen in order to have sufficient power to detect a medically meaningful result at a certain level of statistical significance would normally be adequate evidence that steps had been taken to ensure an appropriate sample size. In the absence of such a statement it may be necessary to seek help from a statistician or an appropriate text (Altman, 1980; Daly, 1991) to establish whether the sample size was adequate. But it is also important to assess the biological representativeness of the sample. Was the sample large enough to encompass the full range of disease? Or was it so small that there was a danger of a biased homogeneous group having a disproportionate effect on the results? It is not uncommon, for example, to read of statistically valid randomized controlled trials containing fewer than 20 patients. Was it likely with such a small number of patients that they were truly representative of all those presenting to clinicians in other centers?

Entry criteria and exclusions: The criteria for entering subjects into a study must be examined carefully; the stage of disease or time of onset, for example, may have a profound effect on the results of treatment or in the detection of aetiological factors. Exclusion criteria should also be defined appropriately. Furthermore, any description of the study participants must be scrutinized in order to assess whether the sample was representative.

Non-respondents: In most studies some subjects do not respond to invitations, some refuse to participate, and others do not attend for examination. The response rate is often viewed as an indicator of the representativeness of participants, but the size of response is only one aspect of sampling and may be less important than the comparability between participants and non-respondents. For example, a response rate of 30% may be satisfactory if there is good evidence that participants do not have atypical characteristics which might affect the results of the research. Thus comparisons should be sought between participants and the non-respondents or the total study population.

C. Control Group Acceptable?

Definition of controls: In studies using a comparison or control group it is important to assess whether this group was adequate for the purpose under study. In a case-control study, for example, were the criteria for defining controls appropriate and was the control group checked to ensure that it did not contain cases?

Comparable characteristics: In controlled trials random allocation to intervention and control groups usually leads to comparability, but not necessarily so, and the distributions of age, sex, and other prognostic variables should therefore be compared between the two groups. Similarly, in case-control and cohort studies matching or other methods of selecting controls are not infallible and the comparability of the groups must be assessed.

Matching and randomization: In case-control studies cases and controls are often matched for certain characteristics, such as age and sex. Did the matching process seem to have been carried out correctly? In controlled trials, on the other hand, subjects are often randomly allocated to intervention and control groups. The method of randomization should be assessed to ensure that the subjects were truly randomized - for example, by use of computer generated random numbers.

Source of controls: In case-control and cohort studies the source of controls should be such that the distributions of characteristics (not under direct investigation) are similar to those in the cases or study cohort. For example, in a study of cerebral atrophy of schizophrenic patients the source of controls should be of the same education levels and socioeconomic status as the patients because higher education often is associated with larger brain mass.

D. Quality of Measurements and Outcomes?

Quality control: Overall, the extent to which the researchers have instituted quality control measures for the examination of subjects, collection of data, and laboratory tests should give some idea of the likely quality of data. Measures might include testing the accuracy and repeatability of observers, checking the calibration and accuracy of instruments, and random checks for errors in data recording. Laboratories often participate in external quality control schemes, but many clinical researchers do not give adequate attention to this concept.

Validity: It is important to assess the validity of measurements made in a research study - that is, the extent to which they reflect the true situation. Dietary questionnaires, for example, are notoriously inaccurate in obtaining a true picture of a person's regular nutritional intake. When a single test is used as a proxy measure of disease the validity of the test (sensitivity and specificity) should be stated in the article. In a randomized controlled trial the results may depend on the measurement of one outcome and it is thus essential that this is an important end point which is sensitive to change.

Blindness: During data collection a common source of bias is that the subjects or those collecting the data are not blind to the purpose of the research. The problems that may occur in controlled trials are well known: subjects, observers, and researchers, by wishing the intervention to succeed, produce an unrealistically good success rate. Inadequate blindness may be a problem in other studies. In case-control studies, for example, patients (cases) who are aware of a possible relation between a risk factor and the disease may over report the risk factor in themselves. Similarly, an observer may make greater efforts to detect a possible risk factor in cases than in controls, or may even unconsciously slant the questions in questionnaires to obtain the desired response. Clearly in many studies total blindness is not feasible, but for the purposes of appraisal it is necessary to consider how this might put the results in doubt.

Reproducibility: In the interests of expediency many research projects pay too little attention to the reproducibility of the measurements. Would the same results have been obtained if the measurements had been taken by a different observer or on a different day? In many larger projects repeatability checks are made at intervals to assess the consistency of measurement. For example, split blood samples may be sent to the laboratory without an indication that they are from the same subject. Evidence on the repeatability of the principal measurements should be sought in the article.

E. Completeness?

Compliance: The end results of a study may be incomplete in relation to the number of subjects who were first enrolled. This need not necessarily lead to bias in the results, but careful assessment is required. In controlled trials continuing compliance of subjects with a regimen may be a serious problem and, although this may partly be overcome by carrying out an "intention to treat" analysis (in which the outcomes of all subjects entering the trial are included in the analysis irrespective of compliance with treatment), when appraising the study it may be quite difficult to assess whether the treatment worked.

Drop outs and deaths: In cohort studies as well as in controlled trials drop outs and deaths in the study sample may occur. It is important to assess not only the proportion of drop outs in each group but also why they dropped out, as this may give a clue to possible bias. For example, more healthy people may move and be lost to follow up, so that a cohort study excluding them might produce an unrealistically gloomy outcome.

Missing data: Incomplete results may often occur due to difficulties in obtaining specimens, laboratory tests going awry, and lost data. The extent and nature of the loss must be assessed in order to estimate possible bias. Also, selectivity in reporting of results and the exclusion of data from tables may have an effect on the conclusions that can be drawn from the research. It is worth checking that in addressing the objectives of the study the authors have presented data on the most appropriate measurements and that some have not mysteriously disappeared.

F.   Distorting Influences?

Changes over time: Be wary of studies in which data on a characteristic have been collected from two groups of subjects at different times. Observed differences between the groups might be due to changes in the characteristic or its measurement over time, and not to real differences between the groups.

Confounding factors: Distorting influences may exist in studies examining the association between a risk factor and disease where the purpose is to find out whether the association is real or spurious (caused by a confounding factor influencing both the risk factor and the disease). In such studies it is necessary to account for possible confounding factors. This may be satisfied by matching in the selection of controls or by evidence of comparability between cases and controls.

Contamination: Another problem in controlled trials is contamination, in which one group is affected by another. For example, in a dietary intervention study people in a control group may change their diet because they hear about supposed benefits from dietary changes in the intervention group.

Distortion reduced by analysis: Distorting influences may also be minimized by some form of stratification or adjustment procedure in the analysis. Age and sex are frequent confounding factors and invariably should be accounted for by describing age standardized, sex specific rates. Multiple regression is a statistical technique which is often used to analyze independent associations of variables while taking account of confounding factors. In controlled trials outcome measures may have to be analyzed separately within subgroups - for example, those exposed and not exposed to extraneous treatments

Extraneous treatments: The results of studies are often distorted by outside influences. In controlled trials, for example, a common problem is that subjects may be exposed to treatments in addition to the one being evaluated. Thus in assessing a trial the question has to be asked, "Could there possibly be extraneous treatments which might have influenced the results? Have these been identified in the study and the results interpreted accordingly (Fowkes, 1991) ?"

Preliminary Statistical Concepts in RCTs

Presenting the results of RCTs

P-value - the p-value refers to the probability that any particular outcome would have arisen by chance. A p-value of less than 1 in 20 (p<0.05) is statistically significant.

Confidence interval - the same trial repeated hundreds of times would not yield the same results every time. But on average the results would be within a certain range. A 95% confidence interval means that there is a 95% chance that the true size of effect will lie within this range.

Quantifying the risk of benefit/harm in RCTs

Experimental Event Rate (EER) - in the treatment group, number of patients with outcome divided by total number of patients.

Control Event Rate (CER) - in the control group, number of patients with outcome divided by total number of patients.

Relative Risk or Risk Ratio (RR) - the risk of the outcome occurring in the intervention group compared with the control group. RR= EER/CER

Absolute Risk Reduction or increase (ARR) - absolute amount by which the intervention reduces (or increases) the risk of outcome. ARR= CER-EER

Relative Risk Reduction or increase (RRR) - amount by which the risk of outcome is reduced (or increased) in the intervention group compared with the control group. RRR=ARR/CER

Odds of outcome - in each patient group, the number of patients with an outcome divided by the number of patients without the outcome.

Odds ratio - odds of outcome in treatment group divided by odds of outcome in control group. If the outcome is negative, an effective treatment will have an odds ratio <1; If the outcome is positive, an effective treatment will have an odds ratio >1. (In case control studies, the odds ratio refers to the odds in favour of exposure to a particular factor in cases divided by the odds in favour of exposure in controls).

Number needed to treat (NNT) - how many patients need to have the intervention in order to prevent one person having the unwanted outcome. NNT=1/ARR, Ideal NNT=1; The higher the NNT, the less effective the treatment (UCL, 2015).

Making a judgment: Once you have reviewed all the details of the methods and results of the paper a decision can be made whether to use the information or not. Unfortunately, there is no magic formula in evaluating a journal article and you will have to score the worth of the paper on your own findings. **Codex Alternus provides a comprehensive array of journal citations to evaluate. You be the final judge of the efficacy and safety of the therapies you evaluate.**

CODEX ALTERNUS™

SECTION ONE

Schizophrenia Treatments

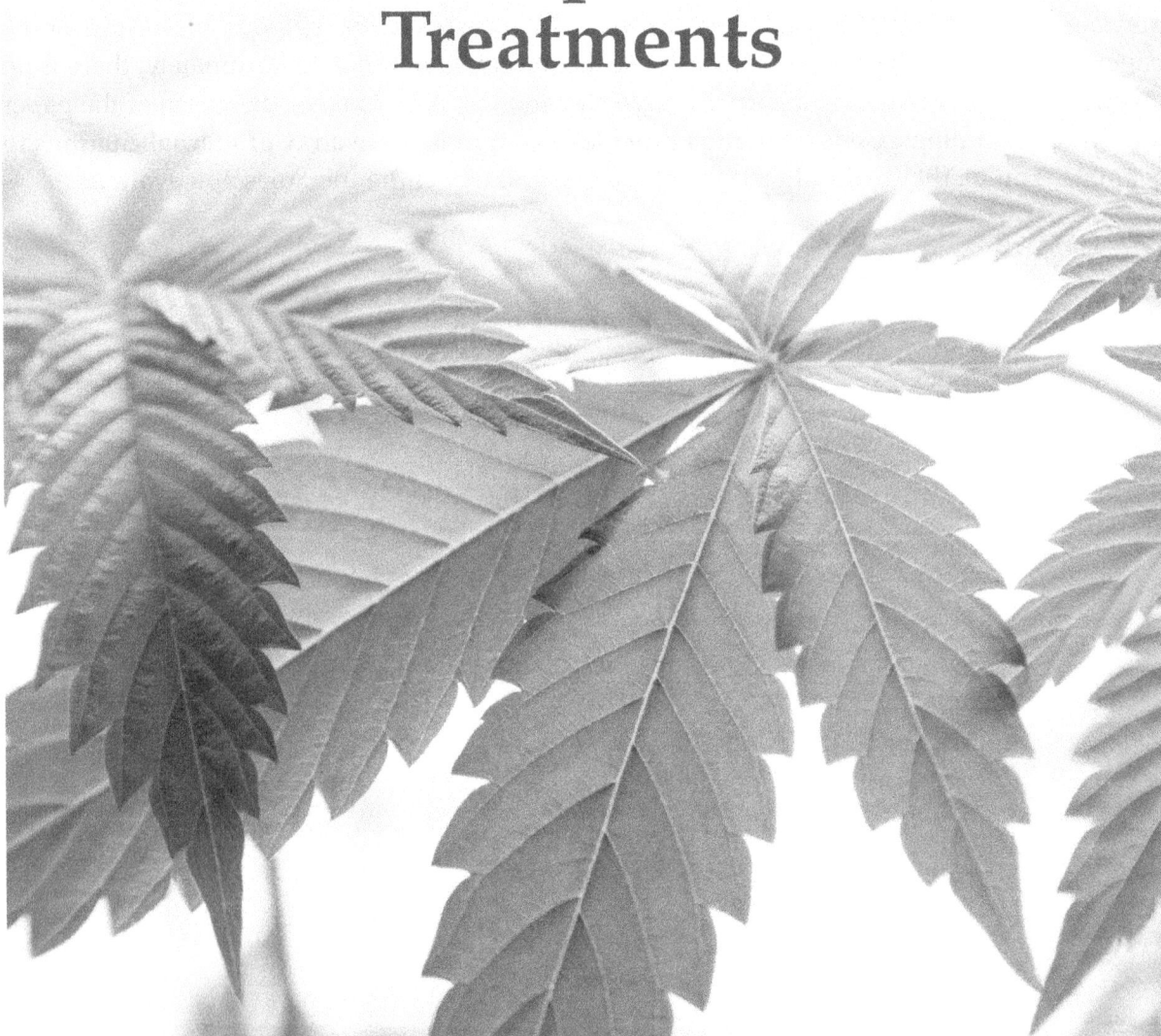

Medical Marijuana, Phytocannabinoids and Cannabidiol

By Will Hall, MA, DiplPW   Reprinted with Permission of Will Hall

Marijuana is now legal in two states, and legal for medical use in 23 states and the District of Columbia. Polls show the majority of Americans support cannabis legalization, and more and more of the country is joining the legalization trend. As a counselor working with people diagnosed with psychosis and mental illness I am often asked about my opinion and clinical experience — as well as my personal experience — with medical cannabis.

The issue is not clear-cut either way, but I think it is time for everyone, especially if you are concerned with the risks of pharmaceutical drugs, to set aside what we think we may know and take a serious look at cannabis as an option for people with serious mental health challenges. Medical use of marijuana has clear potential for reducing psychiatric drug use, drugs that are notorious for their devastating adverse effects. The decision to use cannabis is not simple, and along with the War on Drugs anti-pot propaganda there is also a lot of pro-marijuana fanaticism to wade through, but this is the reality: many people can forgo pharmaceutical drugs and use cannabis instead.

I don't need to reiterate the extensive research on medical use of cannabis available on the internet, and I have already written about cannabis and substance use in counseling practice in a previous post on Mad In America ('The Substance of Substance Use"). But here are some more thoughts about cannabis specifically.

There is now widespread evidence people are already successfully using cannabis to treat psychiatric conditions. Cannabis has long been used as medicine and spiritual tool throughout human history, for far longer than the brief period of prohibition when it's been criminalized. Criminalization didn't come from medical assessment of cannabis' usefulness, but was instead a political decision motivated by racism and suppression of the insurgent youth culture. Extensive studies showing medical benefits — for cancer, Alzheimers, multiple sclerosis, hepatitis C, irritable bowel, Parkinsons, pain management, and other conditions — have driven ballot initiative success around the country. This has begun to convince even longtime opponents, with US President Obama formally acknowledging cannabis as no more dangerous than alcohol, and CNN's chief medical correspondent Dr. Sanjay Gupta, one of the world's most influential opinion leaders on medicine, recently reversing his opposition to medical marijuana. Dr. Gupta even apologized for his previous anti-legalization stance and "not looking hard enough" at the issue.

But what about mental health conditions?

Around the country, medical marijuana cards are routinely given to people suffering anxiety, depression, insomnia, ADHD, trauma, and mental health issues. The internet is replete with a growing number of testimonies of successful symptom alleviation through cannabis, including people diagnosed with psychotic disorders such as bipolar and schizophrenia, These are not just a few anecdotes, these are thousands of people giving firsthand accounts of benefitting from cannabis for mental health conditions. And with the growing number of dispensaries, review websites, and legal cannabis consumers, these testimonies are growing in number.

And at the same time, it is not uncommon for me to receive emails like this:

"Our son was doing so well in school, and then he started smoking marijuana and went psychotic and went into the hospital, where he was diagnosed with schizophrenia."

"Before her delusions began I learned she was experimenting with marijuana…"

So what is going on?

Our culture has been saturated for years with a simplistic prohibition mentality around marijuana. Media reports demonize cannabis, with many scientific studies were twisted and manipulated to support a political agenda. Just one notorious example was the Heath/Tulane study in 1974. which claimed to show marijuana "kills brain cells." These findings, reported by a mainstream research institution with impeccable scientific credentials, were considered gold standard evidence and quickly became part of the mainstream attitudes. "Marijuana kills brain cells" was paraded by President Reagan in his anti-drug propaganda and brought out by frightened parents everywhere when they discovered a joint in their teenager's bedroom. The study even supported extremist media campaigns like the "This is your brain on drugs" television commercial, where a broken egg on a hot griddle became the last word on marijuana dangers.

The Heath/Tulane study was later exposed as pure scientific fraud: researchers were able to show brain cell death only by pumping so much marijuana smoke into the laboratory animals that the animals couldn't breathe. It was asphyxiation from lack of oxygen, not ingesting marijuana, that caused the brain damage. The poltiicization of science continues, and Dr. Gupta writes that of current US marijuana studies, 94% are designed to investigate harm, not potential benefits. Despite countless other studies showing marijuana's benefits and extremely low risk profile compared to either tobacco or alcohol - two very legal and very deadly drugs — we have let prohibition politics, not solid science, shape and continue to determine US drug policy and leadership worldwide.

This corruption is even more true in mental health, where substance use has become synonymous with substance abuse, and the mental health system oversees abstinence-based treatments that are often the criminal punishment for users arrested for possession alone.

No leading mental health organization has publicly expressed opposition to the War on Drugs or presented an honest discussion of the potential value of legalization. Mainstream mental health websites such as National Alliance for the Mentally Ill and the Schizophrenia Society of Canada continue to echo this demonization. Any potentially valuable caution about the role of cannabis use in psychosis - of which I will discuss more in a moment - gets lost and discredited in the general "just say no" message. There is no balanced discussion, not of how cannabis might help some people forgo the risks of psychiatric drugs relative to the possible risks to adolescent brain development. Mainstream opinion makers, driven in part by pharmaceutical and American Medical Association opposition to legalization, have instead elected to emphasize the psychosis-marijuana link research and ignore everything else.

NAMI medical director Dr. Ken Duckworth sums it up on the NAMI website "The overwhelming consensus from mental health professionals is that marijuana is not helpful—and potentially dangerous—for people with mental illness." He doesn't point out that this consensus is a result of politics, not medical science. The rest of the policy document has War on Drugs propaganda on full display. Dr. Duckworth writes, "Approximately one-third of people in America with schizophrenia regularly abuse marijuana." Really? Can we see a study citation for that statement? The answer is no, there is no citation because NAMI made this claim up, there is no research behind it.

Dr. Duckworth also rings the alarm bell of addiction, counting the mental health industry's conflation of use and abuse. He states that "a significant percentage of individuals who use marijuana will become physically dependent on the drug. This means that stopping their marijuana abuse will cause these people to experience a withdrawal syndrome." Dr. Gupta, however, disagrees. Dr. Gupta writes on CNN that "In 1944, New York Mayor Fiorello LaGuardia commissioned research to be performed by the New York Academy of Science. Among their conclusions: they found marijuana did not lead to significant addiction in the medical sense of the word…" He adds, "The physical symptoms of marijuana addiction are nothing like those of the other drugs I've mentioned."

My bet is with Dr. Gupta on this one. As Dr. Gupta's reversal indicates, there is a clear case for legalization of cannabis because there is an undeniable scientific research base — and common sense base - for cannabis' benefits relative to its risks. As a recreational drug there is just no comparing cannabis risks to other drugs such as alcohol and tobacco. But in the context of the War on Drugs' demonization, proponents of marijuana have reacted with a defensive romanticization, adding to the confusion. Left in a vacuum by mental health and medical organizations that should have been providing sound and honest discussion on the issue, the many mainstream research studies on medical benefits of cannabis are often touted and available on aggressively pro-marijuana sites. You feel that you are pulled to one side of the other in this political - and economic - tug of war. (The pro-marijuana sites are after all, now burgeoning with advertising revenue from the surfacing marijuana industry. The message today is "cannabis is good for you," and of course the next message will be "buy some today" and then "from us.")

As a society we are thankfully stepping away from both demonization and romanticization. And this means looking at two important facts about cannabis: dosage and strain.

The cannabis of today isn't the cannabis of yesterday. But the commonplace claim that "marijuana today is stronger than it was in the past" is far from the whole picture. Yes there is a lot more strong marijuana out there, but that also has positive implications for medical use. There is a an increased complexity and sophistication of how cannabis is being used, in many different ways by many different people, that has to be understood.

As far as dosage goes, the importance of understanding this complexity is well illustrated by the experience of New York Times Pulitzer Prize winning columnist Maureen Dowd. In a high-visibility, and influential, act that formed part of Times reporting on growing legalization efforts in Colorado and elsewhere, Dowd got high on pot in Denver. And promptly had a psychotic episode. She presumably didn't go on to be diagnosed bipolar, and did not need to be hospitalized, but her bad trip, replete with delusions of being dead and paranoid fears of the police, for some might be considered proof positive that cannabis is a bad idea for anyone "at risk for psychosis."

Dowd, however, was in effect writing a denunciation of wine by binge drinking on tequila. "Alcohol makes you sick and pass out" says more about how, how much, and what we drink, than it does that we drink alcohol. Simple enough common sense, but that is exactly what has been lost with prohibition propaganda. Without adequate understanding, Dowd apparently downed an entire cannabis infused edible candy. Edibles are notorious for their potency. Then she did what anyone following sensible marijuana use knows not to do - she gobbled up even more of the edible when she didn't feel any effects after a few minutes. She doubled the eventual impact of the drug, and delivered a massive dose to her marijuana-naive self after the slow-onset that is standard for eating marijuana (smoking effects are much faster; eating means the cannabis has to be digested before experiencing amplified effects.). It could be humorous - Dowd was lambasted in the internet for her irresponsibility - if it wasn't so emblematic of the impact of prohibition. Rational discussion by a presumably thoughtful professional journalist turns into nonsense, fuel for more simplistic demonization.

Dosage, including the delivery method (and now there are tinctures, vaporizers and other methods beyond smoking or eating), is an important reality to cannabis consumption. If a drug leads to psychosis at a higher dose, but doesn't at a lower dose, is the problem the drug or its use? If a drug at one dose is useful and at a higher dose is harmful, does that mean the drug is "useful" or "harmful?" So we begin to see one explanation for how a drug that many people find useful for psychosis can be the very drug that causes psychosis for many others. It becomes more understandable that my email inbox has emails from people blaming marijuana for mental illness alongside emails from people who've been helped.

Dowd also didn't chose her strain with any care, and strains can make a huge difference in cannabis use. There are hundreds of strains of crossbred hybrid cannabis, with colorful names like Blue Dream, Girl Scout Cookies, AC/DC, and Lemon Alien Dawg. This diversity isn't just fanciful or aesthetic: strains differ by aroma and flavor, Much more importantly, different strains have drastically different psychoactive effects. Alcohol intoxication might feel a bit different between beer, wine, and spirits, but not by much The different effects between different cannabis strains are like taking completely different substances.

There are 483 currently known compounds in marijuana, and at least 84 different psychoactive cannabinoids. THC is just one. This may explain why some people are using marijuana to alleviate psychosis while others find it makes psychosis worse. Medical marijuana users routinely share information about the qualities of different strains - some good for sleep, some for anxiety, some for depression, etc - to help each user find out what works for them. Of the many alkaloids, cannabidiol (CBD) is associated with tranquilizing response, while THC causes more mind-altering, and is potentially paranoia and anxiety inducing. Similarly, marijuana users have long known that the sativa varieties are different than the indica; sativa is associated with a more energetic high, prone to produce anxiety and paranoid in some people. while indica is more sedating. There is strong evidence that high CBD cannabis can alleviate psychosis for the simple reason that is tranquilizing, in the same way that anti-psychotics are for many people helpful because they are tranquilizing. CBD, however, clearly lacks the devastating side effects of antipsychotic drugs.

(The cannabis industry is still only now emerging from the underground, and with lack of the regulation and quality control of other industries users still have to rely on trial and error. It's not a guarantee that what the dispensary labeled as Blue Dream isn't actually Kali Mist, or there isn't sativa in that tincture marked indica. Medical users will be better served by legalization, which will allow greater testing and reliability of supply, as in the wine industry. The best role of regulation in the legalization process is fiercely debated by growers concerned about issues such as ecological sustainability, labor conditions, and the specter of Big Tobacco-style profiteering. In Sonoma County where I live, there is a huge marijuana industry and vast sums of money moving into the state in anticipation of California following the trend towards full legalization. The legal wine industry in the area is very shady, and has a deserved reputation for greedy disregard for the environmental and local community in its rapid expansion. That might be a cautionary tale: the gentle peace-ecology-love aura of marijuana may, some fear, quickly give way to the cutthroat realities of just another boom industry and agribusiness product.)

Word about CBD is getting out. Along with the emails from people tracing psychosis back to marijuana use, I now routinely encounter people in my work, lucky to be in a legal state or country or able to risk acquiring pot through the underground, who are using cannabis to help with distressing experiences associated with psychosis and mental illness diagnosis. Some have switched strains to high CBD and found different effects, some are using cannabis to help come off psych drugs, some are using cannabis instead of psych drugs, and some - very interestingly - have gotten benefits from cannabis and never gotten on psychiatric medications to begin with. Scientific studies on CBD support what I am seeing: a University of Cologne study from Germany, in a four week trial, found CBD as effective as an anti-psychotic in calming psychotic symptoms. A co-author of the study wrote "Not only was [CBD] as effective as standard antipsychotics, but it was also essentially free of the typical side effects seen with antipsychotic drugs."

A glance through research results on CBD from studies around the world shows evidence to support what we know already: CBD marijuana can help mental health conditions. These users are often careful in dosage, some even using just a few drops or "homeopathic" doses to get the desired effects.

(Other research is also intriguing. Numerous studies show anxiety alleviation, and, consistent with studies on Alzheimers and Parkinsons, one University of Montreal study published in Psychiatry Research even showed cannabis users diagnosed with schizophrenia to have better memory and prefrontal lobe functioning than those not using cannabis. Could cannabis be not only a substitute for psychiatric medications, but a treatment for the harm they caused? And other studies that are more troubling, such as those showing memory impairment and youth development harm, are essential to come to terms with in any benefit/risk assessment, but what do dosage and strain have to do with the results these studies found?)

So the kind of cannabis used, as well as the dosage, may explain part of the puzzle of different reports around cannabis and psychosis. This is in addition to a general principle with all psychoactive substances, a principle that applies to cannabis as well:

Response to cannabis use is widely diverse and individual. The medical marijuana dispensary community is thoroughly familiar with the fact that as a "medicine" cannabis does not provide uniform "treatment." Instead, just as each individual experiences "illness" differently, each individual has their own response, and what is right for one person might not be right for another - including the need to forgo cannabis altogether. Some people find the "high" contributes positively their medical condition and life circumstances, others seek out strains that have helpful effects without the high. Dispensary staff I've met are skilled at helping individuals navigate different strains and dosages for individual needs.

Substance abuse is a serious and devastating problem. Some people find that abstinence is the best strategy, such as following an AA 12 step program. Taking any drug - alcohol, tobacco, or cannabis -- involves risks. Cannabis needs to be subjected to the same caution, but overall cannabis is undoubtedly much safer on the body than alcohol or tobacco (zero marijuana caused deaths compared to many millions of alcohol and tobacco deaths) and much safer than any psychiatric medication. The growing legalization and medicalization of cannabis will no doubt be used by some to rationalize their addiction or avoid facing the fact that the drug is not helping them - but this is true of any substance, including alcohol and psychiatric meds. Once we step outside the demonization/romanticization polarity of the War On Drugs mentality we can engage this complicated reality more clearly. Saying cannabis might be helpful for some people is not to deny it might make others worse.

What about me personally? I found years ago that marijuana only worsens my own anxiety and further disconnects me from reality. I was smoking around the time I was first hospitalized, and though I quit marijuana I still had another psychotic break many years later when I wasn't using and hadn't used marijuana for 8 years. I do believe that pot was a contributing - but in no way a causal - factor in my first crisis, however, and that smoking played a role in the several years on decline that led to that crisis. But tellingly this was all wildly overstated by the hospital doctors who interviewed me. When I moved to Conard House, an outpatient facility in San Francisco, I was sent to a mandatory anti-drug meeting along with every marijuana user at the house, regardless of the frequency of use or whether or not it was abused or a problem. When I challenge the meeting leader by saying that marijuana was much safer than alcohol, I was kicked out of the program. (I was sent to a homeless shelter at 14th and Mission, right next to a thriving street crack market where I passed dealers every day on my way to and from my room. A good friend of mine from a previous program, who had been abstaining from cocaine for several years, was sent to the same shelter, I watched as he gradually lost control of his addiction with the temptation of those dealers; he left the shelter and I never heard from him again.)

I think that CBD strains are promising, and I personally would not hesitate to try a small dose of CBD marijuana in a time of emotional distress where I felt I had run out of other options. I would watch carefully my response, and proceed only if I felt confident I wasn't going to get paranoid or become anxious. Friends, clients, and colleagues who use cannabis have educated me about its potential if I did ever find myself in need, and have introduced me to the California dispensary system. I'm grateful I live in a state where I can learn about these issues and can first try a CBD brownie (gluten free of course) instead of a dose of Seroquel if I ever get out of hand with sleep deprivation or go off the deep end in a psychosis. And when I've seen friends go down to the psychotic vortex and head for the hospital, I wish there was some CBD weed around to try first to help them break the crisis cycle, rather than relying on a psych med as a last resort.

With clients I work with I now feel it is unethical as a therapist to not include cannabis in the list of possible wellness tools for those in legal states. I am pro-choice regarding psych drugs, and if I acknowledge that anti-psychotics, even with the risks, might be a wise choice for some people, I would be completely, well, crazy not to acknowledge that cannabis might be a wise choice for some people as well. I've always welcomed herbal medicine and traditional Chinese and other treatments into the range of possible wellness choices, because they have such a demonstrated history of helping so many people. Cannabis also has such a history, and I believe everyone working in the field as a therapist or psychiatrist needs to consider taking the same stance I have.

From a mental health advocacy standpoint, marijuana legalization also has many other implications that we as mental health professionals should look at. The AMA, APA, NAMI and other groups have failed to meet this issue responsibly. An American Journal of Public Health study by a team of economists, for example, examined states that had legalized marijuana for medical use. The study found there was a 10.8 percent reduction in the suicide rate of men in their 20s and a 9.4 percent reduction in men in their 30s. That is extraordinary - we know that psychiatric drug use can exacerbate suicidality (the drug warning is right there on the label), and alcohol of course can contribute to suicidality. It's not clear exactly why greater availability of medical cannabis might lower suicide rates, but this is a very, very significant finding to study further for anyone who takes suicide prevention seriously. (I recently lost a dear friend to suicide, and I am convinced benzodiazepines and alcohol played a role in killing her. I wish her therapist and doctors had explored cannabis as an alternative - she needed any alternative - and her death is one of the things motivating me to write this blog post and "come out" with my clinical practice decisions around cannabis.)

Studies also show reduction in alcohol use results from legalization, which, again, has enormous implications. Alcohol is an extremely dangerous and socially destructive drug with notorious mental health harms. The National Council on Alcoholism and Drug Dependence reports that alcohol use is a factor in 40 percent of all violent crimes in the United States, including 37 percent of rapes and 27 percent of aggravated assaults. In 1995 alone, college students reported more than 460,000 alcohol-related incidents of violence in the US. A 2011 prospective study found that dating abuse was associated with drinking among college students. A 2014 study found marijuana had clearly lower rates of associated domestic and partner violence. As pro-legalization comedian Bill Hicks remarked, imagine you are at a sporting event and some guy in front of you is screaming and picking a fight: is he high on marijuana or is he drunk on alcohol?

Reducing alcohol use in society will likely reduce violence; reducing violence means reducing trauma in society as a whole. When did we lose sight of ending violence as a way of preventing the cause of so many mental health problems? And legalization has already reduced traffic fatalities associated with drunk driving in states where it is legal - each traffic death sends out shockwaves of trauma and grief, and turns many people to alcohol or psychiatric drugs. (Hicks also said the biggest traffic danger from driving high is hitting the garage door because you forgot to open it.) Marijuana legalization is an upstream solution with huge implications. From a public health standpoint there is really no argument: if we can bring alcohol use down in society, then marijuana legalization is clearly worth it. According to the Centers for Disease Control, abuse of prescription opioids such as Oxy-Contin and Vicodin is a national epidemic that kill 16,000 people annually and devastate lives and families. Cannabis legalization could also reduce the market and illegal demand for opioids, easing this epidemic.

Legalization of cannabis also has important implications for young people and families - once we understand the complexity of substance use. The War on Drugs has devastated the US black community, and it is shameful that white-dominated mental health organizations have not spoken up against prohibition. Prison and the police are a traumatizing factor that directly interfere with mental health recovery. While legalization, according to the Journal of Adolescent Health, has not led to an increase in teen marijuana use, it does give families and youth more flexibility. For young people using cannabis, it might be more realistic to switch the kind of cannabis they are using as a harm reduction approach, rather than giving cannabis up completely. Many young people are committed to cannabis as a lifestyle, a form of religious expression, and a pathway to independence. Under prohibition it is impossible to talk openly about their cannabis experiences, and difficult to differentiate cannabis strains they are consuming. It may be easier for a teen to hear "use CBD strains, not the THC strains" than for them to hear "you have to stop smoking entirely;" "You can smoke pot, but in moderation" might work better than "you can't get high at all."

A harm reduction perspective is best served by legalization. Collaborative relationships require honesty: young people today know that different strains do different things, and they know the hypocrisy of a War On Drugs that sends people to jail for smoking a joint and then sells their lawyer whiskey at the bar next to the courthouse. Overgeneralized associations between marijuana and mental health problems, including psychosis, ignore a complex reality.

Adolescents using marijuana who get into emotional and psychological difficulties are like any adolescents who get into emotional and psychological difficulties, for whatever reason. They need help and support. The family needs help and support. The problem is never "marijuana plus genetics equals psychotic disorder." The marijuana may, or may not, be part of the problem. When families — and doctors —are blaming the marijuana it is usually a sign of a deeper problem being avoided. Prohibition is based on fear, the same fear behind the search for a simplistic answer, something to grab ahold of as the solution in a situation that feels out of control.

Cannabis use then often becomes a power struggle in families. As a therapist I have seen time and time again families where a son or daughter has been psychotic after using marijuana, and the family's response is to ban their son or daughter from using. So what does the young person do? They keep smoking, of course, except now they have a new problem: hiding from the parents, a power struggle with their parents, and the beginning of a cycle of isolation if the power struggle continues. I have to work hard to stay in a trusting relationship with both sides, and that job gets harder the more prohibition fear entrenches intolerance. The solution is to create conversations about the substance; even if the parents are strongly against any marijuana use, it's important to respect all sides, but on an equal playing fiend where the young person can be validated for a choice that has some science on its side. Dismissing one side doesn't help. Doesn't it make more sense to say Let's talk? than to Just Say No?

I have no doubt that marijuana use has played a role in many people's problems with psychosis. I routinely work with people to encourage them to stop smoking when they know it can lead to crisis. I've seen people off marijuana start using again and end up hospitalized. And marijuana can certainly lead to habituation for some people and play a role in substance problems. Educating society about these risks makes the same sense that educating society about alcohol risks makes sense - as long as the risks are not exaggerated. Personally I would like to see cannabis avoid the commercialization of alcohol and be a more accepted - but not promoted or advertised - personal option. We really don't need any more consumerism than we already have. Instead, we need an honesty and smart use that we really don't even have with alcohol, with all the alcohol advertising and the culture of happy hour and spring break.

And of the risks, what about the correlation between first break psychosis with a higher rate of marijuana use? There is in my view validity to that concern — and it also be at least in part misleading. What if the causality is sometimes in the other direction? What if people who end up psychotic are drawn to altered states of consciousness in general, what if they first seek out in marijuana what they eventually end up later seeking in their break to a psychotic reality? Working with young people over many years, I see the need to get "high" comes first, not after, the substance. Few families have honest discussions about the need to get high and get away - how it is a human need that everyone has. And getting high repeatedly may be an escape hatch out of untenable life circumstances and confusing options. Maybe a young person is drawn to cannabis by the same inner need that will eventually draw them to psychosis, correlating the two - but not indicating causality.

As we come to terms with the devastating impact that psychiatric drugs have on society, we face a compelling question: What if there was a substitute? Someone considering a benzo, or an anti-psychotic, or an anti-depressant, is about to embark on a risky treatment option that might work out fine, or might end up destroying their life. That is the reality of the risks of psychiatric drugs. The Soteria House alternative and the Open Dialogue approach, it should be remembered, do rely on psychiatric drugs as a last resort. What if everyone had, on a wide scale, the option of choosing something with a lower side effect profile, and perhaps thereby could be diverted from a risky pathway? That may be what the US is on the brink of with legalization. And what exactly do we know of Pharma's influence in opposing marijuana legalization? The American Medical Association and APA have long opposed legalization; does medical cannabis represent a threat to Pharma markets?

These social implications have not gone unnoticed by the web of financial interests benefitting from cannabis prohibition. The same public policy corruption driving psychiatric drug use is also evident in efforts to block legalization. Dr. Herbert Kleber of Columbia University, an impeccably credentialed academic, is widely quoted in the press warning against marijuana - and also serves as a paid consultant to leading prescription drug companies. Oxy-Contin manufacturer Purdue Pharma and Vicodin manufacturer Abbott Laboratories are among the leading funders of the Community Anti-Drug Coalition of America and Partnership for Drug Free Kids - both fierce prohibition advocates. (Other funders include Janssen and Pfizer.) When Patrick Kennedy's so-called Project SAM (Smart Approaches to Marijuana) worked against Alaska's legalization initiative, activists counterattacked by pointing out the organizations extensive financial ties to the liquor and beer lobby. Dr. Stuart Gitlow, President of the American Society Of Addiction Medicine, another legalization opponent, went on the media circuit disputing President Obama's statement that marijuana is no more dangerous than alcohol: Gitlow serves as medical director for pharma company Orexo, an opioid manufacturer. Former Drug Enforcement Administration head Peter Bensinger and former White House drug czar Robert DuPont (yes that was his title) now run a commercial firm that specializes in the market for workplace drug testing.

While some police have come out against the War on Drugs, many police are lobbying in favor of it. Is it because they receive millions in funds to use under drug money seizure and assets forfeiture laws? One Florida sheriff who led opposition to legalization went so far as to state openly that drug asset forfeitures were important for county law enforcement resources. California legalization was opposed by another police lobbyist who made a career of funneling federal War on Drugs grants to state law enforcement. This is corruption in the crudest form : a mandate for serving public good diverted to individual gain.

As Los Angeles Police Department Deputy Chief Stephen Downing told The Nation, "The only difference now compared to the times of alcohol prohibition is that, in the times of alcohol prohibition, law enforcement—the police and judges—got their money in brown paper bags. Today, they get their money through legitimate, systematic programs run by the federal government. That's why they're using their lobbying organizations to fight every reform." Legalization means challenging economies of influence and politics of corruption that have made drug policy and criminalization big business. Importantly, ending alcohol Prohibition in 1933 involved a vast clearing out of this corruption from the federal to the local level; hopefully the grassroots drive for cannabis policy reform will likewise have wide anti-corruption implications.

Even when we support cautious consideration and avoid making any blanket endorsement, cannabis is a powerful psychoactive plant that involves risks. Small controlled doses - a few drops of tincture, a small puff from a cigarette, a single edible candy - are still unpredictable, and might launch someone onto an unpleasant altered state, make working or relating in public difficult, trigger insomnia, interfere with driving, set someone down a path to addiction, or worse. Harms to memory and cognition development among adolescents might reveal themselves after long term heavy use. There are risks: it's not a one size fits all solution. It will take some time to sort out studies and research honestly and get a realistic sense of the social impact in the wake of a politicized and corrupted research legacy.

And this underscores one of the central problems with the cannabis policy discussion. Legalization activists wisely chose to emphasize medical uses on a pathway towards greater marijuana acceptance. But in practice, as a plant medicine, cannabis has never been and probably never will be a targeted medical treatment. It is a plant, not a pill. Cannabis is a choice to introduce a substance into one's body that will have unique and unpredictable effects on consciousness. It's a life decision. It changes you, in subtle ways or dramatic ways, to ingest a substance.

Like regularly taking alcohol, drinking coffee daily, smoking cigarettes, and the use of food and herbal medicines in traditional cultures, marijuana is really best understood as a relationship. The human body and mind have receptors uniquely designed to interact with cannabis, which helps explain the broad range of consciousness and physical health effects now bing studied and experienced. Specific uses and strains might target symptoms associated with a diagnosis, but cannabis is not like penicillin. Only the individual knows how perception and consciousness are altered, and whether that is experienced as a plus or a minus in life. Some people will choose to be high if it goes along with reduction of some other discomfort; others will prefer to avoid getting high in any form. From food to movies to wine to sexuality, "self-medicating" is after all a widespread social practice and should be acknowledged: we all, to some degree, medicate ourselves just as we all, to some degree, get high. And this is what we have overlooked in our understanding of psychiatric drugs - they too are very powerful mind altering substances that get us "high." It's not what we think of as a high, we are still altered when we take our Zyprexa or our Prozac, and some psychiatric drugs, such as the benzodiazepines and the stimulants, are widely used recreationally. The psychiatric drugs have clear toxicities to the body; cannabis has extremely few, and a wide profile of benefits. That's why it's been used around the world as medicine since prehistoric times. It is also mind altering, despite the emphasis on "medical" use, and we need to recognize that altering our minds is part of what we do as humans.

We need the freedom, especially when we are facing extreme distress and crisis, to choose what risks we want to take and what substances we want to introduce, or not introduce, into our bodies and minds. We are bombarded by physical and psychological stresses in virtually every aspect of our lives today. Some of us choose alcohol, Some of us choose yoga, running, and organic food. Some us will choose cannabis. We need to take a principled and ethical look at that choice, and we need to ensure that people exploring this option aren't put in jail for it (madinamerica.com, 2015).

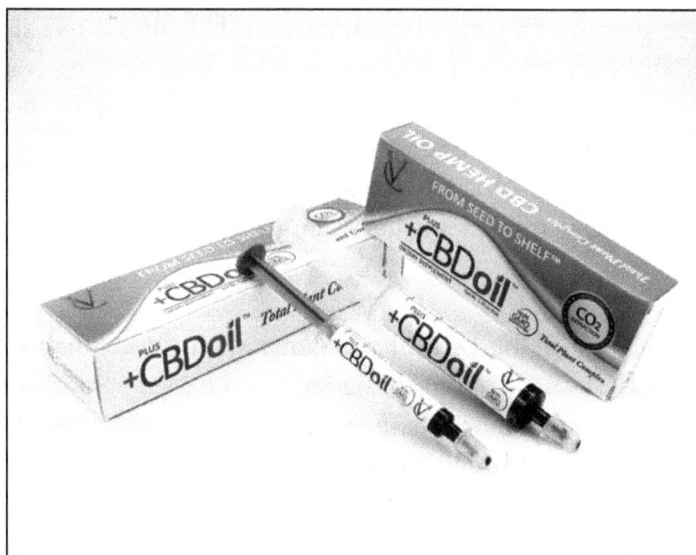

CannaVest™
PLUSCBD OIL™ Green Oral Applicator

CODEX ALTERNUS

Vitamin Therapy

Megavitamin Therapy

Those on Megavitamin Therapy had a 50% Lower Hospital Readmission Rate Than the Control Group in This Study of 160 Patients Diagnosed with Schizophrenia

Hawkins, D. R. et al., "Orthomolecular Psychiatry: Niacin and Megavitamin Therapy." *Psychosomatics* 11, no. 5 (October 1970): 517–21. Publisher: AMERICAN PSYCHIATRIC PUBLISHING, INC. doi:10.1016/S0033-3182(70)71622-8. PMID: 5470684

> ➤ This study covered a two-year period during which 160 patients were followed up following discharge from the hospital. In all of these patients the diagnosis o schizophrenia was clearcut. The sample consisted of 94 female and 66 male patients with the median age of 28. While in the hospital all patients received phenothiazines plus megavitamins which included pyridoxine at minimum daily dose of 50 mgs, ascorbic acid 4 grams daily and either niacin or niacinamid in daily doses of 4 to 10 grams. At the time of discharge the megavitamins were discontinued in 85 cases and the remaining patients took the megavitamins for either three months, six months or one year. During the course of the study of the 85 patients in whom megavitamins were discontinued at time of discharge 30 patients were hospitalized (35%). Those patients in whom the medication was continued for three to ten months had a readmission rate of 25%. Of those patients who were continued on the megavitamins for one year over (57 patients) only 9 patients were readmitted (16%). The X_2 score value for this comparison is in the excess of 5.99 reqired for significance at the 0.05 level. This study establishes a defintite correlation between the continuation of megavitamin therapy and a 50% lower readmission rate than patients in the control group.

Vitamin B₁ (Thiamine)

Malnutrition-induced Wernicke-Korsakoff Syndrome Should Be Treated with Thiamine

McCormick, Laurie M., et al., "Beyond Alcoholism: Wernicke-Korsakoff Syndrome in Patients with Psychiatric Disorders." *Cognitive and Behavioral Neurology: Official Journal of the Society for Behavioral and Cognitive Neurology* 24, no. 4 (December 2011): 209–16. Publisher: LIPPINCOTT WILLIAMS & WILKINS; doi:10.1097/WNN.0b013e31823f90c4., PMID: 22134191

> ➤ In summary, physicians should be aware of preventable vitamin deficiency-related neuropsychiatric syndromes, and should consider new signs and symptoms in patients with known psychiatric disorders as potential harbingers of reversible WE and

irreversible WKS. Physicians should ask patients, relatives, and caregivers specifically about what patients have been eating—and not eating—and should thoroughly review the medical record for warning signs of nutritional deficiency. Physicians must exclude somatoform disorders, characterized by symptoms that mimic disease or injury but for which there is no identifiable physical cause; however, a patient with a psychiatric diagnosis can still develop serious medical conditions. If physicians assume that a patient's symptoms stem wholly from a psychiatric disorder, they can miss the life-threatening emergency of WE. If they delay treating this reversible condition, the patients who survive may be left with long-term physical and cognitive sequelae. Patients at highest risk of developing non-alcoholic WE and WKS have a history of malnutrition, delusions related to food, or vomiting lasting longer than a week. These patients should be treated prophylactically with thiamine, especially before refeeding.

Malnutrition-induced Wernicke's Encephalopathy in Patient with Schizophrenia Responds Well to IV Thiamine Administration

Harrison, Rebecca A. et al., "Wernicke's Encephalopathy in a Patient with Schizophrenia." *Journal of General Internal Medicine* 21, no. 12 (December 2006): C8–11. Publisher: SPRINGER NEW YORK; doi:10.1111/j.1525-1497.2006.00600.x. PMID: 16925799

> ➤ Clinically, we most often associate Wernicke's encephalopathy (WE) with an alcohol abusing population. However, it is important to consider other causes of malnutrition and vitamin deficiency as risk factors for the development of this disorder. We present a case of a 51-year-old man with schizophrenia and malnutrition who presented with delirium, ophthalmoplegia, and seizures. He responded rapidly to the administration of IV thiamine. Because of the high rate of mortality and morbidity, WE should be high on the differential of any patient at risk for malnutrition or with ophthalmoplegia, regardless of alcohol history. This is particularly important in psychiatric patients where the syndrome may be masked and thus treatment delayed.

Intravenous Vitamin B1 Supplementation Resolves Deficiency and Psychotic Symptoms

Sasaki, Takeshi, et al., "[A case of thiamine deficiency with psychotic symptoms--blood concentration of thiamine and response to therapy]." *Seishin Shinkeigaku Zasshi = Psychiatria Et Neurologia Japonica* 112, no. 2 (2010): 97–110., PMID: 20384190

> ➤ We report the case of a 63-year-old woman with thiamine deficiency who showed auditory hallucinations, a delusion of persecution, catatonic stupor, and catalepsy but no neurological symptoms including oculomotor or gait disturbance. Brain MRI did not show high-intensity T2 signals in regions including the thalami, mamillary bodies, or periaqueductal area. Her thiamine concentration was 19 ng/mL, only slightly less than the reference range of 20-50 ng/mL. Her psychosis was unresponsive to antipsychotics or electroconvulsive therapy, but was ameliorated by repetitive intravenous thiamine administrations at 100-200 mg per day. However, one month after completing

intravenous treatment, her psychosis recurred, even though she was given 150 mg of thiamine per day orally and her blood concentration of thiamine was maintained at far higher than the reference range. Again, intravenous thiamine administration was necessary to ameliorate her symptoms. The present patient indicates that the possibility of thiamine deficiency should be considered in cases of psychosis without neurological disturbance and high-intensity T2 MRI lesions. Also, this case suggests that a high blood thiamine concentration does not necessarily correspond to sufficient thiamine levels in the brain. Based on this, we must reconsider the importance of a high dose of thiamine administration as a therapy for thiamine deficiency. The validity of the reference range of the thiamine concentration, 20-50 ng/mL, is critically reviewed.

Vitamin B₃ (Niacin, Nicotinic Acid)

Niacin Deficiency is a Important Contributor to the Development of Schizophrenia and Supplementation May Help a Subset of Patients

Xu, X. J., et al., "Niacin-respondent subset of schizophrenia–a therapeutic review." *European Review for Medical and Pharmacological Sciences* 19, no. 6 (2015): 988-997. , Publisher: VERDUCI EDITORE SRL

> ➤ Niacin deficiency seems to be an important contributor in the development of the clinical picture of schizophrenia. Studies and sparse case reports indicate that niacin augmentation could help a subset of patients suffering from schizophrenia. These patients could benefit from an early intervention of addition of therapeutic doses to schizophrenia in addition to ongoing treatment.

Niacin Megavitamin Therapy Cures Young Schizophrenic Woman

Hoffer, A. "A Neurological Form of Schizophrenia." *Canadian Medical Association Journal* 108, no. 2 (January 20, 1973): 186 passim., Publisher: CANADIAN MEDICAL ASSOCIATION; PMID: 4684627

> ➤ A case is described of a young woman who first showed manifestations of schizophrenia in childhood. At the age of 13 years evidence was present of what was authoritatively diagnosed as a progressive degenerative cerebellar syndrome and her condition continued to deteriorate. Improvement commenced shortly after the institution of megavitamin therapy, notably nicotinic acid 3 grams daily. Her subsequent educational progress was satisfactory and her social rehabilitation is now complete. No medication other than nicotinic acid is required.

Nicotinic Acid Reduces Hospital Readmission Rate

Hoffer, A. "TREATMENT OF SCHIZOPHRENIA WITH NICOTINIC ACID. A TEN YEAR FOLLOW-UP." *Acta Psychiatrica Scandinavica* 40 (1964): 171–89, Publisher: BLACKWELL MUNKSGAARD; PMID: 14235254

> "The group which received nicotinic acid had the best record which showed most clearly in the total days of rehospitalization, i.e. about 11 days per patient per year. The comparison group required about 19 days per patient per year."

Hoffer, A. "Nicotinic Acid: An Adjunct in the Treatment of Schizophrenia." *The American Journal of Psychiatry* 120 (August 1963): 171–73., Publisher: AM PSYCHIATRIC ASSN; PMID: 13963912

> Of the first 16 patients treated in 1952, 75% have not required any further readmissions, 4 have between them had 6 brief readmissions and none now in the hospital. A comparison group of 27 did not fare so well. Of them 17 have required readmission 63 times. These 27 patients required 34 years of admissions over a ten-year period. The nicotinic acid group required only 1.4 years.

Osmond, H., et al., "Massive Niacin Treatment in Schizophrenia. Review of a Nine-Year Study." *Lancet* 1, no. 7224 (February 10, 1962): 316–19. Publisher: LANCET PUBLISHING GROUP; PMID: 14482545

> Table IV shows the effect of niacin and other treatments on the time spent in the hospital. One way of summarizing this table would be to say that, during the four-year follow-up, patients who had never had nicotinic acid spent two-fifths of a year in hospital, while for those who received it the average was only a sixth of a year.

> …Schizophrenics treated in Saskatchewan without niacin or nicotinamide had an equally gloomy prognosis (table III): over half were readmitted at least once within five years of discharge. But of those receiving this vitamin only about a sixth required readmission during the same period.

Adequate Doses of Niacin Contribute to Recovery in Schizophrenic Patients

Hoffer, A. "Treatment of Schizophrenia with Nicotinic Acid and Nicotinamide." *Journal of Clinical and Experimental Psychopathology* 18, no. 2 (June 1957): 131–58., Publisher: MEDICAL DIGEST INC [L]; PMID: 13439009

> "When used in adequate dosages, nicotinic acid and nicotinamide materially contribute to the recovery of schizophrenic patients."

Niacin Augmentation Therapy for Rapid Resolution of Delusional Parasitosis

Prakash, Ravi, et al., "Rapid Resolution of Delusional Parasitosis in Pellagra with Niacin Augmentation Therapy." *General Hospital Psychiatry* 30, no. 6 (December 2008): 581–84. Publisher: ELSEVIER INC. doi:10.1016/j.genhosppsych.2008.04.011., PMID: 19061687

> We report a case of pellagra manifesting with delusional parasitosis in a man whose delusion resolved rapidly after he started niacin-augmentation therapy. This case may

provide clues to the biological underpinnings of delusional parasitosis as well as niacin treatment as treatment option in similar cases.

Vitamin B₅ (Pantothenic Acid)

Pantothenate May Play a Role in Causation of Schizophrenia and Therapeutic Role in Those Who Have the Deficiency

Bou Khalil, Rami, et al., "Pantothenate's Possible Role in Schizophrenia Pathogenesis." *Clinical Neuropharmacology* 35, no. 6 (December 2012): 296. doi:10.1097/WNF.0b013e3182711faf., PMID: 23151470

> ➤ ...pantothenic acid or pantothenate or Vitamin B₅ is essential for synthesis of CoA. Pantothenate kinase 2 mutation is responsible for the appearance of psychotic symptoms in patients carrying it. Accordingly, pantothenate may play a role in the pathogenesis of a least some presentations of schizophrenia, and its subsequent therapeutic role in patients with schizophrenia should be further evaluated.

Adrenal Failure May Be Due to Pantothenic Deficiency Which is Sometimes Found in Schizophrenia and Should Be Treated with Pantothenate to Alleviate Some Symptoms

Monro, J., "Pantothenic Acid in Schizophrenia." *Lancet (London, England)* 1, no. 7797 (February 3, 1973): 262–63., PMID: 4119403

> ➤ "Adrenal impairment, which is concomitant of many severe chronic diseases, may occur in schizophrenia, and the pigmentation may be partly to adrenal failure. It is not suggested that calcium pantothenate will correct the schizophrenic process, but only that it may alleviate some symptoms."

Vitamin B₆ (Pyridoxine)

After Several Weeks on Neuroleptic—Pyrodoxine Therapy Patients Reported Significant Improvement

Bucci, L., et al., "Pyridoxine and Schizophrenia." *The British Journal of Psychiatry: The Journal of Mental Science* 122, no. 567 (February 1973): 240. Publisher: ROYAL MEDICO-PSYCHOLOGICAL ASSOCIATION; PMID: 4714839

> ➤ After 4 to 6 weeks of this neuroleptic-pyridoxine therapy, 8 out of 15 patients reported a certain degree of subjective improvement, claiming to feel more alert and responsive, more active and less anergic. The improvement was only subjective and it was acknowledged only as such, since no noticeable clinical change could be elicited by the

the physician of their mental status became slowly but progressively more and more apparent, and 8 to 10 weeks after the beginning of the new drug regimen the patients appeared no longer blunted in their affect, nor indifferent to their personal habits and their environment. While in the past most of them had shown complete lack of interest in becoming involved in conversation, now they were willing to talk about themselves and their illness. At the end of the third month of therapy the lack of drive and motivation and the blunted affect had been replaced in 8 patients by feeling of well-being, and they agreed to be referred either to occupational therapy or to a vocational and rehabilitation programme, and in brief became active participants.

Potentiation of Therapeutic Effects of Nicotinic Acid by Pyridoxine (vitamin B6) in Schizophrenia

> **Ananth, J. V.,** et al., "Potentiation of Therapeutic Effects of Nicotinic Acid by Pyridoxine in Chronic Schizophrenics." *Canadian Psychiatric Association Journal* 18, no. 5 (October 1973): 377–83., Publisher: CANADIAN PSYCHIATRIC ASSOCIATION; PMID: 4147710

➢ "Based on these findings it was hypothesized that the administration of pyridoxine will enhance the therapeutic effect of nicotinic acid in schizophrenic patients by opening up kynurenine cycle of tryptophan metabolism and thereby decreasing the formation of indoles.

➢ In this 48-week placebo-controlled study, the therapeutic effect of a combination of nicotinic acid and pyridoxine was compared with that of treatment with either nicotinic acid or pyridoxine alone. Of the three indices of therapeutic effects, global improvement in psychopathology (BPRS and NOSIE) scores was seen in all three groups; the number of days of hospitalization during the period of the clinical study was lower in both the nicotinic acid and combined treatment group; and only in the combined treatment group was the daily average dosage of phenothiazine medication decreased. Thus, improvement in all three indices was noted in the combined treatment group."

Pyridoxine has an Antidepressant Effect (vitamin B6) in Schizophrenic Patients with Co-morbid Minor Depression

> **Shiloh, R.,** et al., "[Antidepressive effect of pyridoxine (vitamin B6) in neuroleptic-treated schizophrenic patients with co-morbid minor depression--preliminary open-label trial]." *Harefuah* 140, no. 5 (May 2001): 369–73, 456., Publisher: HA-HISTADRUT; PMID: 11419053

➢ "Two of nine patients (22%), characterized by higher initial HAM-D and SANS scores, and by older age and longer duration of illness, experienced marked improvements in depressive symptoms (23% and 28% decrease in HAM-D scores) following 4 weeks of pyridoxine administration. In one of these two, the improvement in depressive symptoms was accompanied by a parallel decrease in SANS scores."

Vitamin B6 is Effective Monotherapy for Certain Types of Catatonic Schizophrenic-like Cases

> **Brooks, S. C., et al.,** "An Unusual Schizophrenic Illness Responsive to Pyridoxine HCl (B6) Subsequent to Phenothiazine and Butyrophenone Toxicities." *Biological Psychiatry* 18, no. 11 (November 1983): 1321–28., Publisher: ELSEVIER INC., PMID: 6652165

> ➤ This report describes the treatment of an 18-year-old male diagnosed (DSM II) as having an acute schizophrenic reaction, catatonic type (APA, 1968) in association with multiplex psychological findings which were partially congruous with several neuropsychobehavioral disorders. The patient did not demonstrate classical symptoms, in constellation, which could support a definitive diagnosis of an organic brain syndrome. The patient did demonstrate classical psychiatric symptoms supporting the clinical diagnosis of a schizophrenic disorder, however. Treatment with haloperidol (buturophenone) from 1-5 mg TID and, alternatively, trifluoperazine (phenothiazine) at 2 mg TID was unsuccessful because of the extrapyramidal side effects and the respective hepatotoxicities which occurred with both drugs. Pyridoxine HCI (vitamin B6) at 500 mg daily was therapeutically effective in eliminating the major schizophrenic reaction. Clinical relapse resulted with dose reduction to 250 mg daily, following full clinical recovery for 1 year, but was reinstituted again at 500 mg daily. The complex findings and clinical success with pyridoxine HCI in this case parallel a previously unreported case of an 11 year-old female with schizophrenia, catatonic type and minimal brain dysfunction who demonstrated initial trifluperazine and thiothixene intolerance but sequent responsiveness to pyridoxine HCI at 500 mg daily. Experience with both cases estimated the effective dosage of pyridoxine HCI at 500 mg daily to be 5-10 mg/kg per day.

Vitamin B9 (Folate, Folic Acid, and Methylfolate)

Methylfolate Significantly Improved Clinical and Social Recovery of Schizophrenic Patients

> **Godfrey, P. S., et al.,** "Enhancement of Recovery from Psychiatric Illness by Methylfolate." *Lancet* 336, no. 8712 (August 18, 1990): 392–95., Publisher: LANCET PUBLISHING GROUP; PMID: 1974941

> ➤ 41 (33%) of 123 patients with acute psychiatric disorders (DSM III diagnosis of major depression or schizophrenia) had borderline or definite folate deficiency (red-cell folate below 200 micrograms/l) and took part in a double-blind, placebo-controlled trial of methylfolate, 15 mg daily, for 6 months in addition to standard psychotropic treatment. Among both depressed and schizophrenic patients methylfolate significantly improved clinical and social recovery. The differences in outcome scores between methylfolate and placebo groups became greater with time. These findings add to the evidence implicating disturbances of methylation in the nervous system in the biology of some forms of mental illness.

Folate Supplementation May Be Good Management Modality for Clinical Improvement in Some Schizophrenic Patients with Genetic Defect

Kim, Tae Ho, et al., "Serum Homocysteine and Folate Levels in Korean Schizophrenic Patients." *Psychiatry Investigation* 8, no. 2 (June 2011): 134–40. Publisher: Korean Neuropsychiatric Association; doi:10.4306/pi.2011.8.2.134., PMID: 21852990

> ➤ "Some schizophrenia patients with high serum homocysteine levels may have the genetic defect of having low folate serum levels. In such cases, folate ingestion may be a good management modality for clinical improvement."

Vitamin B₁₂ (Cobalamin)

Chronic Psychosis Improves Dramatically with Short-term Antipsychotic Medication and Intramuscular Cobalamin Injections

Rajkumar, A. P., et al., "Chronic Psychosis Associated with Vitamin B12 Deficiency." *The Journal of the Association of Physicians of India* 56 (February 2008): 115–16., Publisher: ASSOCIATION OF PHYSICIANS OF INDIA; PMID: 18472513

> ➤ B12 deficiency is widely prevalent and usually presents with haematologic and neuropsychiatric manifestations. Psychiatric symptoms seldom precede anaemia and present as the principal manifestation of B12 deficiency. A report an unusual presentation of long standing psychotic symptoms without anaemia in a 31 year old male, who presented to a tertiary care psychiatric facility. His physical examination revealed hyper pigmentation of extremities and posterior column involvement. Laboratory investigations confirmed normal haemoglobin and low serum B12 levels. He recovered dramatically with short term antipsychotic medication and intramuscular cobalamin supplementation. He remained asymptomatic and functionally independent at two years follow up.

Three Patients Recovered Only on a Combination of B12 Supplementation and Psychiatric Medication

Bhat, Amritha S., et al., "Psychiatric Presentations of Vitamin B 12 Deficiency." *Journal of the Indian Medical Association* 105, no. 7 (July 2007): 395–96., Publisher: INDIAN MEDICAL ASSOCIATION; LTD; PMID: 18178994

> ➤ Vitamin B12 deficiency has been implicated in various psychiatric conditions for a long time. The association could be primary, secondary to the psychiatric disorder, or even just coincidental. However, left untreated, the deficiency can delay or preclude recovery. Hence early recognition is important, especially when the traditional manifestations of B12 deficiency like anaemia, macrocytosis or spinal cord symptoms are not prominent.

CODEX ALTERNUS

Three cases are presented here where vitamin B12 deficiency and psychiatric symptomatology were coexistent, and the patients recovered only on a combination of B12 supplementation and psychiatric medication.

Patient Recovers from Schizophrenia-like Psychotic Episode with Oral Cobalamin Supplementation and Short Course Antipsychotic Treatment

Kuo, Shin-Chang, et al., "Schizophrenia-like Psychotic Episode Precipitated by Cobalamin Deficiency." *General Hospital Psychiatry* 31, no. 6 (December 2009): 586–88. doi:10.1016/j.genhosppsych.2009.02.003., Publisher: ELSEVIER INC.; PMID: 19892219

> Although cobalamin deficiency is widely known and usually presents with hematologic and neuropsychiatric manifestations, the psychiatric symptoms are not usually the predominant manifestation. We describe a young single male vegetarian who developed a cobalamin-induced psychotic episode without preceding neurologic manifestations and without any hematologic symptoms. He recovered after a short course of antipsychotics and oral cobalamin supplementation and remained asymptomatic and functionally independent at 1 year of follow-up.

Psychosis is Eliminated by Vitamin B12 Replacement Therapy

Masalha, R., et al., "Cobalamin-Responsive Psychosis as the Sole Manifestation of Vitamin B12 Deficiency." *The Israel Medical Association Journal:* IMAJ 3, no. 9 (September 2001): 701–3., Publisher: ISRAEL MEDICAL ASSOCIATION; PMID: 11574992

> Treatment for vitamin B12 deficiency is described as simple, uncomplicated and very helpful, especially when the deficiency is diagnosed early and the appropriate treatment instituted promptly. Our patients were treated with anti-psychotic drugs for 2 months with- out any benefit and the treatment was stopped. After substitution with intra-muscular injections of hydroxycobala-min, the effect was observed within 6±8 weeks after initiation of therapy. Similarly, the two patients described by Evans et al. also showed improvement after several weeks, even though their initial response was more dramatic. Both our patients are currently receiving oral hydroxycobalamin (300 g/day), and after a year of follow-up have maintained their mental health. The therapeutic protocol we used was entirely empirical, as there are no controlled studies or recommendations of optimal therapy for dietary vitamin B12 deficiency. We con- tend however, that prevention would have been the most effective approach.

Vitamin B Complex

Schizophrenic Patients with Hyperhomocysteinemia Benefit from the Addition of B Vitamins

CODEX ALTERNUS

Levine, Joseph, et al., "Homocysteine-Reducing Strategies Improve Symptoms in Chronic Schizophrenic Patients with Hyperhomocysteinemia." *Biological Psychiatry* 60, no. 3 (August 1, 2006): 265–69. doi:10.1016/j.biopsych.2005.10.009., Publisher: ELSEVIER INC. PMID: 116412989

> Homocysteine levels declined with vitamin therapy compared with placebo in all patients except for one noncompliant subject. Clinical symptoms of schizophrenia as measured by the Positive and Negative Syndrome Scale declined significantly with active treatment compared with placebo. Neuropsychological test results overall, and Wisconsin Card Sort (Categories Completed) test results in particular, were significantly better after vitamin treatment than after placebo. A subgroup of schizophrenic patients with hyperhomocysteinemia might benefit from the simple addition of B vitamins.

Correction of Essential Fatty Acids and B vitamin Status Reduces Psychiatric Symptoms and Cardiovascular Disease

Kemperman, R. F. J., et al., "Low Essential Fatty Acid and B-Vitamin Status in a Subgroup of Patients with Schizophrenia and Its Response to Dietary Supplementation." *Prostaglandins, Leukotrienes, and Essential Fatty Acids* 74, no. 2 (February 2006): 75–85. doi:10.1016/j.plefa.2005.11.004., Publisher: CHURCHILL LIVINGSTONE; PMID: 16384692

> We conclude that a subgroup of patients with schizophrenia has biochemical EFA deficiency, omega3/DHA marginality, moderate hyperhomocysteinemia, or combinations. Correction seems indicated in view of the possible relation of poor EFA and B-vitamin status with some of their psychiatric symptoms, but notably to reduce their high risk of cardiovascular disease.

Folate Plus Vitamin B12 Supplementation Can Improve Negative Symptoms of Schizophrenia

Roffman, Joshua L., et al., "Randomized Multicenter Investigation of Folate plus Vitamin B12 Supplementation in Schizophrenia." *JAMA Psychiatry* 70, no. 5 (May 2013): 481–89. Publisher: American Medical Association; doi:10.1001/jamapsychiatry.2013.900., PMID: 23467813

> "Folate plus vitamin B12 supplementation can improve negative symptoms of schizophrenia, but treatment response is influenced by genetic variation in folate absorption. These findings support a personalized medicine approach for the treatment of negative symptoms."

Vitamin C

Vitamin C Improves Outcome of Schizophrenia

Dakhale, G. N., et al., "Supplementation of Vitamin C with Atypical Antipsychotics Reduces Oxidative Stress and Improves the Outcome of Schizophrenia." *Psychopharmacology* 182, no. 4 (November 2005): 494–98. doi:10.1007/s00213-005-0117-1., Publisher: SPRINGER-VERLAG; PMID: 16133138

> ➤ "BPRS change scores at 8 weeks improved statically significant with vitamin C as compared to placebo."

Vitamin C May Help Schizophrenics and an Add-on Treatment

Beaclair, L., et al., "An Adjunctive Role for Ascorbic Acid in Treatment of Schizophrenia?" *J Clin Psychopharmacol* Vol. 7, No.4, Aug 1987, PMID: 3624518

The results from the addition of ascorbic acid to treatment with maintained doses of antipsychotics were better than we had anticipated. A controlled study of this procedure is now justified. The role of acorbic acid in treating schizophrenia has been long controversial; it remains to be seen whether the adjunctive role suggested by the present study will be confirmed.

Vitamin D

Vitamin D Supplementation in Deficient Schizophrenic Patients Should Be Considered

Yüksel, Rabia Nazik, et al., "Correlation between Total Vitamin D Levels and Psychotic Psychopathology in Patients with Schizophrenia: Therapeutic Implications for Add-on Vitamin D Augmentation." *Therapeutic Advances in Psychopharmacology* 4, no. 6 (December 2014): 268–75. Publisher: Sage; doi:10.1177/2045125314553612., PMID: 25489478

> ➤ Even though important factors for vitamin D synthesis were similar, there was severe vitamin D deficiency in patients presenting with an acute episode, significantly different from those in remission. Is vitamin D deficiency the result or the cause of an acute episode? Our results contribute to the idea that vitamin D deficiency and schizophrenia may have interactions with an unknown pathway. Present data points out a possible influence at a genomic level. Future trials may investigate this association with longer follow up. We recommend that, serum vitamin D levels should be measured in patients with schizophrenia especially in long term care. Appropriate further treatment with add-on vitamin D supplements and diets that are rich in vitamin D should be considered

Vitamin D Supplementation is recommended in Schizophrenia Patients, Particularly Those with Elevated Proline

> **Clelland, James D.**, et al., "Vitamin D Insufficiency and Schizophrenia Risk: Evaluation of Hyperprolinemia as a Mediator of Association." *Schizophrenia Research* 156, no. 1 (June 2014): 15–22. Publisher: ELSEVIER BV; doi:10.1016/j.schres.2014.03.017., PMID: 24787057

> ➤ Although definitive causality cannot be confirmed, these findings strongly support vitamin D supplementation in patients, particularly for those with elevated proline, who may represent a large subgroup of the schizophrenia population.

Vitamin D May Be Considered an Anti-aggression Agent in Women with Schizophrenia

> **Cieslak, Kristina**, et al., "Low Vitamin D Levels Predict Clinical Features of Schizophrenia." *Schizophrenia Research* 159, no. 2–3 (November 2014): 543–45. Publisher: ELSEVIER BV doi:10.1016/j.schres.2014.08.031. PMID: 25311777

> ➤ Among females, decreased Vitamin D was associated with lesser hallucinatory behavior and emotional withdrawal, but did predict higher anti-social aggression. Increased aggression is seen among women with schizophrenia, though is not a ubiquitous finding. Ina study of admitted patients with schizophrenia, 53% of women were noted to exhibit aggressive behavior, compared to 75% of men. Should further analyses corroborate this correlation, Vitamin D may be considered as a potential therapy in women who present with aggressive manifestations of schizophrenia.

Vitamin E (Tocopherols, and Tocotrienols)

Vitamin E and Polyunsaturated Fatty Acids May Improve the Antioxidant Defense Reduce Motor Retardation in Schizophrenic Patients

> **Bošković, Marija**, et al., "Vitamin E and Essential Polyunsaturated Fatty Acids Supplementation in Schizophrenia Patients Treated with Haloperidol." *Nutritional Neuroscience*, July 24, 2014. doi:10.1179/1476830514Y.0000000139.

> ➤ Concentration of oxidized glutathione was decreased in patients receiving vitamin E. In addition, compared to placebo a non-significant trend of increased activity of catalase and superoxide dismutase was observed in all three treatment groups. Patients receiving vitamin E experienced less motor retardation. No difference in extrapyramidal symptoms was found. Discussion Our study indicates that supplementation with vitamin E and EPUFAs may improve the antioxidative defense, especially glutathione system, while there is no major effect on symptoms severity. Supplemental treatment with EPUFAs and vitamin E in schizophrenia patients treated with haloperidol is potentially beneficial and a larger independent study appears warranted.

CODEX ALTERNUS

Pyroluria Treatment

Pyroluric Schizophrenia Requires Large Doses of Vitamin B6 and Zinc for Treatment

C. PFEIFFER, Ph.D., et al., "Treatment of Pyroluric Schizophrenia (Malvaria) With Large Doses of Pyridoxine and a Dietary Supplement of Zinc." *Journal of Orthomolecular Psychiatry*, 1974 http://www.orthomolecular.org/library/jom/1974/pdf/1974-v03n04-p292.pdf

> ➤ A syndrome is described in the mauve-positive, urinary kryptopyrrole-ex-creting patient which has many distinguishing features, namely: (1) white spots in nails; (2) failure to remember dreams; (3) sweetish breath odor; (4) left upper quadrant abdominal pain; (5) dysperceptive schizophrenia and neurological-metabolical symptoms. These patients excrete urinary pyrroles at a level above 20 mcg percent. The usual age of onset is 15 to 20 years of age when the patient encounters the stress of senior year high school or first year of college. Kryptopyrrole has been shown to combine chemically with pyridoxal which then complexes with zinc to produce symptoms of vitamin B6 and zinc deficiency. The incidence is 30 to 40 percent in schizophrenics and 5 to 10 percent in normals. The disorder is familial and is responsible for the high incidence of "schizophrenia" in families. Adequate doses of 86 (up to 3.0 gm/day) and zinc will relieve the symptoms and reduce the urinary excretion of kryptopyrrole to the normal range. Discontinuation of the B6 - zinc results in a rapid return of serious symptoms within 48 hours. Work is progressing on the biochemical nature of stress-induced formation of kryptopyrrole.

Dietary and Nutrition

Detoxification

Juicing and Coffee Enemas May Be an Effective Detoxification Method for Schizophrenics

R. G. Green, M.D., CM., "Carrots, Coffee and Chronic Schizophrenia." *Journal of Orthomolecular Psychiatry*, 1979, http://www.orthomolecular.org/library/jom/1979/pdf/1979-v08n02-p118.pdf

> ➤ What has all this to do with carrot juice, coffee and schizophrenia? It is the root of all therapy if we will but admit it to ourselves. I use carrots in the sense of giving freshly made juices, vegetables and fruit which provide the building blocks or nutrients for the body. The fresher the juice and the greater the variety, the better it is for the body. Fresh juice contains the enzymes and nutrients needed by the body to let the cells replace and replenish themselves. Juice is easily assimilated and does not require the pancreas or the digestive tract to work too hard to make these nutrients available. If the juice comes in cans, bags or bottles, it is not nearly so effective. Gerson claims juice should be made

and drunk within ten minutes for the best results. I suggest 10 to 14 glasses of juice a day to detoxify a patient. These are 8 oz. glasses so we talk of 80 to 120 oz. of juice a day to supply nutrients and flush out waste products. This flushing action is very important. As you loosen up the accumulated cellular waste products, you must get them first into circulation, then out of the body. It does no good to drink that much and not get rid of the cellular detritus. If you do, the patient gets sicker, not better, and you wonder why. I liken juice therapy to flushing out a septic tank with a hose. The water under pressure stirs up the sediment which is what you want, but then it must be drained off or it will pack on the bottom again. This is where coffee enemata comes into play. Use three tablespoons of coffee, the percolator variety, to each quart of pure water per enema. Pure means no chlorine, no fluorine, no salt; I use well water, spring water or distilled water. I sense ionized water is not useful for my purpose. I now use caffeine capsules, 250mg. per quart. It is cheaper,, easier and works just as well. How strict we have to be about the water depends on the conditions being treated. The more severe the illness, the greater the need for good water. Cancer is the ultimate in degenerative disease. Caffeine has the ability to dilate the small ductules of the biliary system in the liver. It then becomes possible for the liver to discharge the accumulated cellular debris brought to it by the circulating blood. Juice therapy loosens it up, the blood carries it to the liver where it is processed, then it is discharged into the biliary system. By dilating these little ductules the poisons are carried to the larger branches of the tree and finally into the common duct which empties into the small bowel. From there it passes out of the body. This is the purpose of doing enemas. Gerson used one every two hours day and night in very toxic patients. This sounds like cruel and unusual treatment. It is nothing of the sort. It works when all else fails. This is the reason why the patient must have the fullest support physically, mentally and spiritually from his family. Detoxification is very trying for the patient and the family, but it can be rewarding for all concerned too."

Dietitian Management

Dietitian Management Program Helps Schizophrenic Patients Learn Needed Food Preparation Skills and Save Money on Meals

> **Johnson, C. A.**, et al., "Dietitians Help Mental Patients 'Make It on the Outside.'" *Journal of the American Dietetic Association* 70, no. 5 (May 1977): 513–15., PMID: 853202

> ➤ A nutrition program was inaugurated by the coordinator of the Day Treatment Center and Chief Dietetics for Salem VA Hospital. The purpose of the first phase was to provide clients with basic knowledge of nutrition and the handling of foods, while the second objective was to develop client's skills in actual preparation of foods. The program helped schizophrenic patients save money on home preparations of meals compared to eating out and some expressed the desire to work in food service.

CODEX ALTERNUS

Fasting

Preplanned Fasting Dietary Treatment of Schizophrenia Results in Complete Disappearance on Symptoms

> **Boehme, D. H.**, et al., "Preplanned Fasting in the Treatment of Mental Disease: Survey of Current Soviet Literature." *Schizophrenia Bulletin* 3, no. 2 (1977): 288–96., Publisher: OXFORD UNIVERSITY PRESS; PMID: 887908

> ➤ This constituted the smallest group of patients, eight of whom had suffered from their disease between 5 and 10 years. Four of the eight patients experienced total disappearance of their symptoms during preplanned fasting. Their symptomatology consisted of moderate depression with a background of slight emotional defect. In general it was found that the results in those patients who had experienced significant improvements were quite impressive—after treatment, a majority of such patients were capable of attending institutions of higher learning, working in their specialty, and even of acquiring academic degrees. In 30 percent recurrence was observed within 2 years of treatment; this recurrence, however, responded to a new course of therapy. In the opinion of Nikolajew (19696), treatment should not be repeated earlier than 6 months after termination of the first course.

Fasting Dietetic Therapy Results in Considerable Improvement of Schizophrenic and Manic-depressive Patients

> **Polishchuk, Iu I.**, et al., "[Fasting-diet therapy of elderly patients with borderline mental disorders]." *Zhurnal Nevropatologii I Psikhiatrii Imeni S.S. Korsakova* (Moscow, Russia: 1952) 91, no. 4 (1991): 101–4., Publisher: MEDIA SFERA; PMID: 1650075

> ➤ During the fasting dietetic therapy (FDT), 89 patients aged 46 to 75 years with mental disorders of nonpsychotic character (neurosis-like, neurotic and affective) were examined. The time-course of changes in the clinical status of patients with cerebral atherosclerosis, essential hypertension, slow-progredient schizophrenia, cyclothymia and manic-depressive psychosis, neuroses and lingering neurotic reactions during the FDT is described. The beneficial results in the form of considerable improvement and improvement of the mental status were attained in 83.2% of the patients. The elderly patients were found to tolerate FDT well. Side effects and somatic complications were recorded in 6 patients and were not serious. Based on the data obtained the FDT can be recommended for use on a wider basis in the management of elderly patients with borderline mental disorders.

CODEX ALTERNUS

Fasting Treatment of Schizophrenia is Effective in the Majority of Cases

Allan Cott, M.D., "Controlled Fasting Treatment of Schizophrenia in the U.S.S.R."
Journal of Orthomolecular Psychiatry, 1971
http://www.orthomolecular.org/library/jom/1971/pdf/1971-v03n01-p002.pdf

> ➤ When patients are discharged from hospital, they are advised to take prophylactic fasts of three to five days each, but not to exceed a total of 10 days in one month. Fasting is terminated when the patient's appetite is restored, his tongue becomes clean and symptoms are alleviated.

> ➤ The treatment has been found to be effective in more than 64% of cases of schizophrenia of many years' duration. Forty-seven percent of patients followed for a period of six years maintained their improvement. Those patients who resume eating a full diet and break the prescribed diet relapse. The maximum effects of the treatment are seen two or three months after the recovery period is started and the diet followed closely.

Controlled Fasting is a Valuable and Potent Alternative to Decompensation for Schizophrenics

ALLAN COTT, M.D., "Controlled Fasting Treatment for Schizophrenia." *Journal of Orthomolecular Psychiatry*, 1974, http://www.orthomolecular.org/library/jom/1974/pdf/1974-v03n04-p301.pdf

> ➤ In the U.S.S.R., fasting was first used 25 years ago as a treatment for mentally ill patients by Professor Yuri Nikolaev. His experience now extends to over 6,000 patients, and the reported results are unusually encouraging with those patients who have failed to improve on all other treatment regimens. With the ever-increasing list of psychopharmaco-logical drugs used for their psychotropic activity, there has concomitantly arisen an increasing number of patients resistant to those drugs. Many patients exhibit toxic and allergic complications during pharmacotherapy. For these patients, fasting treatment is a most valuable and potent alternative to decompensation and deterioration.

Fruits and Vegetables

Dietary Improvement in Schizophrenia

McCreadie, Robin G., et al., "Dietary Improvement in People with Schizophrenia: Randomised Controlled Trial." *The British Journal of Psychiatry: The Journal of Mental Science* 187 (October 2005): 346–51. doi:10.1192/bjp.187.4.346., Publisher: ROYAL MEDICO-PSYCHOLOGICAL ASSOCIATION; PMID: 16199794

> ➤ People with schizophrenia make poor dietary choices. Aims were to measure the impact of giving free fruits and vegetables for 6 months on eating habits in

schizophrenia. Conclusions: The diet of people with schizophrenia improved when they were given free fruits and vegetables but this was not sustained after withdrawal of intervention. A support group added no benefit.

Gluten-free Diet

Gluten-free Diet Shows Improvement in Some Schizophrenics in Hospital Setting

> **Rice, J. R.,** et al., "Another Look at Gluten in Schizophrenia." *The American Journal of Psychiatry* 135, no. 11 (November 1978): 1417–18., Publisher: AM PSYCHIATRIC ASSN; PMID: 707651

> ➤ After the gluten phase, 1 patient of 16 demonstrated severe regression below baseline on the Brief Psychiatric Rating Scale and clinical observations. She has had paranoid schizophrenia since she was 15 years old and has been in the South Carolina State Hospital for 14 years. She is now 29 years old. While she was ingesting excess gluten, she became severely agitated, uncooperative, and paranoid. We had to discontinue the gluten drink and give her intramuscular medication for three days because she became uncooperative and refused to take hen oral medications. During the gluten- free diet phase, 2 patients improved in their levels of functioning above baseline on the Brief Psychiatric Rating Scale and clinical observations. One of these patients was the woman already described; she showed improvement in level of functioning and decreased level of paranoid ideation. We were able to reduce her medications substantially. She continued on a gluten-free diet after this study, but despite her improvement she was never able to develop insight into her illness. She discontinued her diet whenever she was not closely observed and therefore had to remain in the hospital. The other patient showed no remark- able regression during the gluten phase, but her level of functioning above baseline improved substantially on the Brief Psychiatric Rating Scale and clinical observations during the gluten-free diet. She had been in a state hospital for over 13 years, with a diagnosis of chronic schizophrenia, undifferentiated type. Because of her improvement we were able to discharge her from the hospital and send her home to her family.

Gluten Free Diet Causes Disappearance of Psychiatric Symptoms

> **De Santis, A.,** et al., "Schizophrenic Symptoms and SPECT Abnormalities in a Coeliac Patient: Regression after a Gluten-Free Diet." *Journal of Internal Medicine* 242, no. 5 (November 1997): 421–23., Publisher: BLACKWELL PUBLISHING LTD. PMID: 9408073

> ➤ A 33 year-old patient, with pre-existing diagnosis of 'schizophrenic' disorder, came to our observation for severe diarrhea and weight loss. Use of SPECT, demonstrated hypoperfusion of the left frontal brain area, without evidence of structural cerebral abnormalities. Jejunal biopsy showed villous atrophy. Antiendomysial antibodies were present. A gluten-free diet was started, resulting in disappearance of psychiatric

symptoms, and normalization of histological duodenal findings and of the SPECT pattern....the SPECT demonstrating a dysfunction of the frontal cortex disappearing after a gluten free diet.

Gluten/Casein Free Diet

Schizophrenics Improve Faster on Gluten Free/Dairy Free Diet

> **Dohan, F. C.** "Relapsed Schizophrenics: More Rapid Improvement on a Milk- and Cereal-Free Diet." *The British Journal of Psychiatry: The Journal of Mental Science* 115, no. 522 (May 1969): 595–96., Publisher: ROYAL MEDICO-PSYCHOLOGICAL ASSOCIATION; PMID: 5820122

> ➤ Relapsed schizophrenic men randomly assigned to a milk-and cereal free diet on admission to a locked ward were released to an open ward considerably more rapidly than those assigned a high-cereal diet. When gluten was secretly added to the cereal-free diet the difference did not occur. Release of non-schizophrenic patients was not related to diet. These findings support the hypotheses that ingestion of cereals may be pathogenic for those with the genotype for schizophrenia.

> **Dohan, F. C.** "Relapsed Schizophrenics: Earlier Discharge from the Hospital after Cereal-Free, Milk-Free Diet." *The American Journal of Psychiatry* 130, no. 6 (June 1973): 685–88., Publisher: AM PSYCHIATRIC ASSN; PMID: 4739849

> ➤ During the first 90 days after admission to the hospital, those schizophrenics assigned to the CFMF diet were discharged more than twice as fast as those in the HC (high cereal) control group. In contrast to the beneficial effects of the CFMF diet, the relapsed schizophrenics on the CFMF diet to which wheat gluten was added (without the knowledge of staff or patients) were not discharged from hospital significantly faster than their temporal controls on the HC diet.

Improvement in Schizophrenic Patients on a Gluten/Milk Free Diet

> **Cade R.** "Autism and Schizophrenia: Intestinal Disorders." *Nutritional Neuroscience*, Vol. 3, pp. 52-72, 2000, Publisher: Maney Publishing

> ➤ ....with a gluten-casein free diet alone. Patients 1 and 6 showed significant improvement after only two months on the diet. After four months on the diet, all seven patients had improved and there was a statistically significant improvement for the group as a whole comparing control with experimental values.

Gluten Free Diet is Found Useful for Improvement of Clinical State of Chronic Schizophrenics

> **KL Reichelt,** et al., "Effect of Gluten Free Diet on Urinary Peptide Excretion and Clinical State in Schizophrenia." *Journal of Orthomolecular Medicine*, 1990

CODEX ALTERNUS

> Some relationship of gluten to the increased urinary secretion of a family of peptides seems probable. A weak but significant effect is possibly seen also by ratings scales for the late changes. The late normalization of the urinary patterns and the simultaneous late appearance of statistically significant changes of the behaviour tests, are probably not accidental. Slow changes are typical for coeliac disease (Davidson and Bridges 1987) also on provocation with gluten (Kumar et al 1979) and in cases of gluten induced dermatitis herpetiformis (Fry et al 1973). Open clinical assessment is that four patients find the treatment useful and three have probably effects, in this rather chronic group of patients. The most important conclusion is that short trials are of very little relevance, and could be the cause of the confusing results obtained in other studies. This is clearly seen in Fig. 4 and 5 where completely normal peptide pattern was only found at 56 weeks. This of course does not preclude faster changes especially in more acute cases.

Ketogenic Diets

Kraft, Bryan D., et al., "Schizophrenia, Gluten, and Low-Carbohydrate, Ketogenic Diets: A Case Report and Review of the Literature." *Nutrition & Metabolism* 6 (2009): 10. Publisher: BIOMED CENTRAL LTD.; doi:10.1186/1743-7075-6-10., PMID: 19245705

> A case report of a 70 year old schizophrenic with severe medical problems who used a ketogenic diet. "Over the course of 12 months, C.D. has continued the low-carbohydrate, ketogenic diet and has had no recurrence of auditory or visual hallucinations. She has also continued to lose weight and experience improvements in her energy level. She acknowledged having 2-3 isolated episodes of dietary non-compliance that lasted several days, where she ate pasta, bread, and cakes around the holidays: however she had no recurrence of her hallucinations.

Pacheco, A., et al., "A PILOT STUDY OF THE KETOGENIC DIET IN SCHIZOPHRENIA." *The American Journal of Psychiatry* 121 (May 1965): 1110–11., Publisher: AM PSYCHIATRIC ASSN; PMID: 14283310

> The average scores showed a statistically significant decrease in symptomology after 2 weeks on the ketogenic diet. The third rating taken one week after discontinuing the diet, showed that in 7 out of 10 patients there was a slight to fairly large increase in symptomology.

Hypocaloric Diet

Hypocaloric Diet Increases BDNF Levels in Schizophrenic Patients

Guimarães, Lísia Rejane, et al., "Serum Levels of Brain-Derived Neurotrophic Factor in Schizophrenia on a Hypocaloric Diet." *Progress in Neuro-Psychopharmacology & Biological Psychiatry* 32, no. 6 (August 1, 2008): 1595–98. Publisher: ELSEVIER INC. doi:10.1016/j.pnpbp.2008.06.004., PMID: 18582525

➤ Serum BDNF levels were significantly higher in patients on the HD (p=0.023). Additional research examining the interaction among patterns of nutritional food behavior and underlying physiopathology may result in insights upon which evidence-based decisions regarding dietary interventions can be made in people identified with major psychiatric disorders, such as schizophrenia.

Hypoglycemic Diet

Treatment of Schizophrenia with Vitamin B3 and Hypoglycemic Diet Provides Prompt Recovery

> **A. COTT, M.D.**, "Treatment of Ambulant Schizophrenics with Vitamin B3 and Relative Hypoglycemic Diet (1967)" . *Journal of Orthomolecular Medicine*, 1999
> http://orthomolecular.org/library/jom/1999/pdf/1999-v14n01-p023.pdf

➤ Summary 1) Hypoglycemia has been found to exist in an unusually high percentage of schizophrenics. Many of the 70 patients in the series could not for various reasons be tested with the 6 hour glucose tolerance test, but of the 33 submitted to the test, 28 (42.8%) were found to be positive. 2) Every patient with schizophrenia should have a 6 hour glucose tolerance test. Niacin should he discontinued one week prior to the test. 3) The hour glucose tolerance test should be interpreted as positive if there is a blood sugar drop of 20 mg.% or more below the fasting blood sugar level. 4) Treatment should consist of niacin or niacinamide and ascorbic acid and a corrective diet high in protein and fat, low in carbohydrate and free of sugar and caffeine. 5) Treatment of the hypoglycemia improves the effectiveness of the niacin therapy so that patients who show a poor initial response improve more rapidly. 6) Hypoglycemia can mimic schizophrenia. 7) Experience with these patients strongly suggests that the hypoglycemia may be an important factor in precipitating schizophrenia in an individual who is genetically predispositioned.

Low Protein, Imbalanced Amino Acid Diet

Treatment of Psychosis and Tardive Dyskinesia with Low Protein, Imbalanced Amino Acid Dietary Intervention

> **Aschheim, E.**, et al., "Dietary Control of Psychosis." *Medical Hypotheses* 41, no. 4 (October 1993): 327–28., Publisher: CHURCHILL LIVINGSTONE; PMID: 8289696

➤ The purposed dietary intervention derives from established animal work dealing with the feeding of diets in which the essential amino acid (EAA) composition has been modified so as to produce a defined imbalance. It has been demonstrated that when animals are kept on a low but adequate protein diet balanced in terms of EAAs the addition of extra amount of single amino acids induces a deficiency of other EEAs…It is likely the biochemical effects of this treatment will become apparent in a matter of hours because amino acids, in contrast to carbohydrates and fats are not stored in the body. Consequently, the change in psychiatric presentation may become noticeable with-in a short time.

Low Tryptophan Diet

Effect of Low Tryptophan Diet as an Adjunct to Neuroleptic Therapy in Schizophrenia

Rosse, R. B., et al., "Effect of a Low-Tryptophan Diet as an Adjuvant to Conventional Neuroleptic Therapy in Schizophrenia." *Clinical Neuropharmacology* 15, no. 2 (April 1992): 129–41., Publisher: LIPPINCOTT WILLIAMS & WILKINS; PMID: 1350512

> "Authors Summary; Dietary manipulations of TRP have been shown to alter levels of 5-HT, kynurenic acid, and quinolinic acid. Conceivably, decreasing dietary ingestion of TRP would (a) diminish central serotonergic transmission due to a reduction of presynaptic stores of 5-HT, (b) relieve antagonism of NMDA-mediated neural transmission by decreasing levels of kynurenic acid, and (c) reduce exitotoxin levels of quinolinic acid. As reviewed above, a reduction in serotonergic transmission and alternation of glutamatergic transmission at a specific receptor subclass may be associated with salutary therapeutic effects in patients with schizophrenia.

> In this investigation, we examined the safety and adjunctive therapeutics effects of 4-day TRP-deficient diet on the behavioral symptomology of schizophrenic patients maintained on a stable dose of their conventional antipsychotic medications.

> Interestingly, however, some of the behavioral rating measures (BPRS, CGI) reached statistical significance in the last 2 days of the diet, suggesting a beneficial adjuvant effect for the low-TRP that was not immediate but delayed a few days.

> Potentially, the most important finding of this study is improved performance on the Stroop Color and Word Test during the diet phase that largely dropped off during the post-diet phase.

Milk with A2 Genetic Variant

Attenuation of Schizophrenic Symptoms Using Milk Containing A2 Genetic Variant

Bell, Stacey J., et al., "Health Implications of Milk Containing Beta-Casein with the A2 Genetic Variant." *Critical Reviews in Food Science and Nutrition* 46, no. 1 (2006): 93–100. doi:10.1080/10408390591001144., Publisher: TAYLOR & FRANCIS INC. PMID: 16403684

> "Furthermore, consumption of milk with A2 variant may be associated with less severe symptoms of autism and schizophrenia"

CODEX ALTERNUS

Modified Cardohydrate Diets

Low Carbohydrate Diets and Diets Low in Glycemic Index May Theoretically Reduce Psychotic Symptoms

Thornley, Simon, et al., "Carbohydrate Reward and Psychosis: An Explanation for Neuroleptic Induced Weight Gain and Path to Improved Mental Health?" *Current Neuropharmacology* 9, no. 2 (June 2011): 370–75. doi:10.2174/157015911795596513.

➢ Our theory provides a parsimonious and testable hypothesis, linking the action of antipsychotic agents with commonly reported side effects. It also explains the common co-occurrence of schizophrenia with addiction, obesity and diabetes. The common link drawn between eating, psychosis and mid-brain dopaminergic reward, logically, suggests that psychosis may be improved, by modifying carbohydrate consumption. We consider that such an idea should be tested in clinical trials.

Nutrition

Dietitians Can Play a Supportive Role in Psychiatric Treatment

Gray, G. E., et al., "Nutritional Aspects of Psychiatric Disorders." *Journal of the American Dietetic Association* 89, no. 10 (October 1989): 1492–98., Publisher: ELSEVIER INC. PMID: 2677098

➢ As most diet therapy texts provide little information about psychiatric illnesses and their treatment, this article is intended as a brief introduction for dietitians. Several psychiatric illnesses, including schizophrenia, mood disorders, eating disorders, and substance abuse, may adversely affect food intake and nutritional status. The drugs used to treat those disorders similarly have effects on appetite and gastrointestinal function and interact with food and nutrients. Antipsychotics, antidepressants, and monoamine oxidase inhibitors (MAOIs) cause dry mouth, constipation, and weight gain. Lithium may cause nausea, vomiting, diarrhea, polydipsia, and weight gain. MAOIs have well-known interactions with foods containing tyramine. Lithium interacts with dietary sodium and caffeine; decreasing dietary intakes of those substances may produce lithium toxicity. Despite claims to the contrary, major psychiatric illnesses cannot be cured by nutritional therapies alone. Dietitians can, however, play an important role as part of a multidisciplinary team in the treatment of patients with psychiatric illness. Such a role includes nutrition assessment and monitoring, nutrition interventions, patient and staff education, and some forms of psychotherapy, including supportive and behavioral therapies for patients with eating disorders.

CODEX ALTERNUS

Phenylalanine Restricted Diet

A Phenylalanine Restricted Diet Could Modify Schizophrenic Behavior

> **SM Saleh, MD.,** "Could Dietary Manipulation Modify Schizophrenic Behavior?" *Journal of Orthomolecular Medicine,* 1991, http://www.orthomolecular.org/library/jom/1991/pdf/1991-v06n01-p023.pdf

> ➢ A diet poor in both PHE and TYR is given to phenylketonuric children and phenylketonuric pregnant mothers. Such a diet will acutely limit the availability of both PHE and TYR to the brain. It has been found to be quite safe and has proved to be without ill effects. If we, therefore, provide such a diet, which is quite safe, to schizophrenic patients, then by limiting their intake of PHE and TYR we should be able to modify their schizophrenic symptoms. A preliminary trial, using such a diet, was done and the results were quite encouraging and warrant further studies.

Probiotics Lactobacillus GG

Culturelle Probiotics Lactobacillus GG Can Significantly Reduce Schizophrenic Symptoms by Reducing Clostridia

> **Shaw, William.** "Increased Urinary Excretion of a 3-(3-Hydroxyphenyl)-3-Hydroxypropionic Acid (HPHPA), an Abnormal Phenylalanine Metabolite of Clostridia Spp. in the Gastrointestinal Tract, in Urine Samples from Patients with Autism and Schizophrenia." *Nutritional Neuroscience* 13, no. 3 (June 2010): 135–43. Publisher: Maney Publishing; doi:10.1179/147683010X12611460763968., PMID: 20423563

> ➢ High doses of the GG strain of Lactobacillus acidophilus have been used to control C. difficile. L. acidophilus therapy has no reported toxicity, and treatment with L. acidophilus GG of individuals with an elevated concentration of 3-(3-hydroxyphenyl)-3-hydroxypropionic acid in their urine markedly reduces the concentration of 3-(3-hydroxyphenyl)-3-hydroxypropionic acid in subsequent urine samples (unpublished data). Bolte reported a marked decrease in symptoms of autism in children treated with antibiotics effective against Clostridia, indicating treatment of abnormal microbial overgrowth may be a promising new therapy for the treatment of autism in individuals with this abnormality. The observation that elevated amounts of this compound in urine samples were associated with mental illnesses in general was made 50 years ago but has been completely ignored since then. Significant decreases in symptoms of schizophrenia, tic disorders, depression, chronic fatigue syndrome, and attention deficit hyperactivity have been reported by the attending physicians (personal communications, see Addendum) following antimicrobial treatment of individuals with elevated urinary concentrations of this compound, indicating that this compound may be of importance to many other mental diseases In addition to autism but also indicating

that these probable Clostridia species are not specific for the etiology of autism or other diseases.

Sugar

Sugar Improves Memory Function of Patients with Schizophrenia

> **Newcomer, J. W.,** et al., "Glucose-Induced Increase in Memory Performance in Patients with Schizophrenia." *Schizophrenia Bulletin* 25, no. 2 (1999): 321–35., Publisher: OXFORD UNIVERSITY PRESS; PMID: 10416734

➤ Previous investigations have found that increasing circulating glucose availability can increase memory performance in rodents, healthy humans, and individuals with dementia of the Alzheimer's type. In this study, patients with schizophrenia, healthy control subjects, and controls with bipolar affective disorder were tested using double-blind treatment with either 50 g anhydrous dextrose plus 4 mg sodium saccharin (for "taste") or 23.7 mg saccharin alone, followed by cognitive testing on a complex battery. At this glucose dose, verbal memory performance on a paragraph recall task was increased during the glucose condition relative to the saccharin condition in the patients with schizophrenia; this effect was not detected in either the psychiatric or normal controls. The results provide preliminary support for the hypothesis that memory performance can be improved in patients with schizophrenia by increasing circulating glucose availability and suggest the importance of further evaluation of therapeutic manipulations of glucose availability.

Fatty Acids

Omega 6 Fatty Acids

The Use of GLA & LA to Differentiate Between Temporal Lobe Epilepsy and Schizophrenia

> **Vaddadi, K. S.,** et al., "The Use of Gamma-Linolenic Acid and Linoleic Acid to Differentiate between Temporal Lobe Epilepsy and Schizophrenia." *Prostaglandins and Medicine* 6, no. 4 (April 1981): 375–79., Publisher: CHURCHILL LIVINGSTONE; PMID: 6269135

➤ Three long-stay, hospitalized schizophrenics who failed to respond adequately to conventional drug therapy were treated with gamma-linolenic acid and linoleic acid in the form of evening primrose oil. They became substantially worse and electroencephalographic features of temporal epilepsy became apparent. In all three the clinical state dramatically improved when carbamazepine, the conventional therapy for temporal lobe epilepsy was introduced. It can be extremely difficult to distinguish on clinical grounds between schizophrenia and temporal lobe epilepsy, and electroencephalographic studies do not always reveal an abnormality in the temporal lobe syndrome, unless additional procedure such as sphenoidal electroencephalography is undertaken. A trial of therapy with gamma-linolenic acid may prove of considerable value in distinguishing between these two states, so allowing specific therapy to be introduced.

Ethyl Eicosapentaenoic Acid (EPA)

EPA Has Procognitive Effects in Patients with Schizophrenia

Reddy, R., et al.,"Reduction in Perseverative Errors with Adjunctive Ethyl-Eicosapentaenoic Acid in Patients with Schizophrenia: Preliminary Study." *Prostaglandins, Leukotrienes, and Essential Fatty Acids* 84, no. 3–4 (April 2011): 79–83. Publisher: CHURCHILL LIVINGSTONE; doi:10.1016/j.plefa.2010.12.001., PMID: 21211955

> ➤ The 27 patients, with a mean duration of illness of 4.2 years, were all receiving atypical antipsychotics; treatment remained unchanged for the study. Perseverative errors - the key measure derived from WCST - were significantly reduced from the baseline mean of 28.2 to 18.4 errors at week 24. Positive symptoms also improved significantly. There were no correlations between EPA levels and any clinical or other neuropsychological measures. These findings suggest that an EPA has procognitive effects for patients with schizophrenia, but controlled trials are required.

Four Out of Five Placebo-controlled Double-blind Studies for Schizophrenia have Given Positive Findings

Peet, Malcolm, et al., "Eicosapentaenoic Acid in the Treatment of Schizophrenia and Depression: Rationale and Preliminary Double-Blind Clinical Trial Results." *Prostaglandins, Leukotrienes, and Essential Fatty Acids* 69, no. 6 (December 2003): 477–85., Publisher: CHURCHILL LIVINGSTONE; PMID: 14623502

> ➤ In depression, there is strong epidemiological evidence that fish consumption reduces risk of becoming depressed and evidence that cell membrane levels of n-3 PUFA are reduced. Four out of five placebo-controlled double- blind trials of eicosapentaenoic acid (EPA) in the treatment of schizophrenia have given positive findings. In depression, two placebo-controlled trials have shown a strong therapeutic effect of ethyl-EPA added to existing medication. The mode of action of EPA is currently not known, but recent evidence suggests that arachidonic acid (AA) if of particular importance in schizophrenia and that clinical improvement in schizophrenic patients using EPA treatment correlates with changes in AA.

CODEX ALTERNUS

Schizophrenics Who Eat More (n-3) Fatty Acids Their Normal Diet have Less Severe Symptoms

Peet, M. "Essential Fatty Acid Deficiency in Erythrocyte Membranes from Chronic Schizophrenic Patients, and the Clinical Effects of Dietary Supplementation." *Prostaglandins, Leukotrienes, and Essential Fatty Acids* 55, no. 1–2 (August 1996): 71–75., Publisher: CHURCHILL LIVINGSTONE; PMID: 8888126

> Furthermore, it appears that changes in diet, which modify membrane levels of fatty acids, can have significant effects upon symptoms of schizophrenia and tardive dyskinesia (TD). Thus, we have found that schizophrenic patients who eat more (n-3) fatty acids in their normal diet have less severe symptoms. In a pilot study of (n-3) fatty acid supplementation we observed significant improvement in both schizophrenic symptoms and tardive dyskinesia over a 6 week period.

EPA was Superior to DHA for Positive Symptoms and EPA Worked Well For Sole Monotherapy Treatment in Schizophrenia

Peet, M. "Two Double-Blind Placebo-Controlled Pilot Studies of Eicosapentaenoic Acid in the Treatment of Schizophrenia." *Schizophrenia Research* 49, no. 3 (April 30, 2001): 243–51. Publisher: ELSEVIER BV; PMID: 11356585

> Forty-five schizophrenic patients on stable antipsychotic medication who were still symptomatic were treated with either EPA, DHA or placebo for 3 months. Improvement on EPA measured by the Positive and Negative Syndrome Scale (PANSS) was statistically superior to both DHA and placebo using changes in percentage scores on the total PANSS. EPA was significantly superior to DHA for positive symptoms using ANOVA for repeated measures. In the second placebo-controlled study, EPA was used as a sole treatment, though the use of antipsychotic drugs was still permitted if this was clinically imperative. By the end of the study, all 12 patients on placebo, but only eight out of 14 patients on EPA, were taking antipsychotic drugs. Despite this, patients taking EPA had significantly lower scores on the PANSS rating scale by the end of the study. It is concluded that EPA may represent a new treatment approach to schizophrenia, and this requires investigation by large-scale placebo-controlled trials.

E-Eicosapentaenoate Has Clinically Important and Statistical Effect PANSS and on all Rating Scales.

Peet, Malcolm "A Dose-Ranging Exploratory Study of the Effects of Ethyl-Eicosapentaenoate in Patients with Persistent Schizophrenic Symptoms." *Journal of Psychiatric Research* 36, no. 1 (February 2002): 7–18., Publisher: PERGAMON, PMID: 11755456

> Patients on 2 and 4 g/day E-E showed significant reductions in triglyceride levels which had been elevated by clozapine. In patients given 2 g/day E-E there were improvements on the PANSS and its sub-scales, but there was also a large placebo effect in patients on

typical and new atypical antipsychotics and no difference between active treatment and placebo. In patients on clozapine, in contrast, there was little placebo response, but a clinically important and statistically significant effect of E-E on all rating scales. This effect was greatest at 2 g/day. There was a positive relationship between improvement on rating scales and rise in red blood cell arachidonic acid concentration.

E-EPA May Accelerate the Treatment Response and Improve the Toleribility to Antipsychotic Drugs

Berger, Gregor E., et al., "Ethyl-Eicosapentaenoic Acid in First-Episode Psychosis: A Randomized, Placebo-Controlled Trial." *The Journal of Clinical Psychiatry* 68, no. 12 (December 2007): 1867–75. Publisher: PHYSICIANS POSTGRADUATE PRESS, INC. PMID: 18162017

> ➢ The findings suggest that E-EPA may accelerate treatment response and improve the tolerability of antipsychotic medications. However, it was not possible to demonstrate a sustained symptomatic benefit of E-EPA in early psychosis, possibly due to a ceiling effect, since a high proportion of first-episode patients already achieve symptomatic remission with antipsychotic medication alone.

Omega 3 Fatty Acids

Omega-3 Fatty Acids as Psychotherapeutic Agent for Pregnant Schizophrenic Patient

Su, K. P., et al., "Omega-3 Fatty Acids as a Psychotherapeutic Agent for a Pregnant Schizophrenic Patient." *European Neuropsychopharmacology: The Journal of the European College of Neuropsychopharmacology* 11, no. 4 (August 2001): 295–99., Publisher: ELSEVIER BV; PMID: 11532384

> ➢ Because of the potential adverse events and teratogenesis of antipsychotic drugs, it is important to find a safe and effective treatment for pregnant women with severe mental illness. The membrane hypothesis of schizophrenia provides a rationale to treat symptoms
> of schizophrenia with omega-3 PUFAs. We report a 30-year-old married woman with chronic schizophrenia, who experienced an episode of acute exacerbation of psychotic symptoms during pregnancy. After entering into an opening trial of omega-3 PUFAs momotherapy, she showed a dramatic improvement in both positive and negative symptoms of schizophrenia and a significant increase of omega-3 composition in erythrocyte membrane. There were no adverse effects in this treatment. Thus, omega-3 PUFAs could be both beneficial and therapeutic to pregnant schizophrenic women.

CODEX ALTERNUS

Omega-3 Fatty Acids Have Much Clinical Potential in the Treatment of Schizophrenia

Emsley, Robin, et al., "Clinical Potential of Omega-3 Fatty Acids in the Treatment of Schizophrenia." *CNS Drugs* 17, no. 15 (2003): 1081–91., Publisher: ADIS INTERNATIONAL LTD. PMID: 14661986

➢ The phospholipids in the neuronal membranes of the brain are rich in highly unsaturated essential fatty acids (EFAs). It has been hypothesized that abnormalities of phospholipid metabolism are present in patients with schizophrenia and that the EFAs omega-3 polyunsaturated fatty acids, and eicosapentaenoic acid (EPA) in particular, may have a role in treating this illness. Considerable preclinical and clinical evidence provides support for this proposal. An epidemiological study reported a better outcome for patients with schizophrenia in countries where the diet is rich in unsaturated fatty acids. Evidence of abnormalities of EFAs has been found in erythrocyte membranes and cultured skin fibroblasts of patients with schizophrenia, and abnormal retinal function and niacin skin flush tests (markers of omega-3 polyunsaturated fatty acid depletion) have also been reported. Case reports and an open-label clinical trial reported efficacy for EPA in schizophrenia. Four randomized, controlled trials of EPA versus placebo as supplemental medication have now been reported. Two of these trials showed significant benefit with EPA on the positive and negative symptom scale total scores, whereas the other two did not show any effects on this primary efficacy measure. One study also reported a beneficial effect on dyskinesia. In the only published trial in which EPA was used as monotherapy versus placebo in schizophrenia, some evidence was found to suggest antipsychotic activity. Taken together, there is considerable evidence to suggest abnormalities of EFAs in cell membranes of patients with schizophrenia, and there is preliminary evidence that EPA is an effective adjunct to antipsychotics.

Omega-3 Fatty Acids May Change Hemispheric Imbalance in Schizophrenic Patients

Richardson, A. J., et al., "Laterality Changes Accompanying Symptom Remission in Schizophrenia Following Treatment with Eicosapentaenoic Acid." *International Journal of Psychophysiology: Official Journal of the International Organization of Psychophysiology* 34, no. 3 (December 1999): 333–39., Publisher: ELSEVIER BV; PMID: 10610057

➢ As measured by the Schedules for the Assessment of Positive Symptoms and Negative Symptoms, a marked reduction in his symptoms was first apparent at 2-month follow-up; further improvement followed, so that at the 6-month point few symptoms remained. Corresponding to his clinical improvement, the patient's performance on the pegboard task at 3-month follow-up had shifted from a strong right-hand advantage to near symmetry, owing to a marked improvement in his left-hand scores. On retest at 6 months this change in asymmetry was also maintained. These findings suggest that treatment with certain fatty acids may have significant benefits in the management of schizophrenia. They are also consistent with existing evidence that an Active syndrome of schizophrenia reflects a left over right hemispheric imbalance which is functional in nature, and can therefore change with symptom remission.

Supplemental Omega-3 Fatty Acids May Increase the Efficacy of Antipsychotics

Jamilian, Hamidreza, et al.,"Randomized, Placebo-Controlled Clinical Trial of Omega-3 as Supplemental Treatment in Schizophrenia." *Global Journal of Health Science* 6, no. 7 Spec No (2014): 38466. Publisher: Canadian Center of Science and Education; PMID: 25363186

> ➤ "We found that supplemental omega-3 might increase efficacy of conventional antipsychotics in decreasing symptoms of schizophrenia. Low price, rare adverse reactions and availability of omega-3 made this substance a potential supplement in improved treatment of schizophrenia."

Omega-3 Fatty Acids Have Low Risk of Harm and Clinicians Should Add Supplements to Drug Regimens

Akter, K., et al., "A Review of the Possible Role of the Essential Fatty Acids and Fish Oils in the Aetiology, Prevention or Pharmacotherapy of Schizophrenia." *Journal of Clinical Pharmacy and Therapeutics* 37, no. 2 (April 2012): 132–39. Publisher: BLACKWELL PUBLISHING LTD. doi:10.1111/j.1365-2710.2011.01265.x., PMID: 21501206

> ➤ "Despite the limited evidence that supplements ameliorate symptoms of schizophrenia, given the low risk of harm, some clinicians might opt to add omega-3 polyunsaturated fatty acid to current drug regimens in hope of better symptomatic control in schizophrenia."

Omega-3 Fatty Acid Supplementation Can Improve Behavioral Aspects and Reduce Cognitve Deterioration

Marano, G., et al., "Omega-3 Fatty Acids and Schizophrenia: Evidences and Recommendations." *La Clinica Terapeutica* 164, no. 6 (2013): e529–37., Publisher: SOCIETA EDITRICE/UNIVERSO; PMID: 24424237

> ➤ Schizophrenia is a brain disease that represents a not rare condition, in fact the lifetime risk of developing schizophrenia is widely accepted to be around 1 in 100. Schizophrenia clinically manifests with acute episodes which are associated with hallucinations, delirium, behavioral disorders and a variable range of chronic persistent symptoms, which can be debilitating. The causes of schizophrenia are not clearly understood. It seems that genetic factors may produce a vulnerability to schizophrenia, along with environmental factors that contribute in a different way from individual to individual. In this context schizophrenia constitutes the outcome of a complex interaction between multiple genes and environmental risk factors, none of which on its own causes the disorder itself. Antipsychotic medications represent the first line of

psychiatric treatment for schizophrenia. But there is a growing body of evidence that omega-3 fatty acids can prevent the disease or at least mitigate the course and symptoms. Probably, an appropriate dietary supplementation can play a partially therapeutic effect, even in more severe patients, improving some behavioral aspects and, mainly, reducing the cognitive deterioration. In this context the role of omega-3 fatty acids as a treatment for schizophrenia will strengthen the thrust of researchers and clinicians to the integrated approach to the prevention and cure of a disease that for more than a century challenging researchers.

Amino Acids

D-alanine

D-alanine is a Promising Approach for the Pharmacotherapy of Schizophrenia

Tsai, Guochuan E., et al., "D-Alanine Added to Antipsychotics for the Treatment of Schizophrenia." *Biological Psychiatry* 59, no. 3 (February 1, 2006): 230–34. Publisher: ELSEVIER INC. doi:10.1016/j.biopsych.2005.06.032., PMID: 16154544

> ➤ "The significant improvement with the D-alanine further supports the hypothesis of hypofunction of NMDA neurotransmission in schizophrenia and strengthens the proof of the principle that NMDA-enhancing treatment is a promising approach for the pharmacotherapy of schizophrenia."

Lower Plasma Alanine Levels Correlate to More Severe Positive Symptoms

Hatano, Tokiko, et al.,"Plasma Alanine Levels Increase in Patients with Schizophrenia as Their Clinical Symptoms Improve-Results from the Juntendo University Schizophrenia Projects (JUSP)." *Psychiatry Research* 177, no. 1–2 (May 15, 2010): 27–31. Publisher: ELSEVIER IRELAND LTD; doi:10.1016/j.psychres.2010.02.014., PMID: 20226539

> ➤ Eighty-one Japanese patients with schizophrenia and 50 age- and gender-matched healthy controls were studied. Plasma alanine levels were measured twice, during the acute stage and during the remission stage, using high-performance liquid chromatography. On admission, lower plasma alanine levels in patients with schizophrenia were accompanied by more severe schizophrenic symptoms, especially positive symptoms. The plasma alanine levels in patients with schizophrenia increased significantly from the time of admission to discharge, when they were significantly higher than control levels. An increase in plasma alanine levels from the acute stage to the remission stage of schizophrenia was correlated with improvement in symptoms. Drug-naïve patients did not show a significant difference in plasma alanine levels when compared with healthy controls. The measurement of plasma alanine levels may be a therapeutic marker for schizophrenia.

CODEX ALTERNUS

D-Amino Oxidase Inhibitors (e.g. Sodium Benzoate)

D-Amino Acid Oxidase Inhibitors Could Be Useful for Reducing the Dose of D-serine to Improve Psychosis or Cognitive Deficits

> **Smith, Sean M.,** et al., "The Therapeutic Potential of D-Amino Acid Oxidase (DAAO) Inhibitors." *The Open Medicinal Chemistry Journal* 4 (2010): 3–9. Publisher: Bentham Science Publishers; doi:10.2174/1874104501004020003., PMID: 20648222

> ➢ Nevertheless, these findings suggest that DAAO inhibitors could be useful clinically for reducing the dose of D-serine necessary to improve psychosis or cognitive deficits associated with schizophrenia. As a result, the coadministration of DAAO inhibitors with D-serine could ameliorate some of the side effects associated with the administration of high doses of D-serine, such as nephrotoxicity.

D-Amino Oxidase Inhibitor Could Enhance the Oral Bioavailability of D-alanine

> **Mao, Horio,** et al., "Effects of D-Amino Acid Oxidase Inhibitor on the Extracellular D-Alanine Levels and the Efficacy of D-Alanine on Dizocilpine-Induced Prepulse Inhibition Deficits in Mice" *The Open Clinical Chemistry Journal*, 2009, 2, 16-21 Publisher: Bentham Science Publishers

> ➢ In this study, we found that administration of DAAO inhibitor CBIO could enhance the oral bioavailability of D-alanine in mice, and that co-administration of D-alanine with CBIO significantly increased the extracellular D-alanine levels in the mouse frontal cortex as compared with Dalanine alone group. In conclusion, co-administration of Dalanine and a DAAO inhibitor would be a new approach for the treatment of schizophrenia.

Adjunctive D-Amino Acid Oxidase Inhibitors Increase the Levels of D-serine in the Brain

> **Sacchi, Silvia,** et al., "D-Amino Acid Oxidase Inhibitors as a Novel Class of Drugs for Schizophrenia Therapy." *Current Pharmaceutical Design* 19, no. 14 (2013): 2499–2511., Publisher: BENTHAM SCIENCE PUBLISHERS LTD; PMID: 23116391

> ➢ Several findings have linked low levels of D-serine to schizophrenia: D-serine concentrations in serum and cerebrospinal fluid have been reported to be decreased in schizophrenia patients while human DAAO activity and expression are increased; oral administration of D-serine improved positive, negative, and cognitive symptoms of schizophrenia as add-on therapy to typical and atypical antipsychotics. This evidence indicates that increasing NMDA receptor function, perhaps by inhibiting DAAO-induced degradation of D-serine may alleviate symptoms in schizophrenic patients. Furthermore, it has been suggested that co-administration of D-serine with a human DAAO inhibitor may be a more effective means of increasing D-serine levels in the

brain. Here, we present an overview of the current knowledge of the structure-function relationships in human DAAO and of the compounds recently developed to inhibit its activity (specifically the ones recently exploited for schizophrenia treatment).

Sodium Benzoate is a DAAO Inhibitor that Produced Significant Improvement in PANSS Total Score in Schizophrenic Patients

Lane, Hsien-Yuan, et al., "Add-on Treatment of Benzoate for Schizophrenia: A Randomized, Double-Blind, Placebo-Controlled Trial of D-Amino Acid Oxidase Inhibitor." *JAMA Psychiatry* 70, no. 12 (December 2013): 1267–75. Publisher: American Medical Association doi:10.1001/jamapsychiatry.2013.2159., PMID: 24089054

➢ Benzoate produced a 21% improvement in PANSS total score and large effect sizes (range, 1.16-1.69) in the PANSS total and subscales, Scales for the Assessment of Negative Symptoms-20 items, Global Assessment of Function, Quality of Life Scale and Clinical Global Impression and improvement in the neurocognition subtests as recommended by the National Institute of Mental Health's Measurement and Treatment Research to Improve Cognition in Schizophrenia initiative, including the domains of processing speed and visual learning. Benzoate was well tolerated without significant adverse effects.

D-aspartate

D-Aspartate May Be Benifical in Treating Schizophrenia--Reducing Exictotoxic NMDAR Activation

Errico, Francesco, et al. "D-Aspartate Prevents Corticostriatal Long-Term Depression and Attenuates Schizophrenia-Like Symptoms Induced by Amphetamine and MK-801." *The Journal of Neuroscience* 28, no. 41 (October 8, 2008): 10404–14. doi:10.1523/JNEUROSCI.1618-08.2008.

➢ In conclusion, the present work supports a central neuromodulatory role for D-aspartate and provides, for the first time, evidence that increased levels of this molecule may have beneficial effects in treating SCZ. It should be noted that persistent NMDAR activation triggers excitotoxic processes. Although Ddo–/– animals showed a lifespan comparable to their Ddo+/+ littermates, future studies are necessary to determine the existence of possible side effects associated with a long-term D-aspartate exposure.

D-Aspartate May Be Benifical During Neurodevelopment

Errico, F., et al. "A Role for D-Aspartate Oxidase in Schizophrenia and in Schizophrenia-Related Symptoms Induced by Phencyclidine in Mice." *Translational Psychiatry* 5, no. 2 (February 17, 2015): e512. doi:10.1038/tp.2015.2.

> In conclusion, our data suggest that increased expression of DDO mRNA in the PFC of SCZ patients can result in a corresponding excessive degradation of d-Asp. We also demonstrate in a preclinical model that constitutive high levels of d-Asp exert a putative protective effect against the SCZ-like symptoms induced by the NMDAR antagonist PCP. Taken together, these findings support a role for d-Asp as a potential vulnerability factor in SCZ. Consistent with a neurodevelopmental hypothesis of SCZ, a putative precocious downregulation of d-Asp levels, associated to abnormal metabolism of this molecule, may have a much greater impact during critical phases of brain development, when d-Asp levels are physiologically high.

Glycine

Glycine Augmentation May Ameliorate Depressive and Extrapyramidal Symptoms in Schizophrenic Patients

Strzelecki, Dominik, et al., "[Augmentation of antipsychotics with glycine may ameliorate depressive and extrapyramidal symptoms in schizophrenic patients--a preliminary 10-week open-label study]." *Psychiatria Polska* 47, no. 4 (August 2013): 609–20., Publisher: PANSTWOWY ZAKAD WYDAWNICTW LEKARSKICH.; PMID: 24946468

> "Glycine augmentation of antipsychotic treatment may reduce the severity of depressive and extrapyramidal symptoms. Glycine use was safe and well tolerated."

High Dose Glycine Results in Significant Reduction in Negative Symptoms

Heresco-Levy, U., et al., "Efficacy of High-Dose Glycine in the Treatment of Enduring Negative Symptoms of Schizophrenia." *Archives of General Psychiatry* 56, no. 1 (January 1999): 29–36., Publisher: AMERICAN MEDICAL ASSOCIATION; PMID: 2892253

> Glycine treatment was well tolerated and induced increased glycine (P=.001) and serine (P=.001) serum levels. Glycine administration resulted in (1) a significant (P<.001) 30%+/-16% reduction in negative symptoms, as measured by the PANSS, and (2) a significant (P<.001) 30%+/-18% improvement in the BPRS total scores. The improvement in negative symptoms was unrelated to alterations in extrapyramidal effects or symptoms of depression. Low pretreatment glycine serum levels significantly predicted (r= 0.80) clinical response.

Adjunctive Glycine Therapy Induced a Significant Reduction in Negative, Depression, and Cognitive Symptoms

Heresco-Levy, U., et al., "Double-Blind, Placebo-Controlled, Crossover Trial of Glycine Adjuvant Therapy for Treatment-Resistant Schizophrenia." *The British Journal of Psychiatry: The Journal of Mental Science* 169, no. 5 (November 1996): 610–17., Publisher: ROYAL MEDICO-PSYCHOLOGICAL ASSOCIATION; PMID: 8932891

> ➢ Glycine was well tolerated, resulted in significantly increased serum glycine levels and induced a mean 36 (7%) reduction in negative symptoms ($P < 0.0001$). Significant improvements were also induced in depressive and cognitive symptoms. The greatest reduction in negative symptoms was registered in the patients who had the lowest baseline serum glycine levels.

Glycine Treatment May Be Effective for Neuroleptic-resistant Negative Symptoms in Schizophrenia

Javitt, D. C., et al., "Amelioration of Negative Symptoms in Schizophrenia by Glycine." *The American Journal of Psychiatry* 151, no. 8 (August 1994): 1234–36., Publisher: AM PSYCHIATRIC ASSN; PMID: 8037263

> ➢ Phencyclidine induces a psychotomimetic state by blocking neurotransmission at N-methyl-D-aspartic acid (NMDA) receptors. In a double-blind, placebo-controlled fashion, 14 medicated patients with chronic schizophrenia were treated with glycine, a potentiator of NMDA-receptor-mediated neurotransmission. Significant improvement in negative symptoms occurred in the group given glycine but not in the group given placebo, suggesting that potentiation of NMDA-receptor-mediated neurotransmission may represent an effective treatment for neuroleptic-resistant negative symptoms in schizophrenia.

Glycine Therapy Reduced Muscle Stiffness and Extrapyramidal Dysfunction in Schizophrenic Patients on Conventional Neuroleptics

Rosse, R. B., et al., "Glycine Adjuvant Therapy to Conventional Neuroleptic Treatment in Schizophrenia: An Open-Label, Pilot Study." *Clinical Neuropharmacology* 12, no. 5 (October 1989): 416–24., Publisher: LIPPINCOTT WILLIAMS & WILKINS ; PMID: 2611765

> ➢ In an open-label study, glycine was administered orally (10.8 g/day in three divided doses) to six chronically psychotic patients, as an adjunct to conventional neuroleptic therapy, for periods extending from 4 days to 8 weeks. Glycine was administered in an effort to facilitate endogenous glutamatergic transmission at the level of the N-methyl-D-aspartate (NMDA) receptor complex, since a glutamatergic deficiency in the pathophysiology of schizophrenia has been postulated. Therapeutic efficacy was

assessed with standardized psychiatric rating scales. Beneficial effects on behavioral symptomatology were observed in two patients, whereas two others worsened. In one of the two responders, clinical deterioration occurred after glycine withdrawal consistent with a positive adjuvant effect in this patient. However, glycine rechallenge in this patient was not associated with the clinical improvement seen during the initial glycine period. Clinical worsening was not observed after glycine discontinuation in the second responder. Glycine administration reduced neuroleptic-induced muscle stiffness and extrapyramidal dysfunction in three of the six patients. All patients tolerated the clinical trial. The limited penetrability of glycine across the blood-brain barrier is a major limitation of this approach to facilitating glutamatergic transmission at the level of the NMDA receptor complex.

Glycine Administration Reduces Positive and Negative Symptoms Significantly

Strzelecki, Dominik , et al., "[Changes in positive and negative symptoms, general psychopathology in schizophrenic patients during augmentation of antipsychotics with glycine: a preliminary 10-week open-label study]." *Psychiatria Polska* 45, no. 6 (December 2011): 825–37., Publisher: PANSTWOWY ZAKAD WYDAWNICTW LEKARSKICH; PMID: 22335126

> "After 6 weeks of glycine administration we observed statistically significant improvement in positive (PANSS P subscale, -7.8%, $p < 0.05$), negative symptoms (N subscale, -16.1%, $p < 0.001$), general psychopathology (G subscale, -12.2%, $p < 0.001$) and PANSS total score (T, -12.8%, $p < 0.001$). 2 weeks after the end of glycine augmentation mental status remained stable."

Glycine was Associated with Reduced Symptoms and Improved Cognitive Function

Woods, Scott W., et al., "Glycine Treatment of the Risk Syndrome for Psychosis: Report of Two Pilot Studies." *European Neuropsychopharmacology: The Journal of the European College of Neuropsychopharmacology* 23, no. 8 (August 2013): 931–40. Publisher: Elsevier doi:10.1016/j.euroneuro.2012.09.008., PMID: 23089076

> "We conclude that glycine was associated with reduced symptoms with promising effect sizes in two pilot studies and a possibility of improvement in cognitive function. Further studies of agents that facilitate NMDA receptor function in risk syndrome patients are supported by these preliminary findings."

Adjunctive High-Dose Glycine Provides a Significant Reduction in Negative Symptoms

Javitt, D. C., et al., "Adjunctive High-Dose Glycine in the Treatment of Schizophrenia." *The International Journal of Neuropsychopharmacology / Official Scientific Journal of the Collegium Internationale Neuropsychopharmacologicum* (CINP) 4, no. 4 (December 2001): 385–91. Publisher: CAMBRIDGE UNIVERSITY PRESS; doi:10.1017/S1461145701002590.,

PMID: 11806864

> Glycine treatment was associated with an 8-fold increase in serum glycine levels, similar to that observed previously. A significant 34% reduction in negative symptoms was observed during glycine treatment. Serum antipsychotic levels were not significantly altered. Significant clinical effects were observed despite the fact that the majority of subjects were receiving atypical antipsychotics (clozapine or olanzapine). As in earlier studies, improvement persisted following glycine discontinuation.

High-Dose Glycine Significantly Improves Negative Symptoms in Schizophrenia

Heresco-Levy, Uriel, et al., "High-Dose Glycine Added to Olanzapine and Risperidone for the Treatment of Schizophrenia." *Biological Psychiatry* 55, no. 2 (January 15, 2004): 165–71., Publisher: ELSEVIER INC. PMID: 14732596

> "The negative symptoms improvement remained significant even following covariation for changes in other symptom clusters and extrapyramidal side effects."

D-phenylanine

D-phenylanine is a Enkephalinase Inhibitor Which Can Treat Endorphin Deficiency States in Schizophrenia

Ehrenpreis, S., et al., "D-phenylalanine and Other Enkephalinase Inhibitors as Pharmacological Agents: Implications for Some Important Therapeutic Application." *Acupuncture & Electro-Therapeutics Research* 7, no. 2–3 (1982): 157–72., Publisher: COGNIZANT COMMUNICATION CORPORATION; PMID: 6128872

> A number of compounds have been shown to inhibit the degradation of enkephalins. As expected, these compounds produce naloxone reversible analgesia and potentiate the analgesia produced by enkephalins and by acupuncture. One of these, D-phenylalanine, is also anti-inflammatory. D-phenylalanine has proven to be beneficial in many human patients with chronic, intractable pain. It is proposed the enkephalinase inhibitors may be effective in a number of human "endorphin deficiency diseases" such as depression, schizophrenia, convulsive disorders and arthritis. Such compounds may alleviate other conditions associated with decreased endorphin levels such as opiate withdrawal symptoms.

D-serine

High Dose D-serine is Effective for Both Persistent Symptoms and Neurocognitive Dysfunction

CODEX ALTERNUS

> **Kantrowitz, Joshua T.,** et al., "High Dose D-serine in the Treatment of Schizophrenia." *Schizophrenia Research* 121, no. 1–3 (August 2010): 125–30. Publisher: ELSEVIER BV doi:10.1016/j.schres.2010.05.012., PMID: 20541910

> ➤ "These findings support double-blind investigation of D-serine at doses> or =60 mg/kg/d, and suggest effectiveness in treatment of both persistent symptoms and neurocognitive dysfunction."

D-serine Resulted in Significant Improvements as an Add-on Pharmacotherapy for Schizophrenia

> **Heresco-Levy, Uriel,** et al., "D-Serine Efficacy as Add-on Pharmacotherapy to Risperidone and Olanzapine for Treatment-Refractory Schizophrenia." *Biological Psychiatry* 57, no. 6 (March 15, 2005): 577–85. Publisher: ELSEVIER INC. doi:10.1016/j.biopsych.2004.12.037., PMID: 15780844

> ➤ "D-serine administration induced increased serine serum levels and resulted in significant improvements in negative, positive, cognitive, and depression symptoms, as measured by the Positive and Negative Syndrome Scale."

D-serine as an Adjunct to Antipsychotic Therapy

> **Nunes, Emerson A.,** et al., "D-serine and Schizophrenia: An Update." *Expert Review of Neurotherapeutics* 12, no. 7 (July 2012): 801–12. Publisher: FUTURE DRUGS LTD. doi:10.1586/ern.12.65., PMID: 22853788

> ➤ A summary of the relevant animal data, as well as genetic studies and clinical trials examining D-serine as an adjunct to standard antipsychotic therapy, is provided in this article. Together, the evidence suggests that research on the next generation of antipsychotic agents should include studies on increasing brain levels of D-serine or mimicking its action on the NMDA receptor.

Adjunctive D-serine Revealed Significant Improvements in Positive, Negative, and Cognitive Symptoms

> **Tsai, G.,** et al., "D-serine Added to Antipsychotics for the Treatment of Schizophrenia." *Biological Psychiatry* 44, no. 11 (December 1, 1998): 1081–89., Publisher: ELSEVIER INC.; PMID: 9836012

> ➤ Patients who received D-serine treatment revealed significant improvements in their positive, negative, and cognitive symptoms as well as some performance in WCST. D-serine levels at week 4 and 6 significantly predicted the improvements. D-serine was well tolerated and no significant side effects were noted.

CODEX ALTERNUS

L-carnosine

L-carnosine Merits Further Consideration as Adjunctive Treatment to Improve Executive Dysfunction in Schizophrenia

Chengappa, K. N. Roy, et al., "A Preliminary, Randomized, Double-Blind, Placebo-Controlled Trial of L-Carnosine to Improve Cognition in Schizophrenia." *Schizophrenia Research* 142, no. 1–3 (December 2012): 145–52. Publisher: ELSEVIER BV doi:10.1016/j.schres.2012.10.001., PMID: 23099060

> ➢ The L-carnosine group performed significantly faster on non-reversal condition trials of the set-shifting test compared with placebo but reversal reaction times and errors were not significantly different between treatments. On the strategic target detection test, the L-carnosine group displayed significantly improved strategic efficiency and made fewer perseverative errors compared with placebo. Other cognitive tests showed no significant differences between treatments. Psychopathology scores remained stable. The carnosine group reported more adverse events (30%) compared with the placebo group (14%). Laboratory indices remained within acceptable ranges. These preliminary findings suggest that L-carnosine merits further consideration as adjunctive treatment to improve executive dysfunction in persons with schizophrenia.

L-lysine

L-Lysine is a Therapeutic Adjunctive Therapy in Patients with Chronic Schizophrenia

Zeinoddini, Atefeh, et al., "L-Lysine as an Adjunct to Risperidone in Patients with Chronic Schizophrenia: A Double-Blind, Placebo-Controlled, Randomized Trial." *Journal of Psychiatric Research,* September 6, 2014. Publisher: PERGAMON doi:10.1016/j.jpsychires.2014.08.016., PMID: 25227564

> ➢ "The present study demonstrated that l-lysine can be a tolerable and efficacious adjunctive therapy for improving negative and general psychopathology symptoms in chronic schizophrenia. However, the safety and efficacy of higher doses of l-lysine and longer treatment periods still remain unknown."

L-lysine Patients Showed a Significant Decrease in Positive Symptoms

Wass, Caroline, et al., "L-Lysine as Adjunctive Treatment in Patients with Schizophrenia: A Single-Blinded, Randomized, Cross-over Pilot Study." *BMC Medicine* 9 (2011): 40. Publisher: BIOMED CENTRAL LTD; doi:10.1186/1741-7015-9-40., PMID: 21501494

> ➢ Four-week L-lysine treatment of 6 g/day caused a significant increase in blood concentration of L-lysine that was well tolerated. Patients showed a significant decrease in positive symptoms as assessed by PANSS in addition to self-reported symptom

improvement by three patients. The NO signaling pathway is an interesting, potentially new treatment target for schizophrenia; however, the effects of L-lysine need further evaluation to decide the amino acid's potentially beneficial effects on symptom severity in schizophrenia.

L-theanine

L-theanine Relieves Positive, Activation, and Anxiety Symptoms in Patients with Schizophrenia

> **Ritsner, Michael S.,** et al., "L-Theanine Relieves Positive, Activation, and Anxiety Symptoms in Patients with Schizophrenia and Schizoaffective Disorder: An 8-Week, Randomized, Double-Blind, Placebo-Controlled, 2-Center Study." *The Journal of Clinical Psychiatry* 72, no. 1 (January 2011): 34–42. Publisher: PHYSICIANS POSTGRADUATE PRESS, INC. doi:10.4088/JCP.09m05324gre., PMID: 21208586

> ➤ 40 patients completed the study protocol. Compared with placebo, L-theanine augmentation was associated with reduction of anxiety (P= .015; measured by the HARS scale) and positive (P= .009) and general psychopathology (P<.001) scores (measured by PANSS 3-dimensional model). According to the 5-dimension model of psychopathology, L-theanine produced significant reductions on PANSS positive (P= .004) and activation factor (P= .006) scores compared to placebo." ….L-theanine augmentation of antipsychotic therapy can ameliorate positive, activation and anxiety symptoms in schizophrenia and schizoaffective disorder patients.

L-theanine has Antipsychotic-like and Possibly Antidepressant Effects

> **Wakabayashi, Chisato,** et al., "Behavioral and Molecular Evidence for Psychotropic Effects in L-Theanine." *Psychopharmacology* 219, no. 4 (February 2012): 1099–1109. Publisher: SPRINGER-VERLAG ; doi:10.1007/s00213-011-2440-z. , PMID: 21861094

> ➤ "Our results suggest that L-theanine has antipsychotic-like and possibly antidepressant-like effects. It exerts these effects, at least in part, through induction of BDNF in the hippocampus and the agonistic action of L-theanine on the NMDA receptor."

L-theanine Produces Significant Improvements in Positive Symptoms and Better Sleep Quality

> **Ota, Miho**, et al., "Effect of L-Theanine on Glutamatergic Function in Patients with Schizophrenia." *Acta Neuropsychiatrica*, April 21, 2015, 1–6. doi:10.1017/neu.2015.22.

> ➤ There were significant improvements in the PANSS positive scale and sleep quality after the l-theanine treatment. As for MRS, we found no significant differences in Glx levels before and after the 8 week l-theanine treatment. However, significant correlations were observed between baseline density of Glx and change in Glx density by l-theanine.

L-tryptophan (Tryptophan)

Tryptophan May Be Useful in the Treatment of Aggressive Schizophrenics

Morand, C., et al., "Clinical Response of Aggressive Schizophrenics to Oral Tryptophan." *Biological Psychiatry* 18, no. 5 (May 1983): 575–78., Publisher: ELSEVIER INC. PMID: 6860730

> ➤ However, tryptophan may be useful in treating aggressive symptoms in patients with poor impulse control who were characterized in this study as having high Buss-Durkee scores, high lifetime aggression frequency, and normal GSRs. Although aggressive behavior has been linked to many neurotransmitters the present study indicates that 5HT can be manipulated in a simple way through administration of the nontoxic dietary 5HT precursor, tryptophan, to modulate aggressive symptomology. We are reporting these preliminary results now in the hope of encouraging other further studies.

Tryptophan Has a Beneficial Effect on Memory in Schizophrenia

Levkovitz, Yechiel, et al., "Effect of L-Tryptophan on Memory in Patients with Schizophrenia." *The Journal of Nervous and Mental Disease* 191, no. 9 (September 2003): 568–73. Publisher: LIPPINCOTT WILLIAMS & WILKINS doi:10.1097/01.nmd.0000087182.29781.e0., PMID: 14504565

> ➤ "Compared with placebo, l-tryptophan had a beneficial effect on memory functions but not on the patients' psychotic state or on the side effects of medications. These preliminary results suggest the possibility of using serotonin precursor to enhance memory function in schizophrenia."

5-hydroxtryptophan (5-HTP)

L-5HTP Attenuates Amphetamine Induced Positive Psychotic Symptoms

Irwin, M. R., et al., "L-5-Hydroxytryptophan Attenuates Positive Psychotic Symptoms Induced by D-Amphetamine." *Psychiatry Research* 22, no. 4 (December 1987): 283–89., Publisher: ELSEVIER IRELAND LTD; PMID: 3501597

> ➤ "Pre-administration with 5HTP significantly antagonized amphetamine-elicited elevations in thought disturbance, activation, and hallucinations."

Peptides

Amylin Peptide

Amylin Peptide May Be a Potential Target for Antipsychotic Medication Research

> **Baisley, Sarah K.,** et al., "Antipsychotic-like Actions of the Satiety Peptide, Amylin, in Ventral Striatal Regions Marked by Overlapping Calcitonin Receptor and RAMP-1 Gene Expression." *The Journal of Neuroscience: The Official Journal of the Society for Neuroscience* 34, no. 12 (March 19, 2014): 4318–25. Publisher: SOCIETY FOR NEUROSCIENCE doi:10.1523/JNEUROSCI.2260-13.2014., PMID: 24647952

> ➢ Coinfusion of AC187 (20 µg), an antagonist for AMY1-R, blocked the ability of amylin to normalize AMPH-induced PPI disruption, showing the specificity of AcbSh amylin effects to the AMY1-R. Intra-AcbSh AC187 on its own disrupted PPI in a haloperidol-reversible manner (0.1 mg/kg). Thus, AMY1-R may be a potential target for the development of putative antipsychotics or adjunct treatments that oppose metabolic side effects of current medications. Moreover, AMY1-Rs may represent a novel way to modulate activity preferentially in ventral versus dorsal striatum.

Caerulein Diethylamine

Ceruletide Has Long Acting Antipsychotic Effects on Schizophrenics

> **Moroji, T.,** et al., "Antipsychotic Effects of Ceruletide (caerulein) on Chronic Schizophrenia." *Archives of General Psychiatry* 39, no. 4 (April 1982): 485–86., Publisher: AMERICAN MEDICAL ASSOCIATION; PMID: 7039550

> ➢ "Our clinical observations indicate that ceruletide—whatever its mechanism—may have a long-acting antipsychotic effect in schizophrenia and, as they differ from conventional neuroleptics, CCK-like peptides could be a useful and effective antipsychotic drug."

Caerulein Has Rapid Action and Long Lasting Effects in Certain types of Schizophrenia

> **Moroji, T.,** et al., "Antipsychotic Effects of Ceruletide in Chronic Schizophrenia. An Appraisal of the Long-Term, Intermittent Medication of Ceruletide in Chronic Schizophrenia." *Annals of the New York Academy of Sciences* 448 (1985): 518–34., Publisher: NEW YORK ACADEMY OF SCIENCES. PMID: 3927809

> ➢ Based on the above findings, caerulein, a decapeptide chemically related to CCK-8, may have therapeutic efficacy in certain types(s) of chronic schizophrenia with rapidity of action and long duration. Caerulein also appears to be applicable to clinical practice with high safety. Before classed as a therapeutic agent, however, there are a great number of urgent problems to be resolved, like the confirmation of clinical utility in double-blind controlled trials and the safety of long-term administration.

CODEX ALTERNUS

Caerulein Diethylamine Has Therapeutic Value in the Treatment of Schizophrenia

Itoh, H., et al., "Clinical Study on the Psychotropic Effects of Caerulein--an Open Clinical Trial in Chronic Schizophrenic Patients." *The Keio Journal of Medicine* 31, no. 3 (October 1982): 71–95., Publisher: SCHOOL OF MEDICINE, KEIO UNIVERSITY; PMID: 6764226

> ➢ An open clinical trial of caerulein diethylamine, a cholecystokinin analogue, was performed in a total of 58 chronic schizophrenic patients maintained on drugs such as antipsychotic agents without dosage modification. The neuro peptide medication by intramuscular route produced a clinical improvement in 20 cases and was eventually assessed to have been of therapeutic value in 23 cases. Clinical responses to the medication observed in the present series included: subjective changes in mood mostly to become feeling "fine" or "refreshed in the head", improvement in contact, increased spontaneity and objective behavioral changes such as restlessness and excitement. These features of clinical responses observed in respect of mental condition seem to indicate that the drug affects emotion and exerts an analeptic effect as its principal clinical effects. The clinical effects were remarkably long sustained for 1-2 weeks after a single i.m. dose in most responders. Feeling of facial warmth and lassitude as well as symptoms of the gastrointestinal system were encountered as attendant symptoms in 6 cases.

Caerulein Has Long Lasting Antipsychotic Activity in Chronic Schizophrenia

Moroji, T., et al., "Antipsychotic Effects of Caerulein, a Decapeptide Chemically Related to Cholecystokinin Octapeptide, on Schizophrenia." *International Pharmacopsychiatry* 17, no. 4 (1982): 255–73., Publisher: S. KARGER. PMID: 7185770

> ➢ Caerulein, a decapeptide chemically related to CCK-8, was administered intramuscularly to 20 patients with chronic schizophrenia in two different doses of 0.3 and 0.6 microgram/kg. BPRS ratings were made before and 3 weeks after the injection. The neuroleptic therapy was not discontinued, but both drug and dose were not changed at least 3 weeks before the first injection and during the study period. Clinically obvious and statistically significant improvement in psychotic symptoms occurred shortly after the injection of caerulein. The greatest change occurred 1--2 weeks later. There was an evident correlation between the observed changes and the dose injected. Our findings suggest that caerulein has a long-acting, antipsychotic activity in chronic schizophrenia. Furthermore, our findings suggest the involvement of CCK-like peptides in the pathogenesis of schizophrenia.

Cholecystokinn-Octapeptide

Cholecystokinin Peptides (CCK-8, CCK-33) Have Shown Therapeutic Effect in Numerous Clinical Trials

> **Nair, N. P.**, et al., "Cholecystokinin Peptides, Dopamine and Schizophrenia--a Review." *Progress in Neuro-Psychopharmacology & Biological Psychiatry* 9, no. 5–6 (1985): 515–24., Publisher: ELSEVIER INC; PMID: 2868491

> ➤ In man there is endrocrinological evidence for an inhibitory effect of CCK-33 and CCK-8 on DA function. However, alternate explanations are possible. CSF CCK-IR is unchanged or decreased in schizophrenia. Autopsy investigations have shown significant decreases, increases or no change in brain CCK-IR concentrations and a decrease in CCK-33 binding in schizophrenia. Eight of 11 clinical trials with CER, CCK-8 or CCK-33 have shown a therapeutic effect in schizophrenia; only two of these eight trials have been double blind studies. The three controlled investigations which have shown no effect have used only small patient populations. None of the trials have used an active placebo.

Cholecystokinn-Octapetide Has Definite Antipsychotic Properties

> **Nair, N. P.**, et al., "Cholecystokinin-Octapeptide in Chronic Schizophrenia: A Double-Blind Placebo-Controlled Study." *Progress in Neuro-Psychopharmacology & Biological Psychiatry* 8, no. 4–6 (1984): 711–14., Publisher: ELSEVIER INC; PMID: 6152344

> ➤ "It is concluded that CCK-8 has definite antipsychotic properties in patients with chronic schizophrenia. Clinical trials in neuroleptic-free patients are warranted."

Desenkephalin-Gamma-Enorphin (DE gamma E)

Desenkephalin-Gamma-Endorphin and Ceruletide were both Effective as Neuroleptics in Schizophrenic Patients

> **Verhoeven, W. M.**, et al., "A Comparative Study on the Antipsychotic Properties of Desenkephalin-Gamma-Endorphin and Ceruletide in Schizophrenic Patients." *Acta Psychiatrica Scandinavica* 73, no. 4 (April 1986): 372–82., Publisher: BLACKWELL MUNKSGAARD; PMID: 3524119

> ➤ The neuropeptides desenkephalin-gamma-endorphin (DE gamma E) and ceruletide were administered intramuscularly to patients with schizophrenic psychoses following a double-blind placebo-controlled design, including a total of 44 subjects. Neuroleptic medication was continued during the experimental period, which was started with one placebo injection for all patients. One week later subjects received a single intramuscular injection with 3 mg DE gamma E, 40 micrograms ceruletide or placebo. After an interval of 10 days, the patients received six similar injections over a period of 2 weeks. Treatment with either peptides resulted in a decrease of psychotic symptomatology as compared to placebo treatment. The beneficial effect of the peptides lasted at least 2 weeks after the experimental treatment period. Of the 14 patients treated with placebo only, three showed a slight response. Of the 30 patients treated with the neuropeptides, eight did not respond (DE gamma E: 3; ceruletide: 5), eight had a slight response (DE

gamma E: 6; ceruletide: 2) and 14 responded moderately or markedly (DE gamma E: 6; ceruletide: 8). No obvious difference between the effects of the two neuropeptides was found, besides a somewhat earlier onset of the effect of ceruletide. Patients presenting relatively less negative psychotic symptoms were particularly susceptible to treatment with either peptide. Apart from slight and short-lasting gastrointestinal complaints after the first injections with ceruletide in some patients, no side effects were observed.

Des-Enkephalin-Gamma-Endorphin has Antipsychotic Properties in Treatment of Schizophrenia

Verhoeven, W. M., et al., "Antipsychotic Properties of Des-Enkephalin-Gamma-Endorphin in Treatment of Schizophrenic Patients." *Archives of General Psychiatry* 39, no. 6 (June 1982): 648–54., Publisher: AMERICAN MEDICAL ASSOCIATION; PMID: 7092498

> ➢ Animal experiments have shown that the gamma-endorphin fragment des-enkephalin-gamma-endorphin (DE gamma E; beta-lipotropin 66-77) is the shortest sequence with neuroleptic-like activity with potency comparable to des-tyrosine-gamma-endorphin. We postulated that DE gamma E may be an endogenous peptide implicated in psychopathologic disease, particularly schizophrenia. To investigate the purported antipsychotic action of DE gamma E, 23 patients with different types of relapsing schizophrenia were treated with DE gamma E dissolved in saline or placebo. Neuroleptic medication was continued during the experimental period. In the first single-blind trial, two patients were treated with 1 mg of DE gamma E and two with 10 mg of DE gamma E intramuscularly (IM) daily for ten days. In the second double-blind placebo-controlled trial 13 patients were treated with 3 mg of DE gamma E IM daily for ten days and six received placebo. Of the 17 patients treated with DE gamma E, two did not respond, 11 had a slight to moderate effect, and four responded markedly. No side effects were observed. The response to DE gamma E appeared to be negatively correlated with the dosage of neuroleptic medication and the duration of the last psychotic episode. These results support the hypothesis that disturbances in gamma-endorphin fragmentation might contribute to the pathogenesis of schizophrenic psychoses.

DTgammaE

DTgammaE has Neuroleptic-like Activity in Schizophrenia

Verhoeven, W. M., et al., "Improvement of Schizophrenic Patients Treated with [des-Tyr1]-Gamma-Endorphin (DTgammaE)." *Archives of General Psychiatry* 36, no. 3 (March 1979): 294–98., Publisher: AMERICAN MEDICAL ASSOCIATION; PMID: 369471

> ➢ It was postulated from animal experiments that gamma-endorphin and, in particular, the nonopiate-like peptide [des-Tyr1]-gamma-endorphin (DTgammaE, beta-lipotropin [beta-LPH]62-77) have neuroleptic-like activity. To test this, 14 patients with long-

lasting, relapsing schizophrenic or schizoaffective psychosis resistant to conventional neuroleptics were treated with DTgammaE. An open design was used first for six patients (study 1) and a double-blind, crossover design for the other eight (study 2). In study 1, all neuroleptic medication was discontinued and 1 mg of DTgammaE zinc phosphate was given daily intramuscularly for about seven days. In study 2, six patients were maintained with neuroleptic therapy and two patients were drug free; all eight received daily intramuscular injections of 1 mg of nonlasting DTgammaE in saline and solution for eight days. There was transient or semi-permanent improvement in both studies in which the psychotic symptoms diminished or even disappeared. In study 2, there was a slight but significant improvement with the first treatment. Improvement continued and by day 4, the psychotic symptoms had almost disappeared. No toxic side effects were noted. These effects of DTgammaE may be a consequence of the normalization of beta-endorphin homeostasis in the brain.

DTgammaE has Effective Pharmalogical Action in Schizophrenic Patients

> **Meltzer, H. Y.,** et al., "Effect of (Des-Tyr)-Gamma-Endorphin in Schizophrenia." *Psychiatry Research* 6, no. 3 (June 1982): 313–26., Publisher: ELSEVIER IRELAND LTD; PMID: 6125982

➤ Des-tyrosine-gamma-endorphin (DT gamma E), a derivative of gamma-endorphin, which has been reported to have some neuroleptic-like properties in man, was administered to eight hospitalized schizophrenic patients (six chronic, one subacute, one acute) in an open study. Following an initial drug-free period, patients were given DT gamma E for 12 days in doses ranging from 1 to 10 mg/day. Two of the patients were markedly improved after receiving DT gamma E. The improvement was sustained for 2 months in one subjects, while the other deteriorated to pretreatment status within 48 hours of the discontinuation of DT gamma E. Of the other six patients, one showed moderate improvement, three showed minimal improvement, and two showed no change. Improvement was mainly in the area of social functioning; change in positive psychotic symptoms was less noticeable. The positive results obtained in this study in some subjects could have been nonspecific effects, rather than pharmacological action, since social functioning, the main area of improvement, may be especially sensitive to expectancy effects in open trials. Nevertheless, further study of DT gamma E in acute schizophrenics for longer periods appears indicated.

Gamma-Endorphin

Pharmacological Actions of Gamma-Type Endorphins are Similar to Neuroleptics

> **Van Praag, H. M.,** et al., "The Treatment of Schizophrenic Psychoses with Gamma-Type Endorphins." *Biological Psychiatry* 17, no. 1 (January 1982): 83–98., Publisher: ELSEVIER INC; PMID: 6174158

> The pharmacological actions of γ-type endorphins show similarities to those of the neuroleptics. Two fragments of γ-endorphin (β-LPH 61-77) were therefore tested in patients with schizophrenic and schizoaffective psychoses who had shown an insufficient response to neuroleptics. The fragments were DTγE (β-LPH 62-77) and DEγE (β-LPH 66-77). Some of the patients studied responded favorably to this treatment.

Glycomacropeptide

Dietary Glycomacropeptide: A Novel Nutritional Treatment for Manic and Psychotic Disorders

Badawy, Abdulla, et al., "Novel Nutritional Treatment for Manic and Psychotic Disorders: A Review of Tryptophan and Tyrosine Depletion Studies and the Potential of Protein-Based Formulations Using Glycomacropeptide." *Psychopharmacology* 228, no. 3 (August 2013): 347–58. Publisher: SPRINGER-VERLAG; doi:10.1007/s00213-013-3191-9., PMID: 23828158

> A palatable alternative lacking Trp, Tyr and Phe has been identified in the whey protein fraction caseino-glycomacropeptide (c-GMP). The absence of these three aromatic amino acids renders GMP suitable as a template for seven formulations for separate and combined depletion or loading and placebo control. The absence of Phe and Tyr enables GMP to provide a unique nutritional therapy of manic and psychotic disorders by inhibition of cerebral dopamine synthesis and release and possibly also by enhancing glutamatergic function, in general, and in patients resistant to antipsychotic medication, in particular.

Thymalin

Thymic Peptide Thymalin was Therapeutic in Schizophrenic Patients with Immune Abnormalities

Govorin, N. V., et al., "[Use of thymic peptide thymalin in the complex treatment of therapy-resistant schizophrenia]." *Zhurnal Nevropatologii I Psikhiatrii Imeni S.S. Korsakova* (Moscow, Russia: 1952) 90, no. 3 (1990): 100–103., Publisher: MEDIA SFERA; PMID: 2163147

> The thymic peptide thymaline combined with psychotropic drugs was used in the treatment of 36 therapeutically resistant patients with pronounced immune abnormalities. Such a policy favoured considerable enhancement of the treatment efficacy which manifested itself by the elimination or amelioration of psychic disorders, appreciable activation of patients and reduction of neuroleptic complications. The positive dynamics in the patients' status always correlated with the normalization of immune abnormalities, with this being seen to a greater degree in cases of the secondary "pharmacogenic" resistance and resistance because of the "pathological ground". On the one hand, the studies demonstrated wide potentialities of the use of thymaline in the

treatment of the resistant patterns of schizophrenia. On the other hand, they showed the heterogeneity of immune abnormalities in patients with different varieties of resistance.

Proteins

Ceruloplasmin

Intravenous Ceruloplasmin Administration Lead to Favorable Clinical Changes in 33 out of 37 Cases of Schizophrenic Patients

> **Martens, S.**, et al., "Continued Studies on the Effect of Ceruloplasmin Administration in Schizophrenic Patients." *Journal of Neuropsychiatry* 2 (June 1961): 238–45., PMID: 13767284

> ➤ The effect of intravenous administration of ceruloplasmin in schizophrenia was studied by the double blind technique. The results were evaluated by the use of standardized rating system. The findings of two independently operating psychiatrists corroborate the impression of the authors –published in previous papers—that favorable clinical changes following ceruloplasmin injections cannot be explained by spontaneous remissions or suggestion, the two most important sources of error in less controlled studies. The results, obtained in this study, however, do not justify any conclusion to the effect that ceuloplasmin effect is specific for schizophrenia.

Hormones

DHEA

DHEA Improves Negative Symptoms in Schizophrenia

> **Strous, Rael D.**, et al., "Dehydroepiandrosterone Augmentation in the Management of Negative, Depressive, and Anxiety Symptoms in Schizophrenia." *Archives of General Psychiatry* 60, no. 2 (February 2003): 133–41., Publisher: AMERICAN MEDICAL ASSOCIATION; PMID: 12578430

> ➤ "Increases in DHEA and DHEA-S levels were correlated with improvement in negative symptoms ($P<.05$), but not with improvement in depressive and anxiety symptoms."

> **Strous, Rael D.**, et al., "Dehydroepiandrosterone (DHEA) Augmentation in the Management of Schizophrenia Symptomatology." *Essential Psychopharmacology* 6, no. 3 (2005): 141–47., Publisher: HATHERLEIGH CO. LTD.; PMID: 15869021

> ➤ "In the authors study, administering DHEA to patients with schizophrenia who had moderate to severe negative symptoms and who were maintained on antipsychotic

medications induced significant improvement, more so in women and corresponding to increased plasma levels of DHEA and DHEA-S."

DHEA Treatment is Associated with Significant Improvement in Cognitive Function

> **Ritsner, Michael S.,** et al., "Improvement of Sustained Attention and Visual and Movement Skills, but Not Clinical Symptoms, after Dehydroepiandrosterone Augmentation in Schizophrenia: A Randomized, Double-Blind, Placebo-Controlled, Crossover Trial." *Journal of Clinical Psychopharmacology* 26, no. 5 (October 2006): 495–99. Publisher: LIPPINCOTT WILLIAMS & WILKINS; doi:10.1097/01.jcp.0000237942.50270.35., PMID: 16974191

➤ Compared to placebo, DHEA administration did not produce significant improvement in clinical symptoms, side effects, and quality-of-life scores. However, 6 weeks of DHEA administration (but not placebo) was associated with a significant improvement in Positive and Negative Symptom Scale ratings compared with baseline. Furthermore, 6 weeks of DHEA treatment was associated with significant improvement in cognitive functions of visual sustained attention and visual and movement skills compared with placebo conditions.

Estrogen (Oestrogen)

Adjunctive Estrogen Treatment Showed a Significant Decrease in Positive and Negative Symptoms

> **Ghafari, Emel,** et al., "Combination of Estrogen and Antipsychotics in the Treatment of Women with Chronic Schizophrenia: A Double-Blind, Randomized, Placebo-Controlled Clinical Trial." *Clinical Schizophrenia & Related Psychoses* 6, no. 4 (January 2013): 172–76. Publisher: WALSH MEDICAL MEDIA; doi:10.3371/CSRP.GHFA.01062013., PMID: 23302446

➤ "The combination of conjugated estrogens with antipsychotic treatment showed a significant decrease in positive (p=0.003), negative (p<0.001), general (p<0.001) and total (p<0.001) PANSS scores over 4 weeks. Estrogen may be an effective adjuvant agent in the treatment of women with chronic schizophrenia."

Further Exploration of Adjunctive Estrogen Treatment in Men in Schizophrenia is Warranted

> **Kulkarni, Jayashri,** et al., "The Role of Estrogen in the Treatment of Men with Schizophrenia." *International Journal of Endocrinology and Metabolism* 11, no. 3 (2013): 129–36. Publisher: Publishing House of Chinese Medical Association; doi:10.5812/ijem.6615., PMID: 24348584

➤ Findings do, however, suggest that further exploration of a therapeutic role for adjunctive estradiol treatment in men with schizophrenia is warranted. The development of the new estrogen compounds - Selective Estrogen Receptor Modulators (SERMs) which do not cause feminisation - opens up the possibility of using a different type of estrogen for a longer period of time at higher doses. Estrogen could therefore prove to be an important component in the treatment of psychotic symptoms in men with schizophrenia. This review explains the scientific rationale behind the estrogen hypothesis and how it can be clinically utilised to address concerns unique to the care of men with schizophrenia.

Kulkarni, Jayashri, et al., "Estrogens and Men with Schizophrenia: Is There a Case for Adjunctive Therapy?" *Schizophrenia Research* 125, no. 2–3 (February 2011): 278–83. Publisher: ELSEVIER BV; doi:10.1016/j.schres.2010.10.009., PMID: 21062669

> ➤ "Results demonstrated for estradiol participants a more rapid reduction in general psychopathology that occurred in the context of greater increases in serum estrogen levels and reductions in FSH and testosterone levels."

Oestrogen to Added to Antipsychotics Reduces Psychosis in Women and Men

Kulkarni, Jayashri, et al., "Oestrogen--a New Treatment Approach for Schizophrenia?" *The Medical Journal of Australia* 190, no. 4 Suppl (February 16, 2009): S37–38., Publisher: AUSTRALASIAN MEDICAL PUBLISHING COMPANY PTY. LTD. PMID: 19220172

> ➤ The oestrogen protection hypothesis proposes that oestrogen has a protective effect against onset of schizophrenia. In support of this: Epidemiological studies have shown that young women are less likely to develop schizophrenia than men of the same age, and women are more likely to develop late-onset schizophrenia after menopause. Clinical studies have shown higher psychotic symptoms in perimenopausal women, and women at the low oestrogen phase of the menstrual cycle. Animal studies provide further evidence in support of the oestrogen protection hypothesis. Three randomised double-blind placebo-controlled trials and an open-label study showed that adding oestradiol to women's usual antipsychotic medications was associated with significant abatement of schizophrenia symptoms. A small study of men with schizophrenia who received oral oestradiol valerate also showed a significant abatement in psychotic symptoms. Although oestrogen appears to be a useful treatment for schizophrenia, further research is required to determine the correct dose and duration of use of oestradiol. New types of oestrogen compounds may provide a safer, non-feminising approach for the treatment of schizophrenia.

Grigoriadis, Sophie, et al., "The Role of Estrogen in Schizophrenia: Implications for Schizophrenia Practice Guidelines for Women." *Canadian Journal of Psychiatry. Revue Canadienne De Psychiatrie* 47, no. 5 (June 2002): 437–42., Publisher: CANADIAN PSYCHIATRIC ASSOCIATION; PMID: 12085678

> ➤ "Estrogen has been used effectively as an adjunctive treatment in women with schizophrenia. Estrogen may also play a preventive role in TD."

CODEX ALTERNUS

Kulkarni, Jayashri "Estrogen in Severe Mental Illness: A Potential New Treatment Approach." *Archives of General Psychiatry* 65, no. 8 (August 2008): 955–60. Publisher: AMERICAN MEDICAL ASSOCIATION; doi:10.1001/archpsyc.65.8.955., PMID: 18678800

> ➤ "Estradiol appears to be a useful treatment for women with schizophrenia and may provide a new adjunctive therapeutic option for severe mental illness."

Hormone Replacement Therapy

Adjunctive Hormone Replacement Therapy May Help Reduce Negative Symptoms in Schizophrenia

Lindamer, L. A., et al., "Hormone Replacement Therapy in Postmenopausal Women with Schizophrenia: Positive Effect on Negative Symptoms?" *Biological Psychiatry* 49, no. 1 (January 1, 2001): 47–51., Publisher: ELSEVIER INC. PMID: 11163779

> ➤ "Our results suggest that the use of hormone replacement therapy in conjunction with antipsychotic medication in postmenopausal women with schizophrenia may help reduce negative, but not positive, symptoms."

Leptin

Leptin Supplementation May Reduce Positive Symptoms in Schizophrenics by Reducing Cortisol and Oxidative Stress

Venkatasubramanian, Ganesan, et al., "Neuropharmacology of Schizophrenia: Is There a Role for Leptin?" *Clinical Chemistry and Laboratory Medicine: CCLM / FESCC* 48, no. 6 (June 2010): 895–96. Publisher: WALTER/DE GRUYTER GMBH & CO. KG doi:10.1515/CCLM.2010.158., PMID: 20518646

> ➤ Thus, it is possible that the magnitude of the central nervous system effects of leptin might be proportionate to its peripheral concentration summarized in (1)x. Moreover, ample evidence supports a neuroprotective effect of leptin (3). Of interest, leptin receptors are found in the cerebral cortex, hippocampus, basal ganglia, hypothalamus, brainstem, and cerebellum (3). In addition, gray matter concentrations in the anterior cingulate gyrus, inferior parietal lobule and cerebellum increased significantly following replacement therapy with leptin in genetically leptin deficient subjects (4). Even in healthy elderly subjects, a significant positive correlation was observed between plasma leptin concentrations and the right hippocampus (5). It is important to note that schizophrenia patients demonstrate deficits in these brain regions summarized in (1)x that have been shown to be influenced by leptin in the above-mentioned studies (3–5). Moreover, these brain regions, especially the limbic brain circuit regions, such as the hippocampus, have been shown to underlie the genesis of positive symptoms in schizophrenia. Hippocampal volume deficits can be caused by high cortisol concentrations and an aberrant hyperactive hypothalamic-pituitary-adrenal (HPA) axis.

The resultant hypercortisolemia has been proposed as one of the contributing factors in the pathogenesis of schizophrenia (6). Interestingly, leptin can potentially reduce HPA axis hyperactivity by inhibiting the release of corticotrophin releasing hormone in the hypothalamus (7). Thus, leptin might have an indirect protective effect on the hippocampus by ameliorating hypercortisolemia (7), as well as a direct protective effect by reducing oxidative stress (8). Critically, both hypercortisolemia as well as oxidative stress have been shown to be associated with positive symptoms in schizophrenia. In this context, the significant positive correlation between baseline serum leptin concentrations and improvements in positive symptoms supports the possibility of a neuroprotective and anti-apoptotic effects of leptin that facilitate clinical improvements in schizophrenia.

Oxytocin

Oxytocin Has Psychotropic Effects Which Can Be Utilized for Psychosis Treatment

Bakharev, V. D., et al., "[Psychotropic properties of oxytocin]." *Problemy Endokrinologii* 30, no. 2 (April 1984): 37–41., PMID: 6718333

➢ Oxytocin neurotropic qualities were investigated in "reserpine depression" tests under ethanol and levomepromazine anesthesia, phenamine depression, haloperidol catatonia and swimming of experimental animals in the cylinder. Twenty seven patients with schizophrenia were treated with the hormone mentioned, injected intravenously and/or intranasally, using a double blind control test. The activating psychotropic oxytocin effects were revealed, allowing one to utilize it as a therapeutic means for psychosis treatment.

Adjunctive Oxytocin Efficaciously Improves Positive Symptoms of Schizophrenia

Modabbernia, Amirhossein, et al., "Intranasal Oxytocin as an Adjunct to Risperidone in Patients with Schizophrenia : An 8-Week, Randomized, Double-Blind, Placebo-Controlled Study." *CNS Drugs* 27, no. 1 (January 2013): 57–65. Publisher: ADIS INTERNATIONAL LTD. doi:10.1007/s40263-012-0022-1., PMID: 23233269

➢ Oxytocin as an adjunct to risperidone tolerably and efficaciously improves positive symptoms of schizophrenia. In addition, effects on negative and total psychopathology scores were statistically significant, but likely to be clinically insignificant. The interesting findings from the present pilot study need further replication in a larger population of patients.

Oxytocin May Represent a Novel Adjunctive Treatment for Patients with Schizophrenia.

De Berardis, Domenico, et al., "The Role of Intranasal Oxytocin in the Treatment of Patients with Schizophrenia: A Systematic Review." *CNS & Neurological Disorders Drug Targets* 12, no. 2 (March 2013): 252–64., Publisher: BENTHAM; PMID: 23469841

➢ Some authors report that intranasal oxytocin administration to schizophrenic patients may reduce symptomatology. The aim of the present paper was to review studies investigating symptomatology, social cognition and emotion recognition changes in DSM-IV-TR schizophrenic patients, after administration of intranasal oxytocin at different doses. Literature search was conducted in March, 2012. PubMed and Scopus databases were used to find studies for inclusion in the systematic review. Oxytocin may represent an important novel adjunctive treatment for patients with schizophrenia. However, some limitations of current studies cannot be overlooked and further investigations are certainly needed.

Oxytocin Enhances the Effectiveness of Cognitive Skills Training When Administered Before Training

Davis, Michael C., et al., "Oxytocin-Augmented Social Cognitive Skills Training in Schizophrenia." *Neuropsychopharmacology: Official Publication of the American College of Neuropsychopharmacology* 39, no. 9 (August 2014): 2070–77. Publisher: NATURE PUBLISHING GROUP; doi:10.1038/npp.2014.68., PMID: 24637803

➢ This study provides initial support for the idea that OT enhances the effectiveness of training when administered shortly before social cognitive training sessions. The effects were most pronounced on empathic accuracy, a high-level social cognitive process that is not easily improved in current social cognitive remediation programs.

Oxytocin Administration Improves Schizophrenic Patients Ability to Recognize Emotions

Averbeck, B. B., et al., "Emotion Recognition and Oxytocin in Patients with Schizophrenia." *Psychological Medicine* 42, no. 2 (February 2012): 259–66. Publisher: CAMBRIDGE UNIVERSITY PRESS; doi:10.1017/S0033291711001413., PMID: 21835090

➢ In the first experiment we found that patients with schizophrenia had a deficit relative to controls in recognizing emotions. In the second experiment we found that administration of oxytocin improved the ability of patients to recognize emotions. The improvement was consistent and occurred for most emotions, and was present whether patients were identifying morphed or non-morphed faces. These data add to a growing literature showing beneficial effects of oxytocin on social-behavioral tasks, as well as clinical symptoms.

Intranasal Oxytocin Exhibits Antipsychotic Properties and Has a Greater Reduction of Symptoms Compared to Placebo

Feifel, David, et al., "Adjunctive Intranasal Oxytocin Reduces Symptoms in Schizophrenia Patients." *Biological Psychiatry* 68, no. 7 (October 1, 2010): 678–80. Publisher: ELSEVIER INC. doi:10.1016/j.biopsych.2010.04.039., PMID: 20615494

> We found that 3 weeks of intranasal oxytocin given adjunctive to standard antipsychotic medications, caused significantly greater reductions in schizophrenia symptoms at the end point compared with placebo. This result supports our hypothesis that oxytocin exhibits antipsychotic properties and validates preclinical studies, case reports, and less well controlled clinical studies suggesting oxytocin's ability to ameliorate symptoms of schizophrenia.

Oxytocin is Effective for Social Cognition Improvements in Schizophrenia

> **Gibson, Clare M.,** et al., "A Pilot Six-Week Randomized Controlled Trial of Oxytocin on Social Cognition and Social Skills in Schizophrenia." *Schizophrenia Research* 156, no. 2–3 (July 2014): 261–65. Publisher: ELSEVIER BV; doi:10.1016/j.schres.2014.04.009., PMID: 24799299

> The current study explored whether oxytocin can improve social cognition and social skills in individuals with schizophrenia using a six-week, double-blind design. Fourteen participants with schizophrenia were randomized to receive either intranasal oxytocin or a placebo solution and completed a battery of social cognitive, social skills and clinical psychiatric symptom measures. Results showed within group improvements in fear recognition, perspective taking, and a reduction in negative symptoms in the oxytocin group. These preliminary findings indicate oxytocin treatment may help improve certain components of functioning in schizophrenia. Implications for the treatment of social functioning in schizophrenia are discussed.

Intranasal Oxytocin Improves Verbal Memory in People with Schizophrenia

> **Feifel, David,** et al., "Adjunctive Intranasal Oxytocin Improves Verbal Memory in People with Schizophrenia." *Schizophrenia Research* 139, no. 1–3 (August 2012): 207–10. Publisher: ELSEVIER BV; doi:10.1016/j.schres.2012.05.018., PMID: 22682705

> We found no evidence for an amnestic effect and, in fact, significantly better performance with oxytocin on several subtests of the CVLT; namely total Recall trials 1-5 (p=0.027), short delayed free recall (p=0.032) and total recall discrimination (p=0.020). In contrast we found no difference between placebo and oxytocin on LNS performance. This is the first report we are aware of documenting a beneficial effect of oxytocin on cognition in schizophrenia. Though from a small sample (n=15), these data both offset past concerns about oxytocin's amnestic effects, and may auger another potential benefit in addition to the already-demonstrated salutary effects on other components of the illness.

Pregnenolone

Pregnenolone Treatment Reduces Severity of Negative Symptoms in Schizophrenia

CODEX ALTERNUS

Ritsner, Michael S., et al., "Pregnenolone Treatment Reduces Severity of Negative Symptoms in Recent-Onset Schizophrenia: An 8-Week, Double-Blind, Randomized Add-on Two-Center Trial." *Psychiatry and Clinical Neurosciences* 68, no. 6 (June 2014): 432–40. Publisher: BLACKWELL PUBLISHING ASIA; doi:10.1111/pcn.12150., PMID: 24548129

> ➢ "Thus, add-on pregnenolone reduces the severity of negative symptoms in recent-onset schizophrenia and schizoaffective disorder, especially among patients who are not treated with concomitant mood stabilizers. Further studies are warranted."

Pregnenolone May Be a Novel Candidate for Treatment of Negative Symptoms in Schizophrenia

Marx, C. E., et al., "Pregnenolone as a Novel Therapeutic Candidate in Schizophrenia: Emerging Preclinical and Clinical Evidence." *Neuroscience* 191 (September 15, 2011): 78–90. Publisher: ELSEVIER BV; doi:10.1016/j.neuroscience.2011.06.076., PMID: 21756978

> ➢ Treatment with adjunctive pregnenolone significantly decreased negative symptoms in patients with schizophrenia or schizoaffective disorder in a pilot proof-of-concept randomized controlled trial, and elevations in pregnenolone and allopregnanolone post-treatment with this intervention were correlated with cognitive improvements [Marx et al. (2009) Neuropsychopharmacology 34:1885-1903]. Another pilot randomized controlled trial recently presented at a scientific meeting demonstrated significant improvements in negative symptoms, verbal memory, and attention following treatment with adjunctive pregnenolone, in addition to enduring effects in a small subset of patients receiving pregnenolone longer-term [Savitz (2010) Society of Biological Psychiatry Annual Meeting New Orleans, LA]. A third pilot clinical trial reported significantly decreased positive symptoms and extrapyramidal side effects following adjunctive pregnenolone, in addition to increased attention and working memory performance [Ritsner et al. (2010) J Clin Psychiatry 71:1351-1362]. Future efforts in larger cohorts will be required to investigate pregnenolone as a possible therapeutic candidate in schizophrenia, but early efforts are promising and merit further investigation. This article is part of a Special Issue entitled: Neuroactive Steroids: Focus on Human Brain.

Low-Dose Pregnenolone Augmentation Demonstrated Significant Reduction of Positive Symptoms and Cognitive Function

Ritsner, Michael S., et al., "Pregnenolone and Dehydroepiandrosterone as an Adjunctive Treatment in Schizophrenia and Schizoaffective Disorder: An 8-Week, Double-Blind, Randomized, Controlled, 2-Center, Parallel-Group Trial." *The Journal of Clinical Psychiatry* 71, no. 10 (October 2010): 1351–62. Publisher: PHYSICIANS POSTGRADUATE PRESS, INC. doi:10.4088/JCP.09m05031yel., PMID: 20584515

> "Low-dose PREG augmentation demonstrated significant amelioration of positive symptoms and EPS and improvement in attention and working memory performance of schizophrenia and schizoaffective disorder patients. Further double-blind controlled studies are needed to investigate the clinical benefit of pregnenolone augmentation."

Pregnenolone May Be a Promising Therapeutic Agent for Negative Symptoms in Schizophrenia

Marx, Christine E., et al., "Proof-of-Concept Trial with the Neurosteroid Pregnenolone Targeting Cognitive and Negative Symptoms in Schizophrenia." *Neuropsychopharmacology: Official Publication of the American College of Neuropsychopharmacology* 34, no. 8 (July 2009): 1885–1903. Publisher: NATURE PUBLISHING GROUP; doi:10.1038/npp.2009.26., PMID: 19339966

> "Pregnenolone may be a promising therapeutic agent for negative symptoms and merits further investigation for cognitive symptoms in schizophrenia."

Pregnenolone Ameliorates Visual Attention Deficits in Schizophrenia

Kreinin, Anatoly, et al., "Adjunctive Pregnenolone Ameliorates the Cognitive Deficits in Recent-Onset Schizophrenia." *Clinical Schizophrenia & Related Psychoses*, February 4, 2014, 1–31. Publisher: WALSH MEDICAL MEDIA; doi:10.3371/CSRP.KRBA.013114., PMID: 24496044

> "Pregnenolone augmentation demonstrated significant amelioration of the visual attention deficit in recent-onset SZ/SA. Long-term, large-scale studies are required to obtain greater statistical significance and more confident clinical generalization."

Secretin (peptide hormone)

Gastrointestinal Peptide Secretin Produces Clinically Meaningful Reductions in Symptoms in Several Schizophrenic Patients

Sheitman, Brian B., et al., "Secretin for Refractory Schizophrenia." *Schizophrenia Research* 66, no. 2–3 (February 1, 2004): 177–81. Publisher: ELSEVIER BV; doi:10.1016/S0920-9964(03)00068-9., PMID: 15061251

> In preliminary uncontrolled studies, intravenous injection of the gastrointestinal peptide secretin produced improvements in the symptoms of autism. Because of the phenotypic overlap between autism and some aspects of schizophrenia, we performed a pilot study of secretin for treatment refractory schizophrenia. Twenty-two patients were randomized to a single intravenous dose of porcine secretin or placebo. Patients were evaluated with the Positive and Negative Symptom Scale for Schizophrenia (PANSS) and the Clinical Global Impression Scale (CGI) at baseline, 2 days after secretin infusion

and weekly for 4 weeks. There were no statistically significant differences between drug- and placebo-treated patients with repeated measures analysis of variance (ANOVA). However, several patients treated with secretin experienced clinically meaningful, but transient, reductions in symptoms and a greater percentage of patients treated with secretin were rated as improved with the CGI. Further study of brain hypocretins and molecules affecting this system are warranted in schizophrenia.

Gastrointestinal Peptide Secretin is a Novel Adjunctive Treatment Strategy in Schizophrenic Patients with Autistic Features

Alamy, Sayed S., et al., "Secretin in a Patient with Treatment-Resistant Schizophrenia and Prominent Autistic Features." *Schizophrenia Research* 66, no. 2–3 (February 1, 2004): 183–86. Publisher: ELSEVIER BV; doi:10.1016/j.schres.2003.07.003., PMID: 15061252

> ➤ Secretin, a gastrointestinal (GI) peptide, may offer therapeutic benefit in autism. Autistic features can also be present in schizophrenia and a recent study suggested a role for adjunctive secretin in treatment-resistant schizophrenia. The current report describes one patient with undifferentiated schizophrenia and prominent autistic features who received a single dose of secretin and demonstrated substantial yet transient improvement. The case illustrates the potential role of secretin as a novel adjunctive treatment strategy in schizophrenic patients with autistic features.

Administration of Gastrointestinal Peptide Secretin Improves Eye-Blink Conditioning in Schizophrenic Patients

Bolbecker, Amanda R., et al., "Secretin Effects on Cerebellar-Dependent Motor Learning in Schizophrenia." *The American Journal of Psychiatry* 166, no. 4 (April 2009): 460–66. Publisher: AM PSYCHIATRIC ASSN; doi:10.1176/appi.ajp.2008.08040597., PMID: 19223439

> ➤ Eye-blink conditioning was significantly improved at 2 and 24 hours after secretin administration but not after treatment with placebo. These results are consistent with evidence of intracellular signaling abnormalities in the pathophysiology of schizophrenia and indicate a possible role for secretin in modulating cerebellar-mediated classically conditioned learning. If cerebellar abnormalities in individuals with schizophrenia are associated with fundamental mechanisms and symptoms of the disorder, as suggested by the cognitive dysmetria model, then cerebellar-targeted treatments may provide a novel approach to treatment for schizophrenia.

Testosterone

Testosterone Gel Augmentation in Male Schizophrenics Improves Depression and Negative Symptoms

CODEX ALTERNUS

Ko, Young-Hoon, et al., "Short-Term Testosterone Augmentation in Male Schizophrenics: A Randomized, Double-Blind, Placebo-Controlled Trial." *Journal of Clinical Psychopharmacology* 28, no. 4 (August 2008): 375–83. Publisher: LIPPINCOTT WILLIAMS & WILKINS; doi:10.1097/JCP.0b013e31817d5912., PMID: 18626263

> ➤ Results indicated a significant improvement of negative symptoms in both the last observation carried forward and the completer analyses and a nonsignificant trend for the improvement of depressive symptoms in completers. There were no significant changes in serum hormone levels except total and free testosterone. The findings of this study suggest that testosterone augmentation may be a potential therapeutic strategy in patients with schizophrenia.

Testosterone Significantly Reduced PANSS and PANSS Subscale Scores

Ceskova, Eva, et al., "Testosterone in First-Episode Schizophrenia." *Neuro Endocrinology Letters* 28, no. 6 (December 2007): 811–14., PMID: 18063925

> ➤ On average the total PANSS and PANSS subscales scores significantly decreased during the acute treatment. In contrast to results in chronic schizophrenia, the mean values of testosterone were within the normal range (15.36 and 22.55 nmol/l respectively) both before and after acute treatment. The range of normal values for the method used is given as 5.76-30.43 nmol/l for males <50 years old. On admission only 6 patients had testosterone values lower than 5.76 nmol/l. No significant correlation between negative symptoms (negative PANSS subscale) at the beginning or at the end of acute treatment or between treatment response and testosterone plasma levels was found.

Thyroid Hormone Treatment

Thyrotropin-Releasing Hormone Shows Some Improvement in Schizophrenic Patients

Kobayashi, K., et al., "Effects of Thyrotropin-Releasing Hormone in Chronic Schizophrenic Patients." *Acta Medica Okayama* 34, no. 4 (September 1980): 263–73., Publisher: OKAYAMA UNIV. MEDICAL SCHOOL. PMID: 6452029

> ➤ The effects of oral and intravenous thyrotropin-releasing hormone (TRH) were studied in 11 male, chronic schizophrenic inpatients in an open trial and a double-blind, crossover design. The general beneficial effects of TRH as assessed on the Brief Psychiatric Rating Scale were not obtained, although improvement of contact, apathy and emotional rapport was observed in a few patients. Serum prolactin, L-triiodothyronine and thyroxine were assayed throughout the study. Since the effects of TRH on behavior were not related to changes in these endocrine factors, the mechanism of action might be independent of its original functions on the pituitary-thyroid axis.

Triiodothyronine May Be Possible Associated with Better Cognitive Function and Less Extrapyramidal Symptoms in Chronic Schizophrenia

Ichioka, Shugo, et al., "Triiodothyronine May Be Possibly Associated with Better Cognitive Function and Less Extrapyramidal Symptoms in Chronic Schizophrenia." *Progress in Neuro-Psychopharmacology & Biological Psychiatry* 39, no. 1 (October 1, 2012): 170–74. Publisher: ELSEVIER INC. doi:10.1016/j.pnpbp.2012.06.008., PMID: 22750309

> ➤ These findings suggest that BDNF, free T_3, and prolactin may be associated with cognitive function and/or extrapyramidal symptoms in patients with chronic schizophrenia. Notably, free T_3 may be possibly associated with better cognitive function and less extrapyramidal symptoms, although our cross-sectional study could not reveal a causal relationship.

Intravenous Protrelin (thyrotropin-releasing hormone) caused a Significant Decrease in Psychotic Symptoms in Schizophrenic Patients

Prange, A. J., et al., "Behavioral and Endocrine Responses of Schizophrenic Patients to TRH (protirelin)." *Archives of General Psychiatry* 36, no. 10 (September 1979): 1086–93., Publisher: AMERICAN MEDICAL ASSOCIATION; PMID: 112944

> ➤ We studied the effects of intravenous protirelin (thyrotropin-releasing hormone) in 17 schizophrenic patients and 17 normal subjects. A total of 12 patients received protirelin, 0.5 mg, and, on another occasion, niacin, 2 mg, in a double-blind, crossover design. Both behavioral and endocrine data were collected. Five patients received protirelin in an open trial; only endocrine data were collected. Protirelin caused about a 50% prompt decrease in psychotic symptoms. Patients then tended slowly to experience a relapse. Side effects were about as infrequent after protirelin as after niacin. We assayed serum prolactin (PRL), growth hormone (GH), thyroid-stimulating hormone (TSH), L-triiodothyronine (T3) and thyroxine (T4). Free T4 (FT4) index was calculated. The values for PRL, GH, and TSH at baseline and after protirelin stimulation were normal. Patients showed lower T3 values at baseline, but a brisker T3 response to protirelin, than controls. Their FT4 indices were higher at baseline. Patients showed diminished T4 binding sites rather than increased total T4. The causes of these alterations in thyroid dynamics are unidentified.

Organotherapy

Adrenal Cortex Extract

Intramuscular Injections of Adrenal Cortex Extract combined with diet, sodium, and calcium show some improvement in mental symptoms.

> **Loehner, Conrad A**. "The Therapeutic Effect of Adrenal Cortex Extract on the Psychotic Patient." *Endocrinology* 23, no. 4 (October 1, 1938): 507–20. doi:10.1210/endo-23-4-507.

> ➢ Eleven patients suffering from mental disease were used in this experiment. Nine of them were treated with a low potassium diet, sodium choride, calcium lactate, and adrenal cortex (eschatin; Parke, Davis & Co.,) by intramuscular injection, and 2 with eschatin alone. The following physiological changes were observed: the blood pressure dropped approximately 10mm of mercury in both systole and diastole, except in 3 cases of hypoadrenalism where it rose to the normal level; reversal of the mood to euphoria and elation; a feeling of warmth, drowsiness, and relaxation was followed by normal, restful sleep without the use of seditives; there were improved bowel movements, and a disappearance of cyanosis of the extremities. One patient showed a remmision of her mental symptoms, 2 were much improved, 6 were somewhat improved, whereas 2 were unimproved.

Brain Extracts

Sheep and Cattle Brain Extracts Show Some Improvement in Dementia Praecox as Well as Other Forms of Insanity

> **Smith, Maule W.,** "On the Use of Brain Extract in the Treatment of Varoious Forms of Insanity" *The British Medical Journal,* 451; November 23, 1912

> ➢ Fourteen cases have been under treatment, and the rule has been that cases of any degree of recency have improved; 8 cases have definitely reacted; and of the remaing 6, 2 are long standing. Of those that have improved, 3 are in an advanced state of convalescence and 2 have passed from a state of emaciation to one of good health. Unfortunatly, the mental symptoms in these two have not altered in the same ratio, but they are manageable without the aid of other treatment. In addition to improved appetites for food and sleep and general health, there is a definite reduction in the degree of katatonia and negativism.

Other Natural Compounds

Alpha-lipoic Acid

Alpha-lipoic Acid plus Clozapine Presents a More Powerful Antipsychotic Profile

CODEX ALTERNUS

Vasconcelos, Germana Silva, et al., "Alpha-Lipoic Acid Alone and Combined with Clozapine Reverses Schizophrenia-like Symptoms Induced by Ketamine in Mice: Participation of Antioxidant, Nitrergic and Neurotrophic Mechanisms." *Schizophrenia Research* 165, no. 2–3 (July 2015): 163–70. doi:10.1016/j.schres.2015.04.017.

> The combination ALA+CLZ2.5 reversed behavioral and some neurochemical parameters. However, ALA+CLZ5 caused motor impairment. Therefore, ALA presented an antipsychotic-like profile reversing KET-induced positive- and negative-like symptoms. The mechanism partially involves antioxidant, neurotrophic and nitrergic pathways. The combination of ALA+CLZ2.5 improved most of the parameters evaluated in this study without causing motor impairment demonstrating, thus, that possibly when combined with ALA a lower dose of CLZ is required.

Alstonine

Indole Alkaloid Alstonine was found to possess an Antipsychotic Profile

Costa-Campos, L., et al.,"Antipsychotic-like Profile of Alstonine." *Pharmacology, Biochemistry, and Behavior* 60, no. 1 (May 1998): 133–41., Publisher: ELSEVIER INC; PMID: 9610935

> An ethnopharmacological study in Nigeria has led to the investigation of a plant-based extract used by traditional psychiatrists with anecdotal antipsychotic-like effects. This extract was later found to bear antipsychotic profile (Elisabetsky et al., unpublished results) using a behavioral approach similar to the present study. Phytochemical studies have identified alstonine as one of the major components of this extract. The following study investigates the putative antipsychotic profile of alstonine using behavioral and neurochemical strategies.

Alstonine is a Potential Innovative Antipsychotic

Linck, Viviane M., et al., "Alstonine as an Antipsychotic: Effects on Brain Amines and Metabolic Changes." *Evidence-Based Complementary and Alternative Medicine: eCAM* 2011 (2011): 418597. Publisher: OXFORD UNIVERSITY PRESS (UK) doi:10.1093/ecam/nep002., PMID: 19189988

> Alstonine is an indole alkaloid identified as the major component of a plant-based remedy used in Nigeria to treat the mentally ill. Alstonine presents a clear antipsychotic profile in rodents, apparently with differential effects in distinct dopaminergic pathways. The aim of this study was to complement the antipsychotic profile of alstonine, verifying its effects on brain amines in mouse frontal cortex and striatum. Additionally, we examined if alstonine induces some hormonal and metabolic changes common to antipsychotics. HPLC data reveal that alstonine increases serotonergic

transmission and increases intraneuronal dopamine catabolism. In relation to possible side effects, preliminary data suggest that alstonine does not affect prolactin levels, does not induce gains in body weight, but prevents the expected fasting-induced decrease in glucose levels. Overall, this study reinforces the proposal that alstonine is a potential innovative antipsychotic, and that a comprehensive understanding of its neurochemical basis may open new avenues to developing newer antipsychotic medications.

Amyloban® 3399 (Lion's Main Extracts)

Amyloban® 3399 Extracts May Help Schizophrenics with Cognitive Functions and Reduce Negative Symptoms

Inanaga, Kazutoyo, et al., "Improvement of Refractory Schizophrenia on Using Amyloban®3399 Extracted from Hericium Erinaceum." *Personalized Medicine Universe* 3 (July 2014): 49–53. doi:10.1016/j.pmu.2014.04.002.

> Amyloban®3399---a product made of amycenone, a standardized extract of HE containing hericenones and amyloban---is currently being tested for safety as a health food supplement. It has been reported that Amyloban®3399 increases mental alertness, encourages positive behavior, and improves mood and attentiveness to one's surroundings, thus, increasing learning and motivation, while promoting interactions with others. Based on these observations, it is hypothesized that Amyloban®3399 may be beneficial for treating primary cognitive deficits and negative symptoms of schizophrenia.

Ampullosporin A

Ampullosporin A has Characteristics of an Atypical Neuroleptic Drug

Berek, I., et al., "Ampullosporin A, a Peptaibol from Sepedonium Ampullosporum HKI-0053 with Neuroleptic-like Activity." *Behavioural Brain Research* 203, no. 2 (November 5, 2009): 232–39. Publisher: ELSEVIER BV; doi:10.1016/j.bbr.2009.05.012., PMID: 19450625

> The potential neuroleptic-like effect of ampullosporin A, a new peptaibol, isolated from the fungus Sepedonium ampullosporum HKI-0053, was characterized using specific behavioural models and methods. Ampullosporin A (amp) disrupted the retrieval of a well-trained conditioned reaction and normalized the behavioural effects of subchronic ketamine treatment in the social interaction test in a dose which showed only inconsiderable side effects. The experiments demonstrated that the substance did not antagonize the apomorphine (apo) induced hyperactivity. On the other hand, the locomotor stimulation induced by the NMDA receptor antagonist MK-801 was nearly completely suppressed by ampullosporin A, supposing interactions with the glutamatergic system. Binding studies demonstrated no interaction with dopaminergic

D(1) and D(2) receptors. However, amp can alter the activity of glutamate receptors. The results resemble characteristics of an atypical neuroleptic drug. But further experiments are necessary to validate the suggested neuroleptic-like activity.

Ampullosporin A Belongs to a Group of Neuroleptic-like Compounds

> **Krügel, Hans,** et al., "Transcriptional Response to the Neuroleptic-like Compound Ampullosporin A in the Rat Ketamine Model." *Journal of Neurochemistry* 97 Suppl 1 (April 2006): 74–81. Publisher: BLACKWELL PUBLISHING LTD. doi:10.1111/j.1471-4159.2005.03621.x., PMID: 16635253

> ➤ Our results suggest the possibility that Ampullosporin A belongs to the group of neuroleptic-like compounds, inducing massive changes in neurotransmitter receptor composition, calcium signaling cascades and second messenger systems, and leading to the plastic reorganization of brain tissue, metabolic pathways and synapses.

Creatine

Creatine Treatment Mildly Improves Schizophrenia Symptomatology

> **Levental, Uri,** et al. "A Pilot Open Study of Long Term High Dose Creatine Augmentation in Patients with Treatment Resistant Negative Symptoms Schizophrenia." *The Israel Journal of Psychiatry and Related Sciences* 52, no. 1 (2015): 6–10., PMID: 25841104

> ➤ "Creatine treatment mildly improved the schizophrenia symptomatology but there were no significant changes in cognitive functions. Several ward behaviors were also improved. Tardive parkinsonism improved numerically by above 40% in 4 out of 6 patients."

Deanol (Deaner)

Deanol Works Well with an Antipsychotic in the Treatment of Schizophrenia

> **Barsa, J. A.,** et al., "Deanol (deaner) in the Treatment of Schizophrenia." *The American Journal of Psychiatry* 116 (September 1959): 255–56., Publisher: AM PSYCHIATRIC ASSN; PMID: 13797141

> ➤ "From this study, it can be concluded that deanol, when combined with a tranquilizer containing a potent antipsychotic action is of definite value in the treatment of schizophrenia. Not only does its stimulating effect counteract the excessive sedation and lethargy produced by the tranquilizer, but its own ant-psychotic effect is additive to that of the tranquilizer."

Deaner Produces Dramatic Responses in Some Cases of Schizophrenia

Toll, N., et al., "Deaner an Adjunct for Treatment of Schizoid and Schzophrenic Patients." *The American Journal of Psychiatry* 115, no. 4 (October 1958): 366–67., Publisher: AM PSYCHIATRIC ASSN; PMID: 13583235

> ➤ Despite the small number of patients included in this study, certain clinical impressions were formed: Deaner appears to merit further study in those conditions where CNS stimulation is needed. Its freedom from serious side-effects, and the dramatic response produced in some cases suggest that the drug is worthy of trial, especially in schizoid and schizophrenic patients who have not responded to other therapies.

Dimethyl Sulfoxide (DMSO)

DMSO has Antipsychotic and Antianxiety Properties and Does Not Produce Major Sedation

Ramírez, E., et al., "Dimethyl Sulfoxide in the Treatment of Mental Patients." *Annals of the New York Academy of Sciences* 141, no. 1 (March 15, 1967): 655–67., PMID: 5342267

> ➤ Preliminary results on 42 severely disturbed psychiatric patients showed DMSO to have antipsychotic and antianxiety properties. It produces emotional calm followed by relief of some psychotic and severe neurotic symptoms. The action differs from so-called tranquilizers mainly in that it does not produce major sedation or central depressant action. On the contrary DMSO produces some mild stimulant effect that makes patients more alert, sociable, and acceptable for psychotherapy and occupational therapy. It does not produce muscle relaxation, autonomic changes or extrapyramidal symptoms. DMSO seems to be useful in the treatment o patients with the following diagnoses: (1) overexcited states (acute schizophrenic reactions, manic phase of manic-depressive psychosis, alcoholic psychosis, symptomatic psychosis); (2) some symptoms of chronic psychosis (autism, sterotypia, negativism, abnormal behavior or the hebephrenic states); (3) severe neurosis (anxiety reactions, obsessives). Tolerance to the drug was judged goodin all the treated patients by clinical and laboratory controls. Inpatient treatment at the hospital was shorter for the acute patients treated with DMSO, as compared with similar control group treated with conventional therapy.

Flavonoids

The Use of Flavonoids in Schizophrenia and Other Neurodegenerative Diseases

Grosso, C., et al., "The Use of Flavonoids in Central Nervous System Disorders." *Current Medicinal Chemistry* 20, no. 37 (2013): 4694–4719., Publisher: BENTHAM SCIENCE PUBLISHERS LTD. PMID: 23834189

> ➤ This review will give emphasis to the benefits of flavonoids found in the diet in the treatment of Alzheimer's disease, Parkinson's disease, epilepsy, depression, and schizophrenia. The antioxidant effect of several flavonoids, as well as their effects not

related with antioxidant activity, in the above mentioned diseases will be reviewed. Aspects concerning structure-activity relationships, but also the bioavailability of these compounds in the brain will be referred.

Folinic Acid

Folinic Acid Treatment Causes Disappearance of Hallucinations in Schizophrenic Patients

Ramaekers, V. T., et al., "Folinic Acid Treatment for Schizophrenia Associated with Folate Receptor Autoantibodies." *Molecular Genetics and Metabolism* 113, no. 4 (December 2014): 307–14. Publisher: ACADEMIC PRESS; doi:10.1016/j.ymgme.2014.10.002., PMID: 25456743

> ➤ Assessment of FR auto-antibodies in serum is recommended for schizophrenic patients. Clinical negative or positive symptoms are speculated to be influenced by the level and evolution of FRα antibody titers which determine folate flux to the brain with up or down-regulation of brain folate intermediates linked to metabolic processes affecting homocysteine levels, synthesis of tetrahydrobiopterin and neurotransmitters. Folinic acid intervention appears to stabilize the disease process.

Galantamine

Galantamine as Adjunctive Treatment is Effective in Resistant Schizophrenia

Allen, Trina B., et al., "Galantamine for Treatment-Resistant Schizophrenia." *The American Journal of Psychiatry* 159, no. 7 (July 2002): 1244–45., Publisher: AM PSYCHIATRIC ASSN; PMID: 12091212

> ➤ Controlled double-blind trials of galantamine as an adjunctive treatment for schizophrenia are currently underway. These two patients were both very heavy smokers and had shown a favorable therapeutic response to clozapine that could not be matched by treatment with any other currently available antipsychotic. Both of these attributes (smoking and clozapine response) may signal that nicotinic pathophysiology contributed to their illnesses and that an agent such as galantamine that can augment nicotinic function may be a useful treatment.

Diminished Expression of Nicotinic Receptors Determine Response to Galantamine in the Treatment of Apathy for Schizophrenia

Arnold, David S., et al., "Adjuvant Therapeutic Effects of Galantamine on Apathy in a Schizophrenia Patient." *The Journal of Clinical Psychiatry* 65, no. 12 (December 2004): 1723–24., Publisher: PHYSICIANS POSTGRADUATE PRESS, INC. PMID: 15641883

> ➤ Conceivably, galantamine's greatest therapeutic benefit will be observed in schizophrenia patients with diminished expression of nicotinic acetylcholine receptors

in selected regions of the brain. Abnormal variants of the promoter region for the α7 nicotinic acetylcholine receptor located on chromosome 15 may be a mechanism for its diminished expression in selected brain areas. Diminished expression of normal receptor protein would encourage exploration of strategies to improve the transduction of the acetylcholine signal, such as galantamine use. Of course, only future double-blind, placebo-controlled trials can substantiate the suggestions of therapeutic efficacy of adjuvant galantmine administration, especially for such targets as negative symptoms, apathy, and mood. It might be informative to randomize subjects in these future studies according to smoking status and genetic profiles of promoter variants that regulate expression of the α7 nicotinic acetylcholine receptor subunit. It is possible that the smoking status of the patient who responded contributed to his therapeutic response to galantamine.

Adjunctive Galantamine Improves Negative Symptoms in Patient with Treatment Refractory Schizophrenia

> **Rosse, Richard B.**, et al., "Adjuvant Galantamine Administration Improves Negative Symptoms in a Patient with Treatment-Refractory Schizophrenia." *Clinical Neuropharmacology* 25, no. 5 (October 2002): 272–75., Publisher: LIPPINCOTT WILLIAMS & WILKINS; PMID: 12410061

➢ Because of the demonstration of a selective alpha nicotinic receptor abnormality in patients with schizophrenia, galantamine was added to the stable regimen of atypical and other antipsychotic medications in a 43-year-old man manifesting severe and persistent positive and negative symptoms, as well as mood disturbance and cognitive dysfunction. Galantamine is an inhibitor of acetylcholinesterase and a positive allosteric modulator of nicotinic cholinergic receptors (with a FDA-approved indication for the treatment of patients with mild to moderate Alzheimer disease (AD) under the trade name Reminyl). Galantamine HBr was initiated at a dose of 4 mg po BID, which was maintained for the first week of adjuvant therapy, and eventually was increased to 12 mg po BID during the final weeks of his 2-month trial. Remarkably, within 1 week of its initiation, there was a dramatic and clinically significant decrease of negative symptoms, as reflected in formal ratings on the Scale for the Assessment of Negative Symptoms. Moreover, within a few days of galantamine discontinuation, negative symptoms worsened, returning to the baseline level of severity. In addition to targeting memory dysfunction in AD, acetylcholinesterase inhibitors may have an expanded range of targets and clinical indications, including behavioral and psychotic symptoms. Galantamine is distinguished from other acetylcholinesterase inhibitors by its positive allosteric modulatory properties, improving the efficiency of transduction of the acetylcholine signal at nicotinic receptors.

Galantamine Shows Some Improvement in Attention and Speech of Schizophrenic Patients with Cognitive Impairment

Ochoa, Enrique L. M., et al., "Galantamine May Improve Attention and Speech in Schizophrenia." *Human Psychopharmacology* 21, no. 2 (March 2006): 127–28. Publisher: JOHN/WILEY & SONS LTD. doi:10.1002/hup.751., PMID: 16482609

➤ "After 34 days the patient showed a remarkable improvement in working memory and delayed recall, though he continued to show impairment in the other examined domains. Negative symptom ratings on the SANS also revealed improvement of attention and speech."

➤ "At the time of his discharge, 20 days after admission, his thought processes were more organized and he was able to maintain a coherent conversation. Speech and attention showed marked improvements with less gains in anhedonia, affective flattening, avolition or apathy."

Adjunctive Galantamine Improves Cognition in Schizophrenic Patients Stabilized on Antipsychotic

Schubert, Max H., et al., "Galantamine Improves Cognition in Schizophrenic Patients Stabilized on Risperidone." *Biological Psychiatry* 60, no. 6 (September 15, 2006): 530–33. Publisher: ELSEVIER INC. doi:10.1016/j.biopsych.2006.04.006., PMID: 16806095

➤ "Adjunctive treatment with galantamine improves memory and attention in patients with schizophrenia who are stabilized on risperidone, providing the opportunity to improve functional outcome in these patients."

Glutamic Acid

Glutamic Acid Has Positive Effect on Some Catatonic Patients, Though Warrants Further Investigation

Kitzinger, H., et al., "A Preliminary Study of the Effects of Glutamic Acid on Catatonic Schizophrenics." *Rorschach Research Exchange and Journal of Projective Techniques* 13, no. 2 (1949): 210–18. doi:10.1080/10683402.1949.10381459.

➤ The results of this preliminary study with twenty-three schizophrenics would indicate that glutamic acid treatment has an effect on' some, although not all such patients. Among those with whom the treatment has effect, the specific changes brought about seem different for different types of individuals. Those catatonics who were, before treatment, functioning at a very low level of reactivity, close to but not having reached muteness, gained a higher level of reactivity, better motor control, and greater capacity for production. Those, on the other hand, who were initially at a level of reactivity more approaching the normal became over reactive, and their motor control and general production suffered under the disrupting effect of extreme tension. It would seem, then, that each patient has a ceiling or maximum capacity to use the energy with which glutamic acid seems to provide him, and that, unless his initial level of reactivity is very low, glutamic acid may quickly raise him to that ceiling, at which point increased energy becomes disruptive rather than productive. It must be admitted that our conclusions make it surprising that the mute catatonics did not show much greater response to the treatment than they did. Unless one considers it possible that real changes may have come about, although still within the range of muteness, and that perhaps, different dosages might have shown observable changes, it must be said that the writers can offer no explanation of this result. Although the small number of cases and limited data necessitate reemphasis of the tentative character of this study, the results seem sufficiently encouraging to warrant further research. A particularly attractive possibility with which future research might be concerned, is that of raising the level of reactivity of near-mute catatonics sufficiently to make other forms of therapy possible.

Guanosine

Guanosine has Potential Antipsychotic Properties

> **Schmidt, André P.**, et al., "Guanosine and Its Modulatory Effects on the Glutamatergic System." European Neuropsychopharmacology: *The Journal of the European College of Neuropsychopharmacology* 18, no. 8 (August 2008): 620–22. Publisher: ELSEVIER BV; doi:10.1016/j.euroneuro.2008.01.007., PMID: 18329859

> ➢ Although the mechanism of action of guanosine and its modulatory effects on MK-801-induced behavioral disturbances are not completely elucidated, these findings point to a potential antipsychotic property of guanosine. This may be especially important in targeting psychotic symptoms that are not generally treated with currently available antipsychotics. Moreover, the neuroprotective and neurotrophic effects of guanosine may also be advantageous for the treatment of schizophrenia and other brain diseases.

Harmine

Harmine a Forgotten Treatment for Catatonic Schizophrenia

> **Hostiuc, Sorin,** et al., "Harmine for Catatonic Schizophrenia. A Forgotten Experiment." *Schizophrenia Research* 159, no. 1 (October 2014): 249–50. Publisher: ELSEVIER BV; doi:10.1016/j.schres.2014.08.006., PMID: 25195064

> ➢ Harmine was found in the 1920's to have a possible use in the treatment of Parkinsonism (Beringer, 1929). As in schizophrenic catatonia muscle rigidity was one of the most important symptoms, Tomescu designed an experiment to test whether Harmine could be used as a potential therapeutic agent for catatonic schizophrenia with it, by using

three patients with this disease. A dosage of 0.03–0.04 cg was found to be optimal. In the first patient injecting 0.03 cg Harmine caused a complete disappearance of the rigidity after an hour, with free passive movements in the upper limbs and only a slight residual rigidity in the lower limbs. Moreover, this dosage had positive effects on negativity, as the patient started saying a few words, and asked for his favorite foods. The patient was able to reveal various information from his past but also information from the time he was admitted (from the time he has been in a catatonic state). The symptoms reemerged gradually a few hours after the treatment; however the patient remained in an ameliorated state for a few days. After this initial success, Tomescu treated the patient for 25 days with Harmine, obtaining the same effects as those from the initial experiment. The patient was cooperative, with an almost complete remission of negativity, no muscle rigidity, and a significant increase in weight. The effects of the drug completely disappeared at 5–6 days after discontinuing it. On the second patient he obtained a complete remission of the muscle rigidity and negativity with a dosage of 0.04 cg. Moreover, the use of the drug on a longer period of time (20 days) had effects on his affectivity as he showed signs of falling in love with a nurse. The effect diminished significantly after 2–3 days. On the third patient similar results were obtained at a dosage of 0.04 cg; the use of the drug on a longer period of time (20 days) caused him to want to leave the hospital and stay with his family. The study concluded that, even if Harmine had a purely symptomatic effect, it Schizophrenia Research 159 (2014) 249–250 did cause significant improvement of the symptoms and of the quality of life. The experiments were not continued due to the prohibitive costs of Harmine (Tomescu and Russu, 1930). The effect disappeared in about five days.

Homeopathy

Homeopathy is Always Helpful in Schizophrenia and in Certain Cases Curative

Smith, Trevor. "A Homoeopathic Approach to Schizophrenia." *British Homoeopathic Journal* 68, no. 1 (January 1979): 20–28. doi:10.1016/S0007-0785(79)80057-5.

> ➤ Homeopathy is always helpful in schizophrenia, in certain cases it is curative. Most of the cases I have treated have shown a lessening of the over-activity. Frequently the sleep disturbances have improved markedly. It is not uncommon to see a rapid lessening of the hallucinations, as the patient begins to take an interest in her self-appearance, frequently neglected in the acute phase of the illness.

There Are a Varity of Homeopathic Remedies for Psychotic Personality

Boericke, C. C. "THE HOMEOPATHIC APPROACH TO THE PSYCHOTIC PERSONALITY." *Journal of the American Institute of Homeopathy* 57 (August 1964): 178–81., PMID: 14178442

> ➤ This article is about 20 different prescriptions of homeopathic remedies that are used to treat psychotic personality.

CODEX ALTERNUS

Huperzine

Huperzine A Demonstrated Beneficial Effects in Treating Cognitive and Negative Symptom Clusters in Schizophrenia

> **Zhang, Zhang-Jin,** et al., "Huperzine A as Add-on Therapy in Patients with Treatment-Resistant Schizophrenia: An Open-Labeled Trial." *Schizophrenia Research* 92, no. 1–3 (May 2007): 273–75. Publisher: ELSEVIER BV; doi:10.1016/j.schres.2007.02.005., PMID: 1738858

> ➢ "In conclusion, this pilot trial demonstrated the beneficial effects of HupA in treating cognitive and negative symptom clusters of schizophrenia and it may deserve to be further tested in larger-scale, controlled trials."

Hydrogen Gas

Hydrogen Gas is a Potential Novel Therapy for Treatment of Schizophrenia and Bipolar Disorder

> **Ghanizadeh, Ahmad,** et al. "Molecular Hydrogen: An Overview of Its Neurobiological Effects and Therapeutic Potential for Bipolar Disorder and Schizophrenia." *Medical Gas Research* 3, no. 1 (2013): 11. doi:10.1186/2045-9912-3-11., PMID: 23742229

> ➢ Hydrogen gas is a bioactive molecule that has a diversity of effects, including anti-apoptotic, anti-inflammatory and anti-oxidative properties; these overlap with the process of neuroprogression in major psychiatric disorders. Specifically, both bipolar disorder and schizophrenia are associated with increased oxidative and inflammatory stress. Moreover, lithium which is commonly administered for treating bipolar disorder has effects on oxidative stress and apoptotic pathways, as do valproate and some atypical antipsychotics for treating schizophrenia. Molecular hydrogen has been studied pre-clinically in animal models for the treatment of some medical conditions including hypoxia and neurodegenerative disorders, and there are intriguing clinical findings in neurological disorders including Parkinson's disease. Therefore, it is hypothesized that administration of hydrogen molecule may have potential as a novel therapy for bipolar disorder, schizophrenia, and other concurrent disorders characterized by oxidative, inflammatory and apoptotic dysregulation.

L-stepholidine (Stepholidine)

Stepholidine Shows Antipsychotic Effects in Animal Model of Schizophrenia

> **Ellenbroek, Bart A.,** et al., "Effects of (-)stepholidine in Animal Models for Schizophrenia." *Acta Pharmacologica Sinica* 27, no. 9 (September 2006): 1111–18. Publisher: BLACKWELL PUBLISHING, INC. doi:10.1111/j.1745-7254.2006.00365.x., PMID: 16923330

> ➢ "The data showed that SPD showed antipsychotic-like effects in both the prepulse inhibition paradigm and in the paw test. Moreover, the results of the paw test suggest

that SPD has an atypical character with relatively small potency to induce extrapyramidal symptoms."

Natesan, Sridhar, et al., "The Antipsychotic Potential of L-Stepholidine--a Naturally Occurring Dopamine Receptor D1 Agonist and D2 Antagonist." *Psychopharmacology* 199, no. 2 (August 2008): 275–89. Publisher: SPRINGER-VERLAG; doi:10.1007/s00213-008-1172-1., PMID: 18521575

> ➤ "Thus, l-stepholidine shows efficacy like an "atypical" antipsychotic in traditional animal models predictive of antipsychotic activity and shows in vitro and vivo D91) agonism, and, if its rapid elimination does not limit its actions, it could provide a unique therapeutic approach to schizophrenia."

Stepholidine Improves both Negative and Positive Symptoms of Schizophrenia

---

Yang, Kechun, et al., "The Neuropharmacology of (-)-Stepholidine and Its Potential Applications." *Current Neuropharmacology* 5, no. 4 (December 2007): 289–94. Publisher: BENTHAM SCIENCE PUBLISHERS LTD. doi:10.2174/157015907782793649., PMID: 19305745

> ➤ (-)-Stepholidine (SPD), a natural product isolated from the Chinese herb Stephania, possesses dopamine (DA) D1 partial agonistic and D2 antagonistic properties in the nigrostriatal and mesocorticolimbic DAergic pathways. These unique dual effects have suggested that SPD can effectively restore previously imbalanced functional linkage between D1 and D2 receptors under schizophrenic conditions, in which, SPD improves both the negative and positive symptoms of schizophrenia. SPD also relieves the motor symptoms of Parkinson's disease (PD) when co-administered with Levodopa. Furthermore, SPD exhibits neuroprotective effects through an antioxidative mechanism and slows down the progression of neuronal degeneration in the substantia nigra (SN) of PD patients and/or animal models. Therefore, SPD is a novel, natural compound with potentially therapeutic roles in the treatment of schizophrenia and/or PD.

L-Stepholidine is a Potential Neurotransmitter Stabilizer and Promising Drug Candidate for Treatment of Schizophrenia

---

Guo, Yang, et al., "Evaluation of the Antipsychotic Effect of Bi-Acetylated L-Stepholidine (l-SPD-A), a Novel Dopamine and Serotonin Receptor Dual Ligand." *Schizophrenia Research* 115, no. 1 (November 2009): 41–49. Publisher: ELSEVIER BV doi:10.1016/j.schres.2009.08.002., PMID: 19744833

> ➤ Taken together, these results indicate that l-SPD-A was not only effective against the hyperactivity, but also improved the sensorimotor gating deficit, social withdrawal and cognitive impairment in an animal model of schizophrenia. The present data suggest

that l-SPD-A, a potential neurotransmitter stabilizer, is a promising novel candidate drug for the treatment of schizophrenia.

L-Stepholidine is a Potential Agent for Treatment of Drug Addiction as Well as Schizophrenia

Mo, Jiao, et al., "Recent Developments in Studies of L-Stepholidine and Its Analogs: Chemistry, Pharmacology and Clinical Implications." *Current Medicinal Chemistry* 14, no. 28 (2007): 2996–3002., Publisher: BENTHAM SCIENCE PUBLISHERS LTD.; PMID: 18220736

> ➤ This unique pharmacological profile made dihydroxyl-THPBs such as l-stepholidine (l-SPD) potential agents in the treatment of drug addiction, Parkinson's disease, and especially, schizophrenia. Clinical studies have shown that co-administration of l-SPD with a typical antipsychotic drug significantly enhances the therapeutic effects and remarkably reduces the tardive dyskinesia induced by the typical antipsychotic drug used with schizophrenic patients. Moreover, l-SPD alone was shown to have therapeutic value without inducing significant extrapyramidal side effects and also seemed to reduce the negative symptoms of schizophrenia. This is confirmed in experimental studies using animal models of schizophrenia, in which l-SPD improved social interaction and cognitive function, inhibited hyperactivity in schizophrenic animals. This review discusses the chemistry, pharmacology and clinical implications of l-THPBs in the drug development for psychosis and neurobiological diseases.

Maganese Chloride

Use of Manganese Chloride Results in Higher Discharge Rate

Reed, G. E. "The Use of Manganese Chloride as Treatment in Dementia Praecox." *Canadian Medical Association Journal* 21, no. 1 (July 1929): 46–49., PMID: 20317414

> ➤ "We have observed a substantially higher discharge rate among the cases with manganese than in similar cases not receiving treatment. However, we feel that more work will be required, and is justified, to determine whether the results are real or apparent."

Manassantin A

Manassantin A is a Potential Neuroleptic Agent form the Plant Saururus Cernuus

Rao, K. V., et al.,"Preliminary Evaluation of Manassantin A, a Potential Neuroleptic Agent from Saururus Cernuus." *Pharmacological Research Communications* 19, no. 9 (September 1987): 629–38., Publisher: PUBLISHED FOR THE ITALIAN PHARMACOLOGICAL SOCIETY; PMID: 289331

CODEX ALTERNUS

> Manassantin A (MNS-A), a novel dineolignan isolated from Saururus cernuus was evaluated for its central depressant effects. Intraperitoneal (IP) administration of MNS-A to mice at nontoxic doses caused a decrease in spontaneous motor activity and inhibition of amphetamine-induced stereotypy, with an ED50 of 0.21 +/- 0.02 mg/kg for its antiamphetamine activity. Doses of MNS-A up to the LD50 did not produce catalepsy and ptosis as were observed with haloperidol used as a reference drug. The compound caused a dose-dependent hypothermia, while haloperidol was not very effective in this test. Potentiation of pentobarbital-sleeping time was observed to be of comparable degree with both drugs. In spite of the higher toxicity (acute LD50 5.4 +/- 0.2 mg/kg, IP) than that shown by haloperidol, the somewhat selective neuroleptic profile of MNS-A makes it an interesting candidate for more detailed studies.

Muscimol

Muscimol at Low Doses Has a Pleasant, Relaxing Effect.

Tamminga, C. A., et al., "Muscimol: GABA Agonist Therapy in Schizophrenia." *The American Journal of Psychiatry* 135, no. 6 (June 1978): 746–47., PMID: 350058

> During high-dose muscimol treatment, all study subjects evidenced diffuse myoclonic twitching or somnolence, and many experienced vivid dreams, dizziness, and confusion. At dose levels below 5 mg, many patients experienced a tranquilizing effect from muscimol. These subjects, when receiving the active drug, reported feeling more relaxed and less anxious and claimed a positive drug experience, despite their lack of relief from psychotic thinking. No significant change in vital signs or routine laboratory studies occurred.

N-acetylcysteine

N-acetylcysteine in Beneficial for Treatment Resistant Schizophrenia

Bulut, Mahmut, et al., "Beneficial Effects of N-Acetylcysteine in Treatment Resistant Schizophrenia." *The World Journal of Biological Psychiatry: The Official Journal of the World Federation of Societies of Biological Psychiatry* 10, no. 4 Pt 2 (2009): 626–28. Publisher: WORLD FEDERATION OF THE SOCIETIES OF BIOLOGICAL PSYCHIATRY doi:10.1080/15622970903144004., PMID: 19735056

> Poor response to antipsychotics is still an important problem in the treatment of many schizophrenia patients. N-acetylcysteine (NAC) is a compound that exerts anti-oxidant and scavenging actions against reactive oxygen species. This paper reports a case of poorly responsive schizophrenia patient who improved considerably with add-on NAC 600 mg/day. The NAC might work through activating cysteine-glutamate antiporters or

reducing in nitric oxide (NO) metabolites, free radicals and cytokines or through both of these mechanisms.

N-acetylcysteine is a Safe and Effective Augmentation Strategy for Schizophrenia

---

Berk, Michael, et al.,"N-Acetyl Cysteine as a Glutathione Precursor for Schizophrenia--a Double-Blind, Randomized, Placebo-Controlled Trial." *Biological Psychiatry* 64, no. 5 (September 1, 2008): 361–68. Publisher: ELSEVIER INC. doi:10.1016/j.biopsych.2008.03.004., PMID: 18436195

> ➤ "Improvement was seen on the CGI-I at 2 weeks and the CGI-S at 4 weeks, while improvement on the PANSS and a trend for improvement on the BAS emerged only toward 24 weeks of treatment."

> ➤ "These data suggest that adjunctive NAC has potential as a safe and moderately effective augmentation strategy for chronic schizophrenia."

N-Acetylcysteine is a Potential Therapeutic Agent for Hallucinations and Psychosis from Hallucinogen use in Schizophrenia

---

Lee, Mei-Yi, et al., "N-Acetylcysteine Modulates Hallucinogenic 5-HT(2A) Receptor Agonist-Mediated Responses: Behavioral, Molecular, and Electrophysiological Studies." *Neuropharmacology* 81 (June 2014): 215–23. Publisher: PERGAMON doi:10.1016/j.neuropharm.2014.02.006., PMID: 24534112

> ➤ "These findings implicate NAC as a potential therapeutic agent for hallucinations and psychosis associated with hallucinogen use and schizophrenia."

N-acetylcysteine is a Safe and Effective Augmentative Strategy for Alleviating Negative Symptoms of Schizophrenia

---

Farokhnia, Mehdi, et al., "N-Acetylcysteine as an Adjunct to Risperidone for Treatment of Negative Symptoms in Patients with Chronic Schizophrenia: A Randomized, Double-Blind, Placebo-Controlled Study." *Clinical Neuropharmacology* 36, no. 6 (December 2013): 185–92. Publisher: LIPPINCOTT WILLIAMS & WILKINS doi:10.1097/WNF.0000000000000001., PMID: 24201233

> ➤ "NAC add-on therapy showed to be a safe and effective augmentative strategy for alleviating negative symptoms of schizophrenia."

Nicotine

Nicotine Has a Greater Cognitive Impact in Schizophrenic Patients than Healthy Controls

AhnAllen, Christopher G., et al., "Early Nicotine Withdrawal and Transdermal Nicotine Effects on Neurocognitive Performance in Schizophrenia." *Schizophrenia Research* 100, no. 1–3 (March 2008): 261–69. doi:10.1016/j.schres.2007.07.030., PMID: 17884348

> ➤ In conclusion, nicotine levels had a greater impact on reaction time and accuracy rates in schizophrenia than in control smokers. Overnight nicotine withdrawal resulted in greater impairment of accuracy in the schizophrenia group while nicotine administration provided greater improvement than that observed in the control group. Nicotine provided greater reaction time benefit in schizophrenia. Despite differences in nicotine levels and a lack of significant group differences in attention network function, these results suggest that cigarette smoking behavior provides ameliorative neurocognitive effects in schizophrenia. Future research on neurocognitive effects of nicotine in schizophrenia will aid in the understanding of increased smoking in this group.

Oleanolic Acid

Oleanolic Acid Could Be a Candidate for the Treatment of Positive Symptoms, Sensorimotor Gating Disruption and Cognitive Impairments in Schizophrenia

Park, Se Jin, et al., "Oleanolic Acid Attenuates MK-801-Induced Schizophrenia-like Behaviors in Mice." *Neuropharmacology* 86C (July 2, 2014): 49–56. Publisher: PERGAMON doi:10.1016/j.neuropharm.2014.06.025., PMID: 24997455

> ➤ "These results suggest that oleanolic acid could be a candidate for the treatment of several symptoms of schizophrenia, including positive symptoms, sensorimotor gating disruption, and cognitive impairments."

Placebo

A Placebo is Effective Treatment and Has Outperformed Antipsychotics in Clinical Trials

Lapierre, Y. D., et al., "Placebo: A Potent but Misunderstood Psychotrope." *Journal of Psychiatry & Neuroscience: JPN* 20, no. 3 (May 1995): 173–74., PMID: 7786877

> ➤ All this is to say that, in any discussion of the role of placebo in the evaluation ofa new treatment, its potency must be recognized. It should be seen as a necessary ingredient in any ethical and honest evaluation of a new treatment. Given that treatments now available are not as effective as we would like them to be, the consistency of their therapeutic value over the placebo factor would often merit an objective reevaluation.

CODEX ALTERNUS

Propentoylline

Propentoylline Has Therapeutic Benefit When Added to Risperidone to Treat Schizophrenia

Salami, Samarand, et al., "A Placebo Controlled Study of the Propentofylline Added to Risperidone in Chronic Schizophrenia." *Progress in Neuro-Psychopharmacology & Biological Psychiatry* 32, no. 3 (April 1, 2008): 726–32. doi:10.1016/j.pnpbp.2007.11.021., PMID: 18096287

> In agreement with our hypothesis, the propentofylline group had significantly greater improvement in the positive symptoms, general psychopathological symptoms and PANSS total scores over 8 weeks trial. No significant differences were observed between the means of the two groups on the negative scores. Moreover, a relatively high dose of risperidone in this study suggests that the extra effect of propentofylline is independent of risperidone's mechanism. In addition, therapy with 900 mg/day of propentofylline was well tolerated, and no clinically important side effects were observed. Gastrointestinal disturbances, dizziness and headache were most common events during the trial with propentofylline.

Rubidium Chloride

Overall Low-dose Effect of Rubidium Chloride was Beneficial in Schizophrenia

Chouinard, G., et al., "The Effect of Rubidium in Schizophrenia." *Communications in Psychopharmacology* 1, no. 4 (1977): 373–83., Publisher: PERGAMON PRESS, INC.; PMID: 28202

> The nature of the dose-response relationship for the BPRS total score suggests that the overall effect of 1g of rubidium on schizophrenia was beneficial. There was evidence, however, that the 2g dose of rubidium was exacerbating the symptoms of anxiety and depression. Since animal studies point to a specific capacity of rubidium to increase norepinephrine turnover, one might hypothesize that the beneficial effect of the 1g dose on withdrawal retardation may be caused by an increase in cerebral norepinephrine. In the same way, the increase in hostile suspiciousness and anxious depression among patients receiving 2g of rubidium may be related to an excess of cerebral norepinephrine. Further investigation is required to determine whether this drug can be of value in the treatment of schizophrenia and, if so, what the therapeutic dose range would be.

SAMe

SAMe Reduces Aggressive Behavior and Increases Quality of Life for Schizophrenic Patients

CODEX ALTERNUS

Strous, Rael D., et al., "Improvement of Aggressive Behavior and Quality of Life Impairment Following S-Adenosyl-Methionine (SAM-E) Augmentation in Schizophrenia." *European Neuropsychopharmacology: The Journal of the European College of Neuropsychopharmacology* 19, no. 1 (January 2009): 14–22. Publisher: ELSEVIER BV doi:10.1016/j.euroneuro.2008.08.004., PMID: 18824331

> ➢ S-adenosyl-methionine (SAM-e), functions as a primary methyl group donor for several metabolic compounds. Since SAM-e is involved in several metabolic processes, its administration may have a role in the amelioration of several disorders. In addition, SAM-e increases catechol-O-methyltransferase (COMT) enzyme activity, which may ameliorate aggressive symptoms in certain patients. We have therefore investigated the efficacy of SAM-e in managing schizophrenia symptomatology in patients with the low activity COMT polymorphism. Eighteen patients with chronic schizophrenia were randomly assigned to receive either SAM-e (800 mg) or placebo for 8 weeks in double-blind fashion. Results indicated some reduction in aggressive behavior and improved quality of life following SAM-e administration. Female patients showed improvement of depressive symptoms. Clinical improvement did not correlate with serum SAM-e levels. Two patients receiving SAM-e exhibited some exacerbation of irritability. This preliminary pilot short-term study cautiously supports SAM-e as an adjunct in management of aggressive behavior and quality of life impairment in schizophrenia.

Sarcosine

Sarcosine Treatment Can Benefit Schizophrenic Patients Treated with Antipsychotics

Tsai, Guochuan, et al., "Glycine Transporter I Inhibitor, N-Methylglycine (sarcosine), Added to Antipsychotics for the Treatment of Schizophrenia." *Biological Psychiatry* 55, no. 5 (March 1, 2004): 452–56. Publisher: ELSEVIER INC. doi:10.1016/j.biopsych.2003.09.012., PMID: 15023571

> ➢ "Sarcosine treatment can benefit schizophrenic patients treated by antipsychotics including risperidone. The significant improvement with the sarcosine further supports the hypothesis of N-methyl-D-aspartate receptor hypofunction in schizophrenia. Glycine transporter-1 is a novel target for the pharmacotherapy to enhance N-methyl-D-aspartate function."

Sarcosine is Supported for Benefit of General Psychiatric Symptoms and Depression in Schizophrenia

Lane, Hsien-Yuan, et al., "Sarcosine or D-Serine Add-on Treatment for Acute Exacerbation of Schizophrenia: A Randomized, Double-Blind, Placebo-Controlled Study." *Archives of General Psychiatry* 62, no. 11 (November 2005): 1196–1204. Publisher: AMERICAN MEDICAL ASSOCIATION; doi:10.1001/archpsyc.62.11.1196., PMID: 16275807

> "The evidence most strongly supports the benefit of sarcosine for general psychiatric symptoms and depression and possible benefit for negative symptoms (blunted effect and alogia) but not for positive symptoms during acute phase."

Sarcosine was Superior to Placebo as an Add-on for the Treatment of Schizophrenia

Lane, Hsien-Yuan, et al., "A Randomized, Double-Blind, Placebo-Controlled Comparison Study of Sarcosine (N-Methylglycine) and D-Serine Add-on Treatment for Schizophrenia." *The International Journal of Neuropsychopharmacology / Official Scientific Journal of the Collegium Internationale Neuropsychopharmacologicum* (CINP) 13, no. 4 (May 2010): 451–60. Publisher: CAMBRIDGE UNIVERSITY PRESS doi:10.1017/S1461145709990939, PMID: 19887019

> Treatment group x treatment duration interaction analysis by multiple linear regression showed that sarcosine was superior to placebo at all four outcome measures of Positive and Negative Syndrome Scale (PANSS)...., Scale for the Assessment of Negative Symptoms (SANS), Quality of Life (QOL) and Global Assessment of Functioning (GAF). However, D-serine did not differ in effect significantly from placebo in any measure.

Sarcosine Works Primarily Well in Antipsychotic-naive Schizophrenic Patients

Lane, Hsien-Yuan, et al., "Sarcosine (N-Methylglycine) Treatment for Acute Schizophrenia: A Randomized, Double-Blind Study." *Biological Psychiatry* 63, no. 1 (January 1, 2008): 9–12. Publisher: ELSEVIER INC; doi:10.1016/j.biopsych.2007.04.038., PMID: 17659263

> "Although patients receiving the 2-g daily dose were more likely to respond, it requires further clarification whether the effect is limited to the antipsychotic-naive population. Future placebo- or active-controlled, larger-sized studies are needed to fully assess sarcosine's effects."

Sulforaphane

Sulforaphane Rich Broccoli Sprout Extract May Improve Cognitive Function for Schizophrenics

Shiina, Akihiro, et al., "An Open Study of Sulforaphane-Rich Broccoli Sprout Extract in Patients with Schizophrenia." *Clinical Psychopharmacology and Neuroscience: The Official Scientific Journal of the Korean College of Neuropsychopharmacology* 13, no. 1 (April 30, 2015): 62–67. doi:10.9758/cpn.2015.13.1.62., PMID: 25912539

> "In conclusion, our pilot study suggests that supplementation therapy of SFN-rich broccoli sprout extract may have the potential to improve cognitive deficits in patients with schizophrenia."

Urea

Urea May Be of Some Therapeutic Value for Psychotic Patients

Grof, P., et al., "Prophylactic Value of Urea in Recurrent Affective Psychoses." *Activitas Nervosa Superior* 10, no. 3 (October 3, 1968): 294–95., PMID: 5705478

> ➤ Additionally, it may be some interest that we used low doses of urea in therapeutic-like trial in seven patients with monotonous chronificated depressive phase. In four of them marked positive or negative shifts and changes in symptomology were observed which seemed to be least partly caused by urea.

Chelation

Penicillamine

Chelation with Penicillamine Produces Effective Results and Reduces Symptomology in Patients with Copper overload from Wilson's Disease

Modai, I., et al., "Penicillamine Therapy for Schizophreniform Psychosis in Wilson's Disease." *The Journal of Nervous and Mental Disease* 173, no. 11 (November 1985): 698–701., PMID: 4056786

> ➤ It appears that penicillamine treatment is much more effective than phenothiazines in amelioration of schizophrenic-like symptomology in Wilson's disease when given at the proper dose. In this case, it was also effective in the treatment of neurological signs which appeared concomitantly. In addition, the relationship between the involvement of CNS copper poisoning, acute psychiatric dysfunction, and the efficiency of penicillamine strengthens the probability that psychosis is correlated to CNS poisoning by copper, and therefore the influence of this chelating agent might be rapid. Signs of mental deterioration as a result of chronic CNS injury, however, might also respond positively to penicillamine, although only after long treatment and with milder results.

Traditional Herbal Remedies (Overview)

Antipsychotic Plants

A Review of 48 Medicinal Antipsychotic Plants

CODEX ALTERNUS

Yadav, Monu, et al., " A Review of Psychosis and Antipsychotic Plants." *Asian Journal of Pharmaceutical and Clinical Research*, Volume 8, Issue 4, 2015

> ➤ The article lists 48 different antipsychotic plants and a few supplements and antioxidants used to treat psychosis.

Bangladesh Medicinal Plants

Formulations of Medicinal Plants used in Bangladesh to Treat Schizophrenia-like Psychosis

Ahmed, Md Nasir, et al., "Traditional Knowledge and Formulations of Medicinal Plants Used by the Traditional Medical Practitioners of Bangladesh to Treat Schizophrenia like Psychosis." *Schizophrenia Research and Treatment* 2014 (2014): 679810. Publisher: Hindawi Publishing Corporation; doi:10.1155/2014/679810., PMID: 25101175

> ➤ The aim of the present study was to conduct an ethnomedicinal plant survey and documentation of the formulations of different plant parts used by the traditional medical practitioners of Rangamati district of Bangladesh for the treatment of schizophrenia like psychosis. It was observed that the traditional medical practitioners used a total of 15 plant species to make 14 formulations. The plants were divided into 13 families, used for treatment of schizophrenia and accompanying symptoms like hallucination, depression, oversleeping or insomnia, deterioration of personal hygiene, forgetfulness, and fear due to evil spirits like genies or ghost. A search of the relevant scientific literatures showed that a number of plants used by the medicinal practitioners have been scientifically validated in their uses and traditional medicinal knowledge has been a means towards the discovery of many modern medicines. Moreover, the antipsychotic drug reserpine, isolated from the dried root of Rauvolfia serpentina species, revolutionized the treatment of schizophrenia. So it is very much possible that formulations of the practitioner, when examined scientifically in their entireties, can form discovery of lead compounds which can be used as safe and effective antipsychotic drug to treat schizophrenia.

Guatemalan Antipsychotic Plants

Two of These Guatemalan Plants Have Potential Antipsychotic Activity

Morales Cifuentes, C., et al., "Neuropharmacological Profile of Ethnomedicinal Plants of Guatemala." *Journal of Ethnopharmacology* 76, no. 3 (August 2001): 223–28., PMID: 11448542

> ➤ We carried out the Irwin's test with some different extracts of the aerial parts of Thidax procumbens L., the leaves of Neurolaena lobata (L.) R. Br., bark and leaves of Byrsonima crassifolia (L.) Kunth. and Gliricidia sepium Jacq. Walp., and root and leaves of Petiveria alliacea L. At dosage of 1.25 g dried plant/kg weight aqueous extracts of bark and leaves

of Byrsonima crassifolia (L.) Kunth. and Gliricidia sepium Jacq. Walp. demonstrated the most activity: decrease in motor activity, back tonus, reversible parpebral ptosis, catalepsy and strong hypothermia. These extracts of both plants were assayed for effects on CNS and they caused very significant reductions in spontaneous locomotor activity, exploratory behavior and rectal temperature and they increased the sodium pentobarbital-induced sleeping time.

Herbal Extracts

Article on Neuroleptic Herbs used in Animal Models of Psychosis

Zhang, Zhang-Jin, et al., "Therapeutic Effects of Herbal Extracts and Constituents in Animal Models of Psychiatric Disorders." *Life Sciences* 75, no. 14 (August 20, 2004): 1659–99. Publisher: ELSEVIER INC. doi:10.1016/j.lfs.2004.04.014., PMID: 15268969

> ➤ "Authors Summary; This article contains a section with numerous neuroleptic herbs that have been tested in animal models of psychosis."

Herbal PAK1 Blockers

Herbal PAK1 Blockers Berberine, Propolis, and Curcumin May Be Therapeutic for the Treatment of Schizophrenia

Maruta, Hiroshi, et al., "Herbal Therapeutics That Block the Oncogenic Kinase PAK1: A Practical Approach towards PAK1-Dependent Diseases and Longevity." *Phytotherapy Research: PTR* 28, no. 5 (May 2014): 656–72. Publisher: JOHN/WILEY & SONS LTD. doi:10.1002/ptr.5054., PMID: 23943274

> ➤ Accordingly, it is presumed that PAK1 is abnormally activated in the brain of schizophrenia patients with DISC1 mutation, and that in principle, anti-PAK1 drugs could suppress schizophrenia as well. In fact, according to a recent review (Kulkarni and Dhir, 2010), among PAK1-blockers, berberine, at least, appears to suppress schizophrenia as well as other PAK1-dependent neuronal disorders such as depression. Thus, it would be worth testing the therapeutic effect on DISC1-induced schizophrenia of other natural PAK1-blockers such as propolis and curcumin.

Mexican Medicine Plants

Mexican Medicine Plants Include Plants with Antipsychotic Properties

Jiménez-Olivares, E., et al., "[Pre-Columbian indigenous psychopharmacology]." *Neurología, Neurocirugía, Psiquiatría* 19, no. 1 (1978): 40–52., PMID: 360092

> ➤ A careful review has been carried out on texts concerning Mexican medicine plants, especially on texts obtained directly from the XVI century Indian reports. The plants

utilized for psychiatric purposes have been separated from the huge group of 1,500 medicine plants used by the prehispanic Indians, and have been found about 150 plants which have been classified in the modern way of antipsychotic, antidepressant, minor tranquilizer, hallucinogens, sedatives, hypnotics, brain tonics, stimulants and anticonvulsants. The intention in making this research is to awake the interest of the people in the experimenting field; as experiments have been effected only on hallucinogen up to now, and if these have proved to possess the effects caused to the Indians, supposedly large part of the other plants have the effects according to the indications they have mentioned.

Traditional Western Herbal Remedies

Cannabis

Cannabis Users Had Better Cognitive Function than Non-users 1 Year After Treatment

Rodríguez-Sánchez, José Manuel, et al., "Cannabis Use and Cognitive Functioning in First-Episode Schizophrenia Patients." *Schizophrenia Research* 124, no. 1–3 (December 2010): 142–51. doi:10.1016/j.schres.2010.08.017., PMID: 20826079

> ➢ Our aim has been to explore the correlates of cannabis use in cognitive and psychopathological features, both cross-sectional and longitudinally, in early phases of schizophrenia. 104 patients with a first episode of non-affective psychosis and 37 healthy controls were studied. Patients were classified according to their use of cannabis prior to the onset of the illness (47 users vs. 57 non-users). They were cross-sectionally and longitudinally studied and compared on clinical and cognitive variables and also on their level of premorbid adjustment. Cannabis user patients had better attention and executive functions than non-cannabis user patients at baseline and after 1 year of treatment. Both groups showed similar improvement in their cognitive functioning during the 1-year follow-up period. We also found that users had a better social premorbid adjustment, particularly during the early periods of life. The amount of cannabis consumed and the length of time of consumption did not significantly relate to cognitive performance. The use of cannabis does not seem to be associated with a negative effect on cognition in a representative sample of first-episode schizophrenia patients. Cannabis user patients appear to comprise a subgroup of patients with a better premorbid adjustment and premorbid frontal cognitive functions.

Cannabinoids

Cannabinoids May Be Useful for the Treatment of Schizophrenia

CODEX ALTERNUS

Coulston, Carissa M., et al., "Cannabinoids for the Treatment of Schizophrenia? A Balanced Neurochemical Framework for Both Adverse and Therapeutic Effects of Cannabis Use." *Schizophrenia Research and Treatment* 2011 (2011): 501726. Publisher: Hindawi Publishing Corporation; doi:10.1155/2011/501726., PMID: 22937266

> ➢ Recent studies have found that cannabinoids may improve neuropsychological performance, ameliorate negative symptoms, and have antipsychotic properties for a subgroup of the schizophrenia population. These findings are in contrast to the longstanding history of adverse consequences of cannabis use, predominantly on the positive symptoms, and a balanced neurochemical basis for these opposing views is lacking. This paper details a review of the neurobiological substrates of schizophrenia and the neurochemical effects of cannabis use in the normal population, in both cortical (in particular prefrontal) and subcortical brain regions. The aim of this paper is to provide a holistic neurochemical framework in which to understand how cannabinoids may impair, or indeed, serve to ameliorate the positive and negative symptoms as well as cognitive impairment. Directions in which future research can proceed to resolve the discrepancies are briefly discussed.

Cannabidiol Alleviates Psychosis by Anadamide Deactivation

Leweke, F. M., et al., "Cannabidiol Enhances Anandamide Signaling and Alleviates Psychotic Symptoms of Schizophrenia." *Translational Psychiatry* 2 (2012): e94. Publisher: Nature Pub. Group; doi:10.1038/tp.2012.15., PMID: 22832859

> ➢ "The results suggest that inhibition of anandamide deactivation may contribute to the antipsychotic effects of cannabidiol potentially representing a completely new mechanism in the treatment of schizophrenia."

Cannabidiol Shows Potential for Antipsychotic Treatment

Schubart, C. D., et al., "Cannabidiol as a Potential Treatment for Psychosis." *European Neuropsychopharmacology: The Journal of the European College of Neuropsychopharmacology* 24, no. 1 (January 2014): 51–64. Publisher: NATURE PUBLISHING GROUP doi:10.1016/j.euroneuro.2013.11.002., PMID: 24309088

> ➢ "Evidence from several research domains suggests that CBD shows potential for antipsychotic treatment."

CODEX ALTERNUS

Cannabidiol a Safe and Well Tolerated Alternative Antipsychotic Drug

---

Zuardi, A. W., et al., "Cannabidiol, a Cannabis Sativa Constituent, as an Antipsychotic Drug." *Brazilian Journal of Medical and Biological Research = Revista Brasileira De Pesquisas Médicas E Biológicas / Sociedade Brasileira De Biofísica* ... [et Al.] 39, no. 4 (April 2006): 421–29. Publisher: ASSOCIACAO BRASIELERA DE DIVULGACAO CIENTIFIC ; doi:/S0100-879X2006000400001., PMID: 16612464

> ➤ A high dose of delta9-tetrahydrocannabinol, the main Cannabis sativa (cannabis) component, induces anxiety and psychotic-like symptoms in healthy volunteers. These effects of delta9-tetrahydrocannabinol are significantly reduced by cannabidiol (CBD), a cannabis constituent which is devoid of the typical effects of the plant. This observation led us to suspect that CBD could have anxiolytic and/or antipsychotic actions. Studies in animal models and in healthy volunteers clearly suggest an anxiolytic-like effect of CBD. The antipsychotic-like properties of CBD have been investigated in animal models using behavioral and neurochemical techniques which suggested that CBD has a pharmacological profile similar to that of atypical antipsychotic drugs. The results of two studies on healthy volunteers using perception of binocular depth inversion and ketamine-induced psychotic symptoms supported the proposal of the antipsychotic-like properties of CBD. In addition, open case reports of schizophrenic patients treated with CBD and a preliminary report of a controlled clinical trial comparing CBD with an atypical antipsychotic drug have confirmed that this cannabinoid can be a safe and well-tolerated alternative treatment for schizophrenia. Future studies of CBD in other psychotic conditions such as bipolar disorder and comparative studies of its antipsychotic effects with those produced by clozapine in schizophrenic patients are clearly indicated.

Cannabidiol is a Well Tolerated Alternative Treatment for Schizophrenia

---

Deiana, Serena, et al., "Medical Use of Cannabis. Cannabidiol: A New Light for Schizophrenia?" *Drug Testing and Analysis* 5, no. 1 (January 2013): 46–51. Publisher: John Wiley & Sons; doi:10.1002/dta.1425., PMID: 23109356

> ➤ Evidence suggests that CBD can ameliorate positive and negative symptoms of schizophrenia. Behavioural and neurochemical models suggest that CBD has a pharmacological profile similar to that of atypical anti-psychotic drugs and a clinical trial reported that this cannabinoid is a well-tolerated alternative treatment for schizophrenia.

Cannabidiol Has Pharmacological Profile Similar to That of Atypical Antipsychotic Drugs

---

Zuardi, Antonio Waldo, et al., "A Critical Review of the Antipsychotic Effects of Cannabidiol: 30 Years of a Translational Investigation." *Current Pharmaceutical Design* 18, no. 32 (2012): 5131–40., Publisher: BENTHAM SCIENCE PUBLISHERS LTD. PMID: 22716160

> Subsequent studies have demonstrated that CBD has antipsychotic effects as observed using animal models and in healthy volunteers. Thus, this article provides a critical review of the research evaluating antipsychotic potential of this cannabinoid. CBD appears to have pharmacological profile similar to that of atypical antipsychotic drugs as seem using behavioral and neurochemical techniques in animal models. Additionally, CBD, prevented human experimental psychosis and was effective in open case reports and clinical trials in patients with schizophrenia with remarkable safety profile.

Emodin Rubarb

Emodin Rubarb Extract Ameliorates Neurobehavioral Deficits and Might Be A Novel Class of Pro-drug for Antipsychotic Medication

Mizuno, M., et al., "The Anthraquinone Derivative Emodin Ameliorates Neurobehavioral Deficits of a Rodent Model for Schizophrenia." *Journal of Neural Transmission* (Vienna, Austria: 1996) 115, no. 3 (2008): 521–30. Publisher: SPRINGER-VERLAG doi:10.1007/s00702-007-0867-5., PMID:18301953

> "We conclude that emodin can both attenuate EGF receptor signaling and ameliorate behavioral deficits. Therefore, emodin might be a novel class of a pro-drug for anti-psychotic medication."

Gentianine

Gentianine Exhibits Significant Antipsychotic Activity with Minimal Toxicity

Bhattacharya, S. K., et al., "Letter: Chemical Constituents of Gentianaceae. XI. Antipsychotic Activity of Gentianine." *Journal of Pharmaceutical Sciences* 63, no. 8 (August 1974): 1341–42., ublisher: JOHN WILEY & SONS, INC. PMID: 4859384

> Gentianine exhibited significant antipsychotic activity in the battery of tests accepted for arriving at such a conclusion . It has the added advantage of its minimal toxicity. The alkaloid, bearing a skeleton (lactonic monoterpene) different from those of known antipsychotic agents, is thus of potential importance as an antipsychotic drug.

Ginseng

Ginseng Significantly Improves Working Memory in Schizophrenic Patients

Chen, Eric Y. H., et al., "HT1001, a Proprietary North American Ginseng Extract, Improves Working Memory in Schizophrenia: A Double-Blind, Placebo-Controlled Study." *Phytotherapy Research: PTR* 26, no. 8 (August 2012): 1166–72. Publisher: JOHN/WILEY & SONS LTD. doi:10.1002/ptr.3700., PMID: 22213250

> Visual working memory was significantly improved in the HT1001 group, but not in the placebo group. Furthermore, extrapyramidal symptoms were significantly reduced after 4 weeks treatment with HT1001, whereas no difference in extrapyramidal effects was observed in the placebo group. These results provide a solid foundation for the further investigation of HT1001 as an adjunct therapy in schizophrenia, as an improvement in working memory and a reduction in medication related side effects has considerable potential to improve functional outcome in this population.

American Ginseng Posses Antipsychotic-like Properties which May Be Beneficial in Negative and Cognitive Symptoms in Schizophrenia

Chatterjee, Manavi, et al., "Evaluation of the Antipsychotic Potential of Panax Quinquefolium in Ketamine Induced Experimental Psychosis Model in Mice." *Neurochemical Research* 37, no. 4 (April 2012): 759–70. Publisher: SPRINGER NEW YORK LLC; doi:10.1007/s11064-011-0670-4., PMID: 22189635

> "Overall our findings suggest that PQ possesses antipsychotic like properties, which may lead to future studies with its specific constitutes which may particularly be beneficial in predominant negative and cognitive symptoms of schizophrenia."

Glory Bower Leaf

Glory Bower Leaf Extract Alleviates Hyperlocomotion and Improve Sensorimotor Gating Deficit Supporting a Therapeutic Role in Schizophrenia

Chen, Hon-Lie, et al., "Clerodendrum Inerme Leaf Extract Alleviates Animal Behaviors, Hyperlocomotion, and Prepulse Inhibition Disruptions, Mimicking Tourette Syndrome and Schizophrenia." *Evidence-Based Complementary and Alternative Medicine: eCAM* 2012 (2012): 284301. Publisher: OXFORD UNIVERSITY PRESS (UK); doi:10.1155/2012/284301., PMID: 22844330

> Previously, we found a patient with intractable motor tic disorder, a spectrum of Tourette syndrome (TS), responsive to the ground leaf juice of Clerodendrum inerme (CI). Here, we examined the effect of the ethanol extract of CI leaves (CI extract) on animal behaviors mimicking TS, hyperlocomotion, and sensorimotor gating deficit. The latter is also observed in schizophrenic patients and can be reflected by a disruption of prepulse inhibition of acoustic startle response (PPI) in animal models induced by methamphetamine and NMDA channel blockers (ketamine or MK-801), based on hyperdopaminergic and hypoglutamatergic hypotheses, respectively. CI extract (10-300 mg/kg, i.p.) dose-dependently inhibited hyperlocomotion induced by methamphetamine (2 mg/kg, i.p.) and PPI disruptions induced by methamphetamine, ketamine (30 mg/kg, i.p.), and MK-801 (0.3 mg/kg, i.p.) but did not affect spontaneous locomotor activity, rotarod performance, and grip force. These results suggest that CI

extract can relieve hyperlocomotion and improve sensorimotor gating deficit, supporting the therapeutic potential of CI for TS and schizophrenia.

Licorice

Licorice Extract is Beneficial for Some Psychotic and Neurotic Patients with Addison's Disease and for Others It May Induce Aggression

Simon, W., et al., "Glycyrrhiza (licorice) in the Treatment of Psychiatric Illness; a Preliminary Clinical Report." *Journal of Clinical and Experimental Psychopathology* 18, no. 1 (March 1957): 79–86., PMID: 24544353

> ➤ In 7 psychiatric patients treated with *Glycyrrhiza*, symptoms of weakness, listlessness, lethargy and lack of energy and stamina were beneficially influenced. Passive-dependent personality traits changed into aggressive behavior. In 2 patients hypotension was altered to a normotensive state. That *Glycrrhiza*, has a potentiating effect on adrenal function is hypothesized, and a review of the applicable literature on *Glycyrrhiza*, as well as on replacement therapy in psychiatric illness, is included.

Maytenus Obtusifola

Maytenus Obtusifola Extract Posses Neuroleptic-like Properties

De Sousa, Damião Pergentino, et al., "Neuroleptic-like Properties of the Chloroform Extract of Maytenus Obtusifolia MART. Roots." *Biological & Pharmaceutical Bulletin* 28, no. 2 (February 2005): 224–25., Publisher: PHARMACEUTICAL SOCIETY OF JAPAN; PMID: 15684473

> ➤ "The results suggest that chloroform extract of Maytenus obtusifolia MART. possesses neuroleptic-like properties."

Mistletoe

Mistletoe has Sedative, Antiepileptic and Antipsychotic Activity in Animals

Gupta, Gaurav, et al., "Sedative, Antiepileptic and Antipsychotic Effects of Viscum Album L. (Loranthaceae) in Mice and Rats." *Journal of Ethnopharmacology* 141, no. 3 (June 14, 2012): 810–16. Publisher: ELSEVIER IRELAND LTD; doi:10.1016/j.jep.2012.03.013., PMID: 22449438

> ➤ "The results obtained in present study suggested that title plant exhibited sedative, antiepileptic and antipsychotic activity in mice and rats."

Myricitrin

Natural Chemical Compound Myricitrin Exerts Antipsychotic-like Effects in Animal Models

Pereira, M., et al.,"Myricitrin, a Nitric Oxide and Protein Kinase C Inhibitor, Exerts Antipsychotic-like Effects in Animal Models." *Progress in Neuro-Psychopharmacology & Biological Psychiatry* 35, no. 7 (August 15, 2011): 1636–44. Publisher: ELSEVIER INC. doi:10.1016/j.pnpbp.2011.06.002., PMID: 21689712

➢ "Thus, myricitrin exhibited an antipsychotic-like profile at doses that did not induce catalepsy, and this effect may be related to nitrergic action."

Ocotea Duckei Tree

Ocotea Duckei Vattimo Possesses Potent CNS Depressant Action and May Be a Potential Candidate for Antipsychotic

Morais, L. C., et al., "Central Depressant Effects of Reticuline Extracted from Ocotea Duckei in Rats and Mice." *Journal of Ethnopharmacology* 62, no. 1 (August 1998): 57–61., PMID: 9720612

➢ Neuropharmacological studies were carried out with reticuline, a benzylisoquinoline alkaloid, isolated from Ocotea duckei Vattimo. It was found that reticuline (50-100 mg/kg i.p.) produced alteration of behaviour pattern, prolongation of pentobarbital-induced sleep, reduction in motor coordination and D-amphetamine-induced hypermotility and suppression of the conditioned avoidance response. These observations suggest that reticuline possesses potent central nervous system depressant action.

Onion

Onions May Posses Antipsychotic Properties

Kadian, Renu, et al., "Evaluation of Antipsychotic Effects of Allium Cepa", *World Journal of Pharmacy and Pharmaceutical Sciences*, Volume 3, Issue 11, 1146-1159, 2014

➢ The results suggest that ACP posse's antipsychotic activity. Further neurochemical investigation can explore the mechanism of action of the plant drug with respect to anti-dopaminergic and anti-serotoninergic functions and help to establish the plant as an antipsychotic agent.

CODEX ALTERNUS

Phytocannabinoid Δ9-Tetrahydrocannabivarin

Phytocannabinoid Δ9-Tetrahydrocannabivarin Has Therapeutic Potential for ameliorating some of the Negative, Cognitive and Positive Symptoms of Schizophrenia

Cascio, Maria Grazia, et al., "The Phytocannabinoid, Δ9-Tetrahydrocannabivarin, Can Act through 5-HT1A Receptors to Produce Anti-Psychotic Effects." *British Journal of Pharmacology,* November 1, 2014, n/a – n/a. Publisher: NATURE PUBLISHING GROUP doi:10.1111/bph.13000.

> ➢ "Our findings suggest that THCV can enhance 5-HT1A receptor activation, and that some of its apparent anti-psychotic effects may depend on this enhancement. We conclude that THCV has therapeutic potential for ameliorating some of the negative, cognitive and positive symptoms of schizophrenia."

Red Cappel

Red Cappel Potentiated Haldol and May Be an Extract with Antipsychotic Potential

Górniak, S. L., et al., "Effects of a Palicourea Marcgravii Leaf Extract on Some Dopamine-Related Behaviors of Rats." *Journal of Ethnopharmacology* 28, no. 3 (March 1990): 329–35., PMID: 2335961

> ➢ The effects of a Palicourea marcgravii leaf extract on some dopamine-related behaviors were studied in rats. The extract given subcutaneously decreased both spontaneous locomotion and rearing frequencies of rats observed in open-field studies and increased their periods of immobility. The extract was also able to produce a rightward displacement of the apomorphine dose-response curve for stereotyped behavior and decrease the maximum response possible. Although the extract (1.87 g/kg subcutaneously) was unable to produce true catalepsy by itself, it potentiated that induced by haloperidol. These results with the extract can be interpreted to be due to a direct blocking action for the extract on a mesostriatal dopamine receptor or to an indirect effect on dopamine pathways through central cholinergic activation.

St. John's Wort

St. John's Wort Extract Reverses Changes in Auditory Evoked Potentials in Humans

Murck, Harald, et al., "Hypericum Extract Reverses S-Ketamine-Induced Changes in Auditory Evoked Potentials in Humans - Possible Implications for the Treatment of Schizophrenia." *Biological Psychiatry* 59, no. 5 (March 1, 2006): 440–45. Publisher: ELSEVIER INC. doi:10.1016/j.biopsych.2005.07.008., PMID: 16165104

> S-ketamine lead to a significant decrease in the N100-P200 peak to peak (ptp) amplitude after the placebo treatment, whereas ptp was significantly increased by S-ketamine infusion in the LI160 treated subjects. The ODT and the cognitive testing revealed no significant effect of ketamine-infusion and therefore no interaction between treatment groups. AEP measures are sensitive means to assess the effect of low dose ketamine. Provided that ketamine mimics cognitive deficits in schizophrenia, LI160 might be effective to treat these symptoms.

St. Johns Wort Shows Potential in Diminishing Catatonic Schizophrenia-like Behaviors

Uma Devi Pongiya, et al. "Protective effect of Hypericum hookerianum in reversing haloperidol induced schizophrenia-like behaviors in Swiss albino mice." *Asian Journal of Biomedical and Pharmaceutical Sciences;* 04 (32); 2014. 14-23.

> Results of pre pulse inhibition, locomotor activity, plus maze performance and stair case tests have showed that the Hypericum hookerianum shows a lot of potential in the treatment of diminishing catatonic schizophrenia related behaviours. The major phytocostituents like flavanoids, polyphenols, saponins etc., present in the plant is believed to have the neuroprotective effect.

Yellow Mombin

Yellow Mombin Has Sedative, Antiepileptic and Antipsychotic Effects

Ayoka, Abiodun O., et al., "Sedative, Antiepileptic and Antipsychotic Effects of Spondias Mombin L. (Anacardiaceae) in Mice and Rats." *Journal of Ethnopharmacology* 103, no. 2 (January 16, 2006): 166–75. doi:10.1016/j.jep.2005.07.019., PMID: 16188408

> The inhibitory effect of the extracts on NIR was not reversed by atropine, yohimbine, naltrexone and flumazenil. However, the extracts blocked the facilitating effect of flumazenil. This suggests that NIR inhibitory effects of extracts of Spondia mombin are not mediated via muscarinic, alpha(2) adrenergic, and mu-opioid receptors, whereas, the extracts appear to facilitate GABAergic transmission. In addition the extracts blocked picrotoxin-induced convulsions. Phenolic compound(s) were present in the ethanolic and methanolic extracts, which exhibited anticonvulsant properties in the picrotoxin-induced convulsions model. The extracts decreased the amphetamine/apomorphine-induced stereotyped behaviour, which suggest that these extracts possess antidopaminergic activity. The effect of the extracts on hexobarbitone-induced sleeping time was blocked by flumazenil a GABA(A) antagonist, indicating that the extracts contain GABA(A) agonists. These results suggest that the leaves extracts of Spondias mombin possess sedative and antidopaminergic effects.

CODEX ALTERNUS

Traditional African Medicine

Black Afara

Evidence Supports Black Afara as a Sedative, Analgesic and Tranquilizer That Has Been Used in the Treatment of Psychosis

Adeoluwa, O. A., et al.,"Neurobehavioural and Analgesic Properties of Ethanol Bark Extract of Terminalia Ivorensis A Chev. (Combrataceae) in Mice." *Drug Research*, December 16, 2014. doi:10.1055/s-0034-1394417., PMID: 25514116

➤ Terminalia ivorensis A. Chev (Combretaceae) is a medicinal plant used in folk medicine in the management of pain, rheumatic condition, gastroenteritis and as a tranquilizer in psychotic disorder. EBETI is sedative and has analgesic effect, thus supporting its folkloric use in pain management and as a tranquilizer in psychosis.

Crassocephalum Bauchiense Leaf

Crassocephalum Bauchiense Leaf Extract Has Antipsychotic and Sedative Properties

Sotoing Taïwe, Germain, et al., "Antipsychotic and Sedative Effects of the Leaf Extract of Crassocephalum Bauchiense (Hutch.) Milne-Redh (Asteraceae) in Rodents." *Journal of Ethnopharmacology* 143, no. 1 (August 30, 2012): 213–20. Publisher: ELSEVIER IRELAND LTD; doi:10.1016/j.jep.2012.06.026., PMID: 22750453

➤ The results show that the antipsychotic and sedative properties of Crassocephalum bauchiense are possibly mediated via the blockade of dopamine D-2 receptors and GABAergic activation, respectively. However, pharmacological and chemical studies are continuing in order to characterize the mechanism(s) responsible for these neuropharmacological actions and also to identify the active substances present in the extracts of Crassocephalum bauchiense.

Fig Tree

Fig Trees Stem Bark Produce Depressant Action on CNS and May Be a Potential Antipsychotic

Wakeel, O.K., et al., "Neuropharmacological Activities of Ficus Platyphylla Stem Bark in Mice." *African Journal of Biomedical Research*, Vol. 7 (2004): 75-78, ISSN: 1119-5096

➤ Methanol Extract Ficus platyphylla stem bark in dosages (17, 40 and 75, 150mg/kg) wasfound to produce a profound decrease in exploratory activity in mice, the extract indicated peripheral and central analgesic effects as shown by significant inhibition of acetic acid -induced writhing, and delayed onset in leptazol induced-convulsion (seizures) in mice respectively. It also decreases the rate of leptazol induced mortality in mice. The totality of these effects showed that the extract possesses depressant action on the central nervous system.

Jobelyn

Jobelyn Exhibits Antipsychotic-like Activity

Omogbiya, Itivere Adrian, et al., "Jobelyn® Pretreatment Ameliorates Symptoms of Psychosis in Experimental Models." *Journal of Basic and Clinical Physiology and Pharmacology* 24, no. 4 (2013): 331–36. Publisher: Freund; doi:10.1515/jbcpp-2012-0073., PMID: 23412872

> ➤ "Taken together, these findings suggest that JB exhibits antipsychotic-like activity, devoid of the adverse effect of cataleptic behavior, and may offer some beneficial effects in the symptomatic relief of psychotic ailments."

Lonchocarpus Cyanescens

Lonchocarpus Cyanescens Extracts Posses Phytochemically Constitutes with Antipsychotic Property

Sonibare, Mubo A., et al.,"Antipsychotic Property of Aqueous and Ethanolic Extracts of Lonchocarpus Cyanescens (Schumach and Thonn.) Benth. (Fabaceae) in Rodents." *Journal of Natural Medicines* 66, no. 1 (January 2012): 127–32. Publisher: Springer Japan KK; doi:10.1007/s11418-011-0562-6., PMID: 21717088

> ➤ "Taken together, these findings suggest that the extracts possess phytochemically active constituents with antipsychotic property. Thus, this investigation provides evidence that may justify the ethnomedicinal applications of Lonchocarpus cyanescens as the major constitute of the recipe used for the management of psychosis in Nigeria."

Arowona, Ismot T., et al., "Antipsychotic Property of Solvent-Partitioned Fractions of Lonchocarpus Cyanescens Leaf Extract in Mice." *Journal of Basic and Clinical Physiology and Pharmacology* 25, no. 2 (May 1, 2014): 235–40. Publisher: Freund; doi:10.1515/jbcpp-2013-0065., PMID: 24356391

> ➤ "These findings suggest that EAF contains the major active constitute(s) mediating the antipsychotic property of LC and further support it use for the management of psychosis in traditional medicine."

Ragleaf

Ragleaf Extract Has Sedative and Antipsychotic Effects

CODEX ALTERNUS

Sotoing Taïwe, Germain, et al., "Antipsychotic and Sedative Effects of the Leaf Extract of Crassocephalum Bauchiense (Hutch.) Milne-Redh (Asteraceae) in Rodents." *Journal of Ethnopharmacology* 143, no. 1 (August 30, 2012): 213–20. Publisher: ELSEVIER IRELAND LTD; doi:10.1016/j.jep.2012.06.026., PMID: 22750453

> ➢ "The results show that the antipsychotic and sedative properties of Crassocephalum bauchiense are possibly mediated via the blockade of dopamine D-2 receptors and GABAergic activation, respectively."

Rauvolfia Vomitoria

Rauvolfia Vomitria is an Effective Antipsychotic Comparable to Synthetic Drugs

Obembe, A., et al., "Antipsychotic Effects and Tolerance of Crude Rauvolfia Vomitoria in Nigerian Psychiatric Inpatients." *Phototherapy Research*, Vol.8, 218-223 (1994)

> ➢ The present report is the first to our knowledge in which suitable tablets from the root powder of Rauvolfia vomitoria have been used in clinical trials. At a clinical Figure2 Therapeutic outcome as measured by mean BPRS total score. level, the claims of the traditional herbal practitioners and earlier observations on the potency of Rauvolfia vomitoria with minimal side effects, absence of depression and suicidal complications appear supported by the following observations. (i) The target symptoms, exhibited by the 10 patients, such as acute excitement, destructive behaviour, restlessness, confusion, severe tension and aggression largely improved on crude Rauvolfia vomitoria tablets. (ii) The consistency of findings from the brief psychiatric rating scale, clinical global impressions and plasma Rauvolfia alkaloid levels testifies to the benefit of the crude Rauvolfia vomitoria tablets in the management of psychiatric patients. (iii) The ability of an antipsychotic agent to interfere with its binding to dopamine receptors correlates with its clinical potency. This agrees with the mechanism of action of reserpine-like alkaloids in having a rapid onset of action (about 1 h following oral administration) measurable by the depletion of catecholamines and serotonin in the brain, attaining maximum depletion in 24 h (Goodman and Gilman, 1980). (iv) Though antipyschotic drugs induce extrapyramidal effects, anticholinergic actions and alpha-adrenergic blocking effects (Lader, 1980), the EPSRS suggest a moderate effect of crude Rauvolfia vomitoria on dopamine mechanisms as in only two patients were the extrapyramidal symptoms severe enough to require antiparkinsonian medication. (v) The consistency of the low mean scores on the Hamilton rating scale for Depression and Beck's depression inventory at least testifies against the assertion that severe depression and even suicide (Kline, 1954) could result from the clinical use of crude Rauvofia vomitoria. (vi) The exact liver involvement and the interpretation of the gradual rise in alkaline phosphatase and transaminases which tend the crude Rauvolfia vomitoria tablets, at the optimum dosage, should be a viable option and comparable antipsychotic drug.

Securinega Virosa Root Bark

Securinega Virosa Root Bark Has Antipsychotic Potential

Magaji, M. G., et al., "Evaluation of the Antipsychotic Potential of Aqueous Fraction of Securinega Virosa Root Bark Extract in Mice." *Metabolic Brain Disease* 29, no. 1 (March 2014): 161–65. Publisher: SPRINGER NEW YORK LLC; doi:10.1007/s11011-014-9483-x., PMID: 24445435

> ➤ "These results suggest that the residual aqueous fraction of methanol root bark extract of Securinega virosa contains biological active principle with antipsychotic potential."

Traditional African Healers

Traditional Healers have a High Rate of Success in Treating Cases of Schizophrenia in African People

Wessels, W. H., et al., "The Traditional Healer and Psychiatry." *The Australian and New Zealand Journal of Psychiatry* 19, no. 3 (September 1985): 283–86., Publisher: BLACKWELL PUBLISHING ASIA; PMID: 3866569

> ➤ Successful psychiatric treatment for rural Africans should incorporate their traditional belief that illness should be viewed in terms of magical, social, physical and religious parameters. Traditional healers divide illness into those of natural causation and those of traditional cultural aetiology which are peculiar to African people. Natural illness includes epilepsy, familial/genetic disorders, mental retardation and schizophrenia. Traditional, cultural disorders often cause difficulties for Western-trained psychiatrists because sorcery, spirit possession and ancestral worship are central to their aetiology and treatment as practised by traditional healers. They, in a state of altered consciousness, use a process of divination to determine why and from whom the misfortune originated. With this in mind, reputable traditional healers were consulted in therapy-resistant cases of culture-bound syndromes in Africans. Their high rate of success in treating these cases was notable. More recognition should be given to the reputable traditional healers.

Violet Tree

Evidence Supports the Violet Tree as a Plant that Can Be used in the Management of Convulsions and Psychosis

Adeyemi, O. O., et al., "Anticonvulsant, Anxiolytic and Sedative Activities of the Aqueous Root Extract of Securidaca Longepedunculata Fresen." *Journal of Ethnopharmacology* 130, no. 2 (July 20, 2010): 191–95. doi:10.1016/j.jep.2010.04.028., PMID: 20435127

> "These findings justify the use of Securidaca longepedunculata in traditional medicine for the management of convulsion and psychosis."

Traditional Ayurvedic Medicine (India)

Alstonia Scholaris and Bacopa Monnieri

Extracts of Alstonia Scholaris and Bacopa Monniera Posses Neuroleptic Activity

Jash, Rajiv, et al., "Ethanolic Extracts of Alstonia Scholaris and Bacopa Monniera Possess Neuroleptic Activity due to Anti-Dopaminergic Effect." *Pharmacognosy Research* 6, no. 1 (January 2014): 46–51. Publisher: Medknow Publications and Media Pvt.Ltd. doi:10.4103/0974-8490.122917., PMID: 24497742

> The result of the study indicated a significant reduction of amphetamine-induced stereotype and conditioned avoidance response for both the extracts compared with the control group, but both did not have any significant effect in phencyclidine-induced locomotor activity and social interaction activity. However, both the extracts showed minor signs of catalepsy compared to the control group. The study also revealed that the neuroleptic effect was due to the reduction of the dopamine concentration in the frontal cortex region of the rat brain. The results largely pointed out the fact that both the extract may be having the property to alleviate the positive symptoms of schizophrenia by reducing the dopamine levels of dopaminergic neurons of the brain. The estimation of dopamine in the two major regions of brain indicated the alteration of dopamine levels was the reason for the anti-psychotic activity as demonstrated by the different animal models.

Ayurvedic Mixtures

Ayurvedic Medicine for Schizophrenia

Agarwal, V., et al., "Ayurvedic Medicine for Schizophrenia." *The Cochrane Database of Systematic Reviews,* no. 4 (2007): CD006867. Publisher: WILEY INTERSCIENCE doi:10.1002/14651858.CD006867, PMID: 17943922

> "....Ayurevedic treatment, in the case a complex mixture of many herbs, is compared with chlorpromazine in acutely ill people with schizophrenia, it is equally, but skewed data seems to favor the chlorpromazine group. Ayurevedic medication may have some effects for treatment of schizophrenia...."

CODEX ALTERNUS

Ayurevedic Formulations for Psychotic Disorders

Kumar, Dileep, et al., Ayurvedic Formulations for the Management of Psychotic Disorders, *International Journal of Research in Ayurveda and Pharmacy* 3(5) Sept-Oct 2012; www.ijrap.net

---

> Ayurveda has many herbal and herbal-mineral formulations in different dosage forms for the treatment of unmade. These drugs need clinical trials and pharmaceutical studies to establish their pharmacokinetic and pharmacodynaminc properties on modern parameters. By using these drugs alone or as adjunct with antipsychotic drugs we can not only control but cure the Unmada.

Ayurvedic Herbs Regulate RGS4 Protein Found in Schizophrenia Establishing a Remedy

---

Preenon Bagchi*, et al., "Establishing an in-silico Ayurvedic Medication Towards Treatment of Schizophrenia". *International Journal of Systems Biology*, ISSN: 0975–2900, Volume 1, Issue 2, 2009, pp-46-50

> ➤ RGS4 protein responsible for Schizophrenia is taken from NCBI's Entrez database; its 3D structure is determined by homology modelling. Ashwagandha, Sarpagandha and Mandukparni (Thankuni) were selected from Indian Ayurvedic medication. Their active component's 3D structures were established. Their combination is found to dock with RGS4 protein, hence establishing a remedy.

Report on Several Ayurvedic Herbs Binding Assays for the NMDA Receptor

---

Preenon Bagchi, et al., "Identification of Novel Drug Leads for NMDA Receptor Implicated In Schizophrenia from Indian Traditional Herbs" *International conference on Intelligent Systems, Data Mining and Information Technology (ICIDIT'2014)*, April 21-22, 2014 Bangkok (Thailand)

> ➤ Schizophrenia is a major debilitating disorder worldwide. Schizophrenia is a result of multi-gene mutation and psycho-social factors. Mutated amino acid sequences of N-Methyl-D- Aspartate (NMDA) have been implicated as factors causing schizophrenia which were retrieved from the National Centre for Biotechnology Information (NCBI). 3D structure of the above receptor was determined by using protein threading technique. Several ayurvedic herbs are implicated as causative factors for schizophrenia. The phyto-compounds information of the above herbs was retrieved from various literature studies. The pharmacophore hypothesis was generated for the reported inhibitors. The phytochemical compounds were screened against the NMDA receptor. Novel ligands were shortlisted based on their fitness & docking score. These shortlisted ligands can be considered for binding assay studies with cell lines with the NMDA receptor in in-vitro.

> "NMDA: The phytocompounds picroside II, wedelolactone, 7-o-methylwogonin and isoformononetin having the best fitness score, docking score and most interactions with the NMDA receptor are considered for binding assay studies with NMDA receptor in-vitro."

Bacopa Monnieri

Bacopa Monnieri May Recover Cognitive Deficit

> **Piyabhan, Pritsana,** et al., "Cognitive Enhancement Effects of Bacopa Monnieri (Brahmi) on Novel Object Recognition and VGLUT1 Density in the Prefrontal Cortex, Striatum, and Hippocampus of Sub-Chronic Phencyclidine Rat Model of Schizophrenia." *Journal of the Medical Association of Thailand = Chotmaihet Thangphaet* 96, no. 5 (May 2013): 625–32., Publisher: MEDICAL ASSOCIATION OF THAILAND. PMID: 23745319

> "Cognitive deficit observed in PCP-administered rats was mediated by VGLUT1 reduction in prefrontal cortex, striatum, CA1 and CA2/3. Interestingly, Brahmi could recover this cognitive deficit by increasing VGLUT1 in CA1 and CA2/3 to normal."

Brahmi (Bacopa Monnieri)

Brahmi (Bacopa monnieri) Resulted in Reduction of Psychopathology in Schizophrenic Patient

> **Sarkar, Sukanto,** et al., "Add-on Effect of Brahmi in the Management of Schizophrenia." *Journal of Ayurveda and Integrative Medicine* 3, no. 4 (October 2012): 223–25. Publisher: Medknow Publications and Media Pvt Ltd; doi:10.4103/0975-9476.104448., PMID: 23326095

> Brahmi (Bacopa monnieri), an Ayurvedic herb has primarily been used to enhance cognitive ability, memory and learning skills. We present a case study of schizophrenia in which add-on Brahmi extracts 500 mg/day for a period of one month resulted in reduction in psychopathology without any treatment-emergent adverse effect. Although preliminary, our case study suggests therapeutic efficacy of add-on Brahmi in schizophrenia, thus opening up a new dimension of its role in alternative medicines.

Brahmyadiyoga

Brahmyadiyoga is an Ayurvedic Drug Compound that is Successful in Treating Schizophrenia

> **Ramu, M. G.,** et al., "A Pilot Study of Role of Brahmyadiyoga in Chronic Unmada(schizophrenia)." *Ancient Science of Life* 2, no. 4 (April 1983): 205–7., Publisher: AVR Educational Foundation of Ayurveda; PMID: 22556983

> Brahmyadiyoga a compound drug was used on fourteen Chronic Unmada patients suffering from 2 years to 8 years between the ago range of 18 to 40 years of either sex.

The dose of the drug was 8 gms. to 16 gms. for three months. Assessments were done independently by Ayurvedic physician, Psychiatrist and Clinical Psychologist. Seven out of 10 patients who underwent treatment for three months and all the four patients who took the drug for two months improved.

Indian Spurgetree Leaves

Indian Spurgetree Leaves Extract Has Anti-anxiety, Antipsychotic and Anti-consultant Activity

Bigoniya, Papiya, et al., "Psychopharmacological Profile of Hydro-Alcoholic Extract of Euphorbia Neriifolia Leaves in Mice and Rats." *Indian Journal of Experimental Biology* 43, no. 10 (October 2005): 859–62., Publisher: SCIENTIFIC PUBLISHERS; PMID: 16235717

> ➤ "These results indicated anti-anxiety, anti-psychotic and anti-convulsant activity of E. neriifolia leaf extract in mice and rats. Phytochemical study showed the presence of steroidal saponin, reducing sugar, tannins, flavonoids in the crude leaf extract"

Kodo Millet

Kodo Millet Extract Has Tranquillizing Effects on Psychotic Patients

Deo, V. R., et al., "STUDY OF PASPALUM SCROBICULATUM EXTRACT IN FORTY PSYCHOTIC PATIENTS." *Psychopharmacologia* 5 (February 12, 1964): 228–33., Publisher: SPRINGER-VERLAG; PMID: 14138758

> ➤ The dried ethanol extract of the husk of Paspalum scrobiculatum grain was given to psychotic patients. The trial was conducted by the double blind control, cross over method. The extract has been found to exert definite tranquillizing effect on patients. The only side effects noticed were tremors and rigidity, which were reversible. However, clinical trial with larger doses and for a longer period is necessary to access its efficacy and safety in psychiatric patients.

Kodo Millet Has Tranquillizing Effect on Acutely Disturbed Schizophrenic Patients

Deo, V. R., et al., "Effect of Paspalum Scrobiculatum Extract on Acutely Disturbed Schizophrenic Patients. A Prelimiinary Report." *Psychopharmacologia* 2 (1961): 295–96., Publisher: SPRINGER-VERLAG; PMID: 13721948

> ➤ As the clinical condition improved within 4 days after starting the extract and mostly relapsed equally rapidly after discontinuing the same, the observed effects cannot be attributed to chance alone. Considering the type of clinical disorder, the short duration of treatment and the expected degree of improvement, double-blind technique was not thought necessary during this initial phase of trial. On the other hand clinical effects of the neuropharmacological agents should be interpreted very cautiously. Thus the

present results appear only to be encouragingly suggestive of the tranquillizing effect of the extract of P. scrobiculatum. Further work in progress.

Kodo Millet Produces Tranquility and Beneficial Effects for Schizophrenic Patients

> **Deo, V. R.**, et al., "Tranquillizing Action of a Crystalline Fraction of Paspalum Scrobiculatum Extract in Fourteen Psychotic Patients." *Indian Journal of Medical Sciences* 25, no. 6 (June 1971): 389–91., Publisher: MEDKNOW PUBLICATIONS; PMID: 4935548

> ➤ A crystalline fraction BZ5 obtained from the dried alcoholic extract of Paspalum scrobiculatum was orally administered for about 11 days to 14 acutely agitated psychotic patients of whom 11 suffered from schizophrenia. It produced tranquility and other beneficial effects in 9 schizophrenic patients. Signs of Parkinsonism were not noticed in this study but reversible hypotension was seen in 3 patients. Like the dried alcoholic ex- tract, BZ5 produced its beneficial effects only in schizophrenic patients.

Neuroleptic Plant Extracts

Mono Ingredient Herbal Neuroleptic Has Similar Effect as Marketed Formulations

> **Samanta M. K.**, et al., "Development of Mono Ingredient Herbal Neuroleptic Tablet for Better Psychiatric Therapy." *Indian J Pharm Sci,* 2005, 67(1):51-56, Publisher: MEDKNOW PUBLICATIONS

> ➤ A tablet containing A. calamus, W. somnifera, and G. glabra" "....three neuroleptic plant extracts were used for the formulation based on ayurvedic neuroleptic formulations and available literatures. ...It was found that these formulations containing three plant extracts were having similar effects as those of marketed formulations. The prepared tablet formulation has not shown any drug induced parkinsonian syndrome or any other relevant side effects, wereas the synthetic drug, chlorpromazine showed maximum pyramidal side effects.

Rauvolfia Serpentina (Snakeroot)

Rauvolfia Serpentina is an Effective Antipsychotic for Treating Psychosis and Mental Illness

> **Dey, Abhijit,** et al.,"Ethobotanical Aspects of Rauvolfia Serpentina (L). Benth. Ex Kurz. In India, Nepal, and Bangladesh." *Journal of Medicinal Plants Research*, Vol. 5 (2), pp. 144-150 18 January 2011

> ➤ The roots of this plant, which is very common in lower and upper Gangetic plains of India, are used in high blood pressure, mental agitation, insomnia, sedative and as hypnotic in Indian Ayurvedic system. Ethnomedical use of this plant as an antihypertensive and tranquilizer (Reserpine, Deserpidine and Rescinnamine) was reported by Fabricant and Farnsworth (2001). The plant is used in insomnia, high blood

pressure and madness in 'Chatara' block of district Sonebhadra, Uttar Pradesh, India (Singh et al., 2010). The Unani formulation Pitkriya capsule contains arsol (R. serpentina). It acts as Musakkin-wo-Munawwim (sedative and hypnotic), Mudir (Diuretic), Musakkin-e-Asab (nervine sedative) and Mukhaddir (anesthetise). This plant is used to treat anxiety, epilepsy and nervous disorders by the Jaunsari tribe of Garhwal Himalaya, Uttaranchal. Root paste is taken either with raw milk or honey in empty stomach twice a day for 21 days to cure mental disorder by the Kandhas of Kandhamal district of Orissa. Mullu kuruma tribe of Wayanad district of Kerala, India uses rhizome of this plant (local name: Amalpori) juice internally to treat high blood pressure and mental disorders. Root powder is given twice a day for two days in case of mental depression as folk medicine in Meerut district, Uttar Pradesh. Roots of this plant are used in mental disorders, nervous disorders and psychosis as a part of forest medicinal plants of Karnataka, India used in primary healthcare. Use of the leaves of this plant (local name: Chandmaruwa) in mental illness in Bantar of Bhaudaha, Morang, Nepal was reported by Acharya and Pokhrel (2006).

"Serpenia" a Total Rauwolfia Alkaloid Product is Free from Side Effects and is Effective for Psychosis

---

Colabawalla, H. M. et al., "A Preliminary Report on the Lack of Toxicity of a Preparation of Tatal Rauwolfia Alkaloids." *Journal of Neurology, Neurosurgery, and Psychiatry* 21, no. 3 (August 1958): 213–15., PMID: 13576173

> ➤ In a group of disturbed psychiatric patients the effects were compared of reserpine and "serpina", a preparation of the total alkaloids of Rauwolfia serpentina Benth. The response to each drug was similar, but " serpina " was free from side-effects. The response to " serpina" and absence of side effects were confirmed in a larger group treated for 22 weeks. Further trial and investigation of this drug are warranted.

Rauwolfia Teraphyllia (Devils Pepper)

Devils Pepper Leaves Show Significant Antipsychotic Activity in Animal Models

---

Gupta, Shikha, et al., "Bioactivity Guided Isolation of Antipsychotic Constituents from the Leaves of Rauwolfia Tetraphylla L." *Fitoterapia* 83, no. 6 (September 2012): 1092–99. doi:10.1016/j.fitote.2012.04.029., PMID: 22579842

> ➤ The findings presented here are important and being reported for the first time from the leaves of R. tetraphylla. The principle results of this study are that the MeOH extract, its alkaloidal fractions and the isolated alkaloids from R. tetraphylla, possess significant atypical antipsychotic-like effect in mice. Out of the six isolated alkaloids, the isomeric mixture of 11-demethoxyreserpiline, and 10- demethoxyreserpiline, α-yohimbine and reserpiline showed significant antipsychotic activity in a dose dependent manner. It would be worth mentioning that none of the extract, alkaloidal fractions or the isolated alkaloids showed any extra pyramidal (EPS) symptoms at the tested doses. It was also observed that MeOH extract behaved similarly to other clinically used novel atypical

antipsychotics and is non toxic hence may be safely used as herbal formulation for treating psychotic conditions in human. Further, this study categorically emphasize that α- yohimbine is a potential innovative antipsychotic and a comprehensive understanding of its neurochemical basis may open new avenues to developing newer antipsychotic medications.

Spikenard

Spikenard May Posses Antipsychotic Activity and Be a Potential Treatment for Schizophrenia

Rajiv, Jash, et al., "Evaluation of Antipsychotic Activity of Ethanolic Extract of Nardostachys Jatamansi on Water Albino Rats." *International Journal of Pharmaceutical Sciences and Research*, 2013, Volume 4, Issue 7, 2730-2736

➢ This study was a trial to evaluate the neuroleptic activity of the ethanolic extracts of Nardostachys Jatamansi with different antipsychotic animal models. Two doses of the extract (100 and 200mg/kg) were used for this study with 5 different animal models. After that, the concentration of the dopamine neurotransmitter was estimated in two different regions of the brain viz. Frontal cortex and Striatum. The result of the study indicated a significant reduction of amphetamine induced stereotype and conditioned avoidance response for the extracts compared with the control group, but did not have any significant effect in phencyclidine induced locomotor activity and social interaction activity. However the extract showed minor signs of catalepsy compared to the control group. The study also revealed that the neuroleptic effect was due to the reduction of the dopamine concentration in the frontal cortex region of the rat brain. The results largely pointed out the fact that the extract may be having the property to alleviate the positive symptoms of Schizophrenia by reducing the dopamine levels of dopaminergic neurons of the brain. The estimation of dopamine in the two major regions of brain indicated the alteration of dopamine levels was the reason for the antipsychotic activity as demonstrated by the different animal models.

Tinospora Cordifolia

Guduchi Standard Extract Has Antipsychotic Activity

Jain, Bindu Nee Giri, et al., "Antipsychotic Activity of Aqueous Ethanolic Extract of Tinospora Cordifolia in Amphetamine Challenged Mice Model." *Journal of Advanced Pharmaceutical Technology & Research* 1, no. 1 (January 2010): 30–33., Publisher: Medknow Publications and Media Pvt. Ltd. PMID: 22247829

➢ The results in SLA showed that the hydro alcoholic extract of the stems of Tinospora cordifolia at a dose level of 250 mg/kg and 500 mg/kg showed no significant antipsychotic activity in amphetamine induced hyperactivity in mice when compared to standard. Extract alone treated group at a dos level of 250 mg/kg and 500 mg/kg showed a decreased in locomotor activity when compared to the control. The plant extract increased the DAD(2) receptor binding in a dose dependent manner in treated mice compared to the control group.

Woodrose

Woodrose Extract Posses Antiepileptic and Antipsychotic Effects

Chitra, KK., et al., "Anti-epileptic and Anti-psychotic Effects of Ipomoea Reniformis (Convolvulanceae) in Experimental Animals." *Journal of Natural Remedies*, Volume 14 (2) July 2014, ISSN:2320-3358

> ➤ In conclusion, methanolic extract of Ipomoea reniformis antagonized MES, INH PTZ-induced seizures and also increased brain GABA levels decreased by INH and PTZ in mice. MEIR also exhibited anti-psychotic activity by inhibiting the apomorphine-induced climbing and stereotyped behaviours in rodents along with normalization of elevated brain neurotransmitters such as dopamine, noradrenaline and serotonin. Further research is warranted to determine the exact mode of its anti-epileptic and anti-psychotic activities.

Traditional Asian/Chinese/Kampo Medicine

Acupuncture

Acupuncture Reduces Hallucinations in Patient with Schizophrenia

Bosch, Peggy, et al., "A Case Study on Acupuncture in the Treatment of Schizophrenia." *Acupuncture in Medicine: Journal of the British Medical Acupuncture Society* 32, no. 3 (June 2014): 286–89. Publisher: THE SOCIETY; doi:10.1136/acupmed-2014-010547., PMID: 24614531

> ➤ This report describes the use of acupuncture as an add on treatment for a patient with chronic schizophrenia. The 63-year-old woman suffered from persistent hallucinations and even physical pain as a result of the hallucination of a black bird that kept pecking her back. The patient received 12 weekly acupuncture treatments. A clinical diagnostic interview and psychological testing (on sleep quality, depression, and on positive and negative symptoms) were conducted before, immediately after and 3 months after the acupuncture treatment. The results of the diagnostic interview gave important insights into the treatment effects. The patient experienced improved daily functioning and noticed a change in hallucinations. Although the hallucinations still occurred, she felt less disturbed by them. Interestingly, pain decreased markedly. In addition, the results showed that the overall score of the positive and negative symptoms did not change immediately; however, a decrease in symptoms occurred 3 months after acupuncture

treatment. Moreover, the patient described an immediate improvement in sleep; this was confirmed by a daytime sleepiness questionnaire. The patient was not able to complete a (longer) test on sleep quality beforehand but did so after the treatment period. Finally, a delayed improvement in the depression scale was found. Although larger clinical intervention studies on acupuncture and schizophrenia are needed, the results of this case study indicate that acupuncture may be beneficial as an add on treatment tool in patients with schizophrenia.

Acupuncture plus Antipsychotic Therapy Shows Significant Effects for Schizophrenia

Lee, M. S., et al., "Acupuncture for Schizophrenia: A Systematic Review and Meta-Analysis." *International Journal of Clinical Practice* 63, no. 11 (November 2009): 1622–33. Publisher: MEDICOM INTL INC; doi:10.1111/j.1742-1241.2009.02167.x., PMID: 19832819

> ➢ Thirteen RTC's, all originating from China, met the inclusion criteria. One RTC reported significant effects of electro-acupuncture plus drug therapy for improving auditory hallucinations and positive symptoms compared to sham EA plus drug therapy. Four RTCs showed significant effects of acupuncture for response rate compared with antipsychotic drugs. Seven RTCs showed significant effects of acupuncture plus antipsychotic therapy for response rate compared with antipsychotic drug therapy. Two RTCs tested laser acupuncture on hallucinations against sham laser acupuncture. One RTC found beneficial effects of laser acupuncture on response rate, Brief Psychiatric Rating Scale and clinical global index compared with sham laser.

Acupuncture (Aricular)

Aricular Acupuncture is Recommended for the Treatment of Auditory Hallucinations

Shi, Z. X., et al., "Observation on the Therapeutic Effect of 120 Cases of Hallucination Treated with Auricular Acupuncture." *Journal of Traditional Chinese Medicine = Chung I Tsa Chih Ying Wen Pan / Sponsored by All-China Association of Traditional Chinese Medicine, Academy of Traditional Chinese Medicine* 8, no. 4 (December 1988): 263–64., Publisher: JOURNAL OF TRADITIONAL CHINESE MEDICINE; PMID: 3246887

> ➢ We have treated auditory hallucination with different kinds of psychosis, mainly using auricular acupuncture and yielding certain cumulative effect. We also noted there is no significant difference in curative effects among groups of simple auricular acupuncture, aricular plus body acupuncture and aricular acupuncture plus chlorpromazine. Therefore, we recommend auricular acupuncture for treating hallucinations.

Acupuncture (Electro)

Electroacupuncture for Treatment of Schizophrenia Has a Higher Clinical Response Rate Than Sham

CODEX ALTERNUS

Jing Cheng, null, et al., "Electro-Acupuncture versus Sham Electro-Acupuncture for Auditory Hallucinations in Patients with Schizophrenia: A Randomized Controlled Trial." *Clinical Rehabilitation* 23, no. 7 (July 2009): 579–88. Publisher: HODDER ARNOLD JOURNALS doi:10.1177/0269215508096172., PMID: 19470551

> ➤ "The clinical response rates in electro-acupuncture and sham electro-acupuncture group were 43.3% and 13.3% respectively."

Electroacupuncture Plus Antipsychotic Shows Higher Compliance in Treating Schizophrenia

---

Feng-Ju, Yao, et al., "[Short-term curative effect of electroacupuncture as an adjunctive treatment on schizophrenia]." *Zhongguo Zhong Xi Yi Jie He Za Zhi Zhongguo Zhongxiyi Jiehe Zazhi = Chinese Journal of Integrated Traditional and Western Medicine / Zhongguo Zhong Xi Yi Jie He Xue Hui, Zhongguo Zhong Yi Yan Jiu Yuan Zhu Ban* 26, no. 3 (March 2006): 253–55., PMID: 16613275

> ➤ "With effect equal to CZ (clonzapine), combination of CZ and EA shows higher compliance in treating schizophrenia…."

Electroacupuncture Plus Antipsychotic Requires less Drug

Zhuge, D. Y., et al., "[Comparison between electro-acupuncture with chlorpromazine and chlorpromazine alone in 60 schizophrenic patients]." *Zhongguo Zhong Xi Yi Jie He Za Zhi Zhongguo Zhongxiyi Jiehe Zazhi = Chinese Journal of Integrated Traditional and Western Medicine / Zhongguo Zhong Xi Yi Jie He Xue Hui, Zhongguo Zhong Yi Yan Jiu Yuan Zhu Ban* 13, no. 7 (July 1993): 408–9, 388., Publisher: Chinese Association of the Integration of Traditional and Western Medicine; PMID: 8251722

> ➤ "The result showed the total curative effects of the two groups were similar. However, the marked effects appeared earlier in combined therapy than using chlorpromazine alone, less chlorpromazine was needed."

Betel Nut

Chewing Betel Nut is Associated with Lower Positive and Negative Symptoms in People with Schizophrenia

---

Sullivan, R. J., et al., "Effects of Chewing Betel Nut (Areca Catechu) on the Symptoms of People with Schizophrenia in Palau, Micronesia." *The British Journal of Psychiatry: The Journal of Mental Science* 177 (August 2000): 174–78., Publisher: ROYAL MEDICO-PSYCHOLOGICAL ASSOCIATION; PMID: 11026959

> ➤ Betel chewers with schizophrenia scored significantly lower on the positive ($P = 0.001$) and negative ($P = 0.002$) sub-scales of the PANSS than did non-chewers. There were no significant differences in extrapyramidal symptoms or tardive dyskinesia. Betel chewing

is associated with milder symptomatology and avoidance of more harmful recreational drugs. These initial results indicate that longitudinal research is merited.

Male High Consumption of Betel Had Significantly Lower Positive Symptoms than Non-betel Users

Coppola, Maurizio, et al., "Potential Action of Betel Alkaloids on Positive and Negative Symptoms of Schizophrenia: A Review." *Nordic Journal of Psychiatry* 66, no. 2 (April 2012): 73–78. Publisher: TAYLOR & FRANCIS LTD; doi:10.3109/08039488.2011.605172., PMID: 21859398

> ➢ "Male high consumption of betel had significantly lower positive symptoms than low consumers or non-betel users."

Schizophrenic Betel Chewers Had Significantly Milder Positive Symptoms than Low Consumption Chewers

Sullivan, Roger J., et al., "The Effects of an Indigenous Muscarinic Drug, Betel Nut (Areca Catechu), on the Symptoms of Schizophrenia: A Longitudinal Study in Palau, Micronesia." *The American Journal of Psychiatry* 164, no. 4 (April 2007): 670–73. Publisher: AM PSYCHIATRIC ASSN; doi:10.1176/appi.ajp.164.4.670., PMID: 17403982

> ➢ Male high-consumption betel chewers had significantly milder positive symptoms than low-consumption chewers over 1 year. Betel chewing was not associated with global health, social functioning, or movement disorders. Betel chewing was associated with tobacco use but not with cannabis or alcohol.

Binding Essays

Binding Essays of Natural Products to Treat Psychotic Illness

Chung, I. W., et al., "Pharmacologic Profile of Natural Products Used to Treat Psychotic Illnesses." *Psychopharmacology Bulletin* 31, no. 1 (1995): 139–45., Publisher: MEDWORKS MEDIA GLOBAL; PMID: 7675978

> ➢ "Authors Summary; in this article there are 31 extracts prepared from natural products frequently used to treat psychotic illnesses were identified from prescriptions in the Korean Tongeuibogam. The screening assays determined the receptor binding of each natural product used to treat psychotic illness."

Blood Stasis Treatments

Chinese Medical Treatment to Relieve Blood Stasis in Schizophrenia

Wang, B., et al., "Traditional Chinese Medical Treatment to Invigorate Blood and Relieve Stasis Treatment of Schizophrenia: Comparison with Antipsychotics Treatment." *Psychiatry and Clinical Neurosciences* 52 Suppl (December 1998): S329–30., Publisher: BLACKWELL PUBLISHING ASIA; PMID: 9895184

> ➤ "Traditional Chinese medicine is superior to antipsychotic drugs in the effects of anti-anxiety-depression and antipsychomotor inhibition, but is less effective in controlling psychomotor excitation compared with antipsychotic drugs"

Zhu, Y. Z., et al., "[Clinical study of shuizhi-dahuang mixture in treating schizophrenics with blood stasis syndrome]." *Zhongguo Zhong Xi Yi Jie He Za Zhi Zhongguo Zhongxiyi Jiehe Zazhi = Chinese Journal of Integrated Traditional and Western Medicine / Zhongguo Zhong Xi Yi Jie He Xue Hui, Zhongguo Zhong Yi Yan Jiu Yuan Zhu Ban* 16, no. 11 (November 1996): 646–48., Publisher: Chinese Association of the Integration of Traditional and Western Medicine; PMID: 9772611

> ➤ A clinical study of 67 female schizophrenics was conducted. Thirty two patients of them treated with Shuizhi (leech)-Dahuang (rhubarb) mixture mainly with low dosage of antipsychotic drugs (combined therapy group). The results showed that their overall therapeutic effects were similar and the combined therapy group could reduce the dosages of antipsychotic drugs and its side effects, and tended to normalize the hemorheologic indices.

Zhang, J. Z., et al., "[Xuefu zhuyu decoction in treating blood stasis syndrome of schizophrenia]." *Zhongguo Zhong Xi Yi Jie He Za Zhi Zhongguo Zhongxiyi Jiehe Zazhi = Chinese Journal of Integrated Traditional and Western Medicine / Zhongguo Zhong Xi Yi Jie He Xue Hui, Zhongguo Zhong Yi Yan Jiu Yuan Zhu Ban* 13, no. 7 (July 1993): 397–401, 387., Publisher: Chinese Association of the Integration of Traditional and Western Medicine; PMID: 8251719

> ➤ The clinical and experimental study of 66 schizophrenics were conducted. Based on mental symptoms, four-diagnostic method of TCM and hemorheology, it presented preliminarily the clinical and experimental criteria for schizophrenia. The combined therapy of Xuefu Zhuyu Decoction and low dosage of antipsychotic drug could relive the mental symptoms and the abnormal hemorhelogic index normalized. Its therapeutic index was higher than that of the control group.

Chinese Herbal Remedies

Chinese Herbal Medicine for Schizophrenia

Rathbone, J., et al., "Chinese Herbal Medicine for Schizophrenia." *The Cochrane Database of Systematic Reviews,* no. 4 (2005): CD003444. doi:10.1002/14651858.CD003444.pub2., Publisher: WILEY INTERSCIENCE; PMID: 16235320

> ➤ "Results suggest that combing Chinese herbal medicine with antipsychotics is beneficial"

Coriariaceae and Loranthaceae

Coriamyrtin and Tutin are used as Herbal Shock Therapies in Southwest China

Okuda, T., et al., "Corianin from Coriaria Japonica A. Gray, and Sesquiterpene Lactones from Loranthus Parasiticus Merr. Used for Treatment of Schizophrenia." *Chemical & Pharmaceutical Bulletin* 35, no. 1 (January 1987): 182–87., PMID: 3594649

> ➤ *Cariaria japonica A. GRAY* (Coriariaceae) is known to produce several sesquiterpene lactones including coriamyrtin (1) and tutin (2) which are the main toxic principles. We have also isolated together with three sesquiterpene lactones, during an investigation of active principles of *Loranthus parasiticus* MERR. (Chinese name: mā sang jìsheng, baso-kiseri in Japanese pronunciation (Loranthaceae), a parasitic plant that grows on the twigs of *Coiaria sinica* MAXIM. (Chinese name: ma sang, baso in Japanese Pronunciation (Coriariaceae), which is distributed in the south and southwest of area of China and is a folk medicine used as a shock therapy for schizophrenia in the southwest of China. In this paper we present a detailed account of the isolation and characterization of sesquiterpene lactones of *L. parasiticus* and the structure of elucidation of corianin.

Daotan

Modified Daotan Decoction Improves Negative Symptoms in Schizophrenia

Liu, Jing-li, et al., "[Clinical observation on effect of modified Daotan Decoction combined with small dose risperidone in treating chronic schizophrenia]." *Zhongguo Zhong Xi Yi Jie He Za Zhi Zhongguo Zhongxiyi Jiehe Zazhi = Chinese Journal of Integrated Traditional and Western Medicine / Zhongguo Zhong Xi Yi Jie He Xue Hui, Zhongguo Zhong Yi Yan Jiu Yuan Zhu Ban* 27, no. 3 (March 2007): 208–10., Publisher: Chinese Association of the Integration of Traditional and Western Medicine; PMID: 17432677

> ➤ "There was no significant difference in the overall efficiency between the two groups, but the improvement of the negative symptoms, illness provocation and general psychopathologic condition was significantly better in the treatment group than that in the control group respectively (P< 0.05)."

Gastrodia Elata

Gastrodia Elata Has Antipsychotic Effects in PCP-induced Schizophrenia-like Psychosis

Shin, E.-J., et al., "Effects of Gastrodia Elata Bl on Phencyclidine-Induced Schizophrenia-like Psychosis in Mice." *Current Neuropharmacology* 9, no. 1 (March 2011): 247–50. Publisher: BENTHAM SCIENCE PUBLISHERS LTD. doi:10.2174/157015911795017263., PMID: 21886599

> ➤ "In conclusion, our finding suggests that 5-HT1A receptor agonistic properties of GE offer potential therapeutic advantages in response to PCP-induced schizophrenia-like psychosis, although many details of the GE-mediated effect(s) remain to be determined."

Ginkgo Biloba (and Shuxening)

Ginkgo Biloba May Enhance the Effectiveness of Antipsychotic Drugs and Reduce Their Extrapyramidal Side Effects

Zhang, X. Y., et al., "A Double-Blind, Placebo-Controlled Trial of Extract of Ginkgo Biloba Added to Haloperidol in Treatment-Resistant Patients with Schizophrenia." *The Journal of Clinical Psychiatry* 62, no. 11 (November 2001): 878–83., Publisher: PHYSICIANS POSTGRADUATE PRESS, INC. PMID: 11775047

> ➤ "EGb treatment may enhance the effectiveness of antipsychotic drugs and reduce their extrapyramidal side effects."

Ginkgo Biloba Was Effective for Positive Symptoms in Refractory Schizophrenia

Knable, Michael B., et al., "Extract of Ginkgo Biloba Added to Haloperidol Was Effective for Positive Symptoms in Refractory Schizophrenia." *Evidence-Based Mental Health* 5, no. 3 (August 2002): 90., Publisher: B M J PUBLISHING GROUP; PMID: 12180457

> ➤ "In patients with chronic, refractory schizophrenia, extract of Ginkgo biloba added to haloperidol was more effective than placebo added to haloperidol in treating positive symptoms."

Ginkgo is Effective as an Add-on Therapy for Schizophrenia

Singh, Vidhi, et al., "Review and Meta-Analysis of Usage of Ginkgo as an Adjunct Therapy in Chronic Schizophrenia." *The International Journal of Neuropsychopharmacology / Official Scientific Journal of the Collegium Internationale Neuropsychopharmacologicum (CINP)* 13, no. 2 (March 2010): 257–71. Publisher: CAMBRIDGE UNIVERSITY PRESS doi:10.1017/S1461145709990654., PMID: 19775502

> ➤ Ginkgo as an add-on therapy to antipsychotic medication produced statistically significant moderate improvement (SMD=-0.50) in total and negative symptoms of chronic schizophrenia. Ginkgo as add-on therapy ameliorates the symptoms of chronic

CODEX ALTERNUS

schizophrenia. The role of antioxidants in pathogenesis of schizophrenia has also been explored.

Ginkgo Biloba Reduces Positive Symptoms in Patients with Schizophrenia

> **Atmaca, Murad,** et al., "The Effect of Extract of Ginkgo Biloba Addition to Olanzapine on Therapeutic Effect and Antioxidant Enzyme Levels in Patients with Schizophrenia." *Psychiatry and Clinical Neurosciences* 59, no. 6 (December 2005): 652–56. Publisher: BLACKWELL PUBLISHING ASIA; doi:10.1111/j.1440-1819.2005.01432.x., PMID: 16401239

> ➤ "At the evaluation of week 8, a significant difference in mean Scale for the Assessment of Positive Symptoms (SAPS) scores but not in Scale for the Assessment of Negative Symptoms between groups was found."

Ginkgo Biloba is Useful for Enhancing the Effect of Clozapine on Negative Symptoms in Schizophrenia

> **Doruk, Ali,** et al., "A Placebo-Controlled Study of Extract of Ginkgo Biloba Added to Clozapine in Patients with Treatment-Resistant Schizophrenia." *International Clinical Psychopharmacology* 23, no. 4 (July 2008): 223–27. Publisher: LIPPINCOTT WILLIAMS & WILKINS; doi:10.1097/YIC.0b013e3282fcff2f., PMID: 18545061

> ➤ "These preliminary data suggested that EGb was found useful for enhancing the effect of clozapine on negative symptoms in patients with treatment resistant schizophrenia"

Shuxening Presented Better Therapeutic Effect for Schizophrenia than Control

> **Luo, H. C.,** et al., "[Therapeutic effect of shuxuening combining neuroleptics for the treatment of chronic schizophrenia--a double blind study]." *Zhongguo Zhong Xi Yi Jie He Za Zhi Zhongguo Zhongxiyi Jiehe Zazhi = Chinese Journal of Integrated Traditional and Western Medicine / Zhongguo Zhong Xi Yi Jie He Xue Hui, Zhongguo Zhong Yi Yan Jiu Yuan Zhu Ban* 17, no. 3 (March 1997): 139–42., Publisher: Chinese Association of the Integration of Traditional and Western Medicine; PMID: 9863076

> ➤ "SXN presented a better therapeutic effect for chronic schizophrenics than the control group when rated with traditional global rating method as well, in which 44.98% marked improvement was obtained in the SXN group compared to 20.98% in the control group."

Huang Qi

Huang Qi Injection Has a Definite Prevention of Hospital Infection in Patients with Chronic Schizophrenia

CODEX ALTERNUS

> **Zhang, Bing-ru,** et al., "[Effects of injection of Huangqi injectio into Zusanli (ST 36) on immune function in the patient of schizophrenia]." *Zhongguo Zhen Jiu = Chinese Acupuncture & Moxibustion* 26, no. 9 (September 2006): 625–28., Publisher: CHINA PUBNS CTR/ GUOJI SHUDIAN; PMID: 17036478

- ➢ "Injection of Huangqi Injectio into Zusanli (ST 36) has definite effect for prevention of the hospital infection in inpatients of chronic schizophrenia, and SIL-2R is a valuable index for investigation of the hospital of infection."

Jieyu Anshen

Jieyu Anshen Decoction has a Definite and Quick Effect in Treating Schizophrenia

> **Zeng, De-zhi,** et al., "[Clinical observation on effect of Jieyu Anshen Decoction combined with aripiprazole in treating chronic schizophrenia]." *Zhongguo Zhong Xi Yi Jie He Za Zhi Zhongguo Zhongxiyi Jiehe Zazhi = Chinese Journal of Integrated Traditional and Western Medicine / Zhongguo Zhong Xi Yi Jie He Xue Hui, Zhongguo Zhong Yi Yan Jiu Yuan Zhu Ban* 27, no. 4 (April 2007): 358–61., Publisher: Chinese Association of the Integration of Traditional and Western Medicine; PMID: 17526180

- ➢ "JAD combined with aripiparazole has definite effect in treating chronic schizophrenia, shows advantages of quickly initiating effect, high safety and with no harm for increasing adverse reactions, so it is better than using aripiprazole alone."

Jinkoh-eremol and Agarospirol

Jinkoh-eremol and Agarospirol from Agarwood is Considered a Neuroleptic

> **Okugawa, H.,** et al., "Effect of Jinkoh-Eremol and Agarospirol from Agarwood on the Central Nervous System in Mice." *Planta Medica* 62, no. 1 (February 1996): 2–6. Publisher: GEORG/THIEME VERLAG; doi:10.1055/s-2006-957784., PMID: 8720378

- ➢ Agarwood (Jinkoh in Japanese), one of the Oriental medicines, is used as a sedative. The benzene extract of this medicine showed a prolonged effect on the hexobarbital-induced sleeping time, and hypothermic effects in terms of rectal temperature, a suppressive effect on acetic acid-writhing, and a reduction of the spontaneous motility in mice. By repeated fractionation, oral administration in mice, and pharmacological screening, the active principles, jinkoh-eremol and agarospirol, were obtained from the benzene extract. They also gave positive effects on the central nervous system by peritoneal and intracerebroventricular administration. They decreased both methamphetamine and apomorphine-induced spontaneous motility. The level of homovanillic acid in the brain was increased by them, while the levels of monoamines and other metabolites were unchanged. Similar results were seen in chlorpromazine administered mice. Therefore, jinkoh-eremol and agarospirol can be considered to be neuroleptic.

CODEX ALTERNUS

Lambertain Acid

Lambertain Acid is Derived from Siberian Pine and Has Antipsychotic and Sedative Effects on the CNS

Tolstikova, T. G., et al., "[Neurotropic activity of lambertian acid and its amino derivatives]." *Eksperimental'naia I Klinicheskaia Farmakologiia* 65, no. 2 (April 2002): 9–11., PMID: 12109303

> The neurotropic activity of the originally synthesized methyl lambertianate (II), as well as lambertianic acid (I) and three amino derivatives (III-V) was studied. All compounds exhibit equally low toxicity, but differ in the type of influence upon CNS. The most pronounced action was observed for esters II and V. Compound II exhibited a strong antidepressant effect with stimulating action. Introduction of the amino group led to an opposite tendency: compound V exhibited an antipsychotic and sedative (calming) effect upon CNS, without any anticonvulsant action.

Kidney Yang

Warm-Supplementing Kidney Yang Enhances Cognitive Performance in Schizophrenia

Guo, Xin, et al., "WSKY, a Traditional Chinese Decoction, Rescues Cognitive Impairment Associated with NMDA Receptor Antagonism by Enhancing BDNF/ERK/CREB Signaling." *Molecular Medicine Reports*, December 12, 2014. Publisher: D. A. Spandidos doi:10.3892/mmr.2014.3086., PMID: 25503442

> "The results of the present study indicated that WSKY enhances cognitive performance via the upregulation of BDNF/ERK/CREB signaling, and that WSKY has potential therapeutic implications for cognitive impairment of schizophrenia."

Warm Supplementing Kidney Yang Capsule Improves Cognitive and Social Function in Schizophrenia

Chen, Zhen-hua, et al., "Effects of Warm-Supplementing Kidney Yang (WSKY) Capsule Added on Risperidone on Cognition in Chronic Schizophrenic Patients: A Randomized, Double-Blind, Placebo-Controlled, Multi-Center Clinical Trial." *Human Psychopharmacology* 23, no. 6 (August 2008): 465–70. Publisher: JOHN/WILEY & SONS LTD. doi:10.1002/hup.958., PMID: 18536066

> "WSKY capsule added on risperidone may improve cognitive function, social function of the chronic schizophrenics patients, and the WSKY safely during treatment"

CODEX ALTERNUS

Noni

Noni Posses Antipsychotic-like Activity Can Be Utilized in the Treatment of Psychiatric Disorders

Pandy, Vijayapandi, et al., "Antipsychotic-like Activity of Noni (Morinda Citrifolia Linn.) in Mice." *BMC Complementary and Alternative Medicine* 12 (2012): 186. Publisher: BIOMED CENTRAL LTD. doi:10.1186/1472-6882-12-186., PMID: 23082808

> ➢ "The present study results demonstrated the antidopaminergic effect of Morinda citrifolia Linn. In mice, suggesting that noni has antipsychotic-like activity which can be utilized in the treatment of psychiatric disorders."

Polygala Tenuifolia

Chinese Senaga Root is a Potential Antipsychotic Agent

Chung, In-Won, et al., "Behavioural Pharmacology of Polygalasaponins Indicates Potential Antipsychotic Efficacy." *Pharmacology, Biochemistry, and Behavior* 71, no. 1–2 (February 2002): 191–95., PMID: 11812522

> ➢ Polygalasaponins were extracted from a plant (Polygala tenuifolia Willdenow) that has been prescribed for hundreds of years to treat psychotic illnesses in Korean traditional medicine. Previous in vitro binding studies suggested a potential mechanism for its antipsychotic action, as polygalasaponin was shown to have an affinity for both dopamine and serotonin receptors [Psychopharmacol. Bull. 31 (1995) 139.]. Polygalasaponin (25-500 mg/kg) was shown to produce a dose-related reduction in the apomorphine-induced climbing behaviour (minimum effective dose [ED(min)] 25 mg/kg ip, 250 mg/kg sc and po), the 5-hydroxytryptamine (5-HTP)-induced serotonin syndrome (ED(min) 50 mg/kg ip) and the MK-801-induced hyperactivity (ED(min) 25 mg/kg ip) in mice. This compound also reduced the cocaine-induced hyperactivity (ED(min) 25 mg/kg ip) in rats. These results demonstrated that polygalasaponin has dopamine and serotonin receptor antagonist properties in vivo. This might suggest its possible utility as an antipsychotic agent.

Schisandria Chinensis (Schizandria)

Schisandria Chinensis showed Effectiveness as Antipsychotic in a Group of Schizophrenics

Panossian, Alexander, et al., "Pharmacology of Schisandra Chinensis Bail.: An Overview of Russian Research and Uses in Medicine." *Journal of Ethnopharmacology* 118, no. 2 (July 23, 2008): 183–212. Publisher: ELSEVIER IRELAND LTD; doi:10.1016/j.jep.2008.04.020., PMID: 18515024

> Galant et. al. (1957) claimed total recovery in psychosis following a trial involving the administration of SSP over a period of ten days (0.5g, three times daily) to 36 patients (19 with schizophrenia, 6 with reactive psychosis, 4 with alcoholic psychosis, 3 with involutional depression, and 4 with psychopathology) presenting astheno-depressive syndrome. However, in the treatment showed no effect in psychopathology, whilst in schizophrenic group, six patients recovered, seven patients improved, and six (the hardest) cases the treatment was ineffective.

Shell Ginger

Shell Ginger May Be a Promising Treatment for Schizophrenia

De Araújo, Fernanda Yvelize Ramos, et al., "Inhibition of Ketamine-Induced Hyperlocomotion in Mice by the Essential Oil of Alpinia Zerumbet: Possible Involvement of an Antioxidant Effect." *The Journal of Pharmacy and Pharmacology* 63, no. 8 (August 2011): 1103–10. Publisher: PHARMACEUTICAL PRESS; doi:10.1111/j.2042-7158.2011.01312.x., PMID: 21718294

> "The results suggest antipsychotic and antioxidant effects for the EOAZ that may have promising efficacy for the treatment of schizophrenia."

Silk Tree

Silk Tree Potentiated Haldol-induced Catalepsy and May Be Considered a Candidate for as a Natural Antipsychotic

Assis, T. S., et al., "CNS Pharmacological Effects of the Total Alkaloidal Fraction from Albizia Inopinata Leaves." *Fitoterapia* 72, no. 2 (February 2001): 124–30., PMID: 11223221

> The total alkaloidal fraction of Albizia inopinata leaves (FLA) was investigated for its central nervous system (CNS) effects. FLA (10 mg/kg, i.p.) significantly reduced (45%) the locomotor activity in mice. In addition, it inhibited the conditioned avoidance response behavior and induced ptosis in rats. On the other hand, FLA did not exert significant effect on catalepsy, but potentiated the haloperidol-induced catalepsy. No effect was observed on sleep induced by sodium pentobarbital or apomorphine-induced stereotypes.

Wendan Decoction

Wendan Decoction Has PANSS Scores Similar to Antipsychotic Drugs, and a Lower Side Effect Profile

CODEX ALTERNUS

Che, Yi-Wen, et al., "Wendan Decoction () for Treatment of Schizophrenia: A Systematic Review of Randomized Controlled Trials." *Chinese Journal of Integrative Medicine*, April 6, 2015. doi:10.1007/s11655-015-2047-z., PMID: 25847776

> Thirteen RCTs (involving 1,174 patients) were included and the methodological quality was evaluated as generally low. The pooled results showed that WDD combined with antipsychotic drugs were more effective in clinical comprehensive effect, Positive and Negative Syndrome Scale (PANSS) scores and Brief Psychiatric Rating Scale scores compared with antipsychotic drugs alone. However, WDD had less effectiveness compared with antipsychotics in clinical comprehensive effect; and WDD was not different from antipsychotic drugs for PANSS scores. The side effects were significantly reduced in the intervention group compared with the control group.

White Mulberry

White Mulberry Extract Posses Antidoparmeinergic Activity

Yadav, Adhikrao V., et al., "Anti-Dopaminergic Effect of the Methanolic Extract of Morbus Alba L. Leaves." *Indian Journal of Pharmacology* 40, no. 5 (October 2008): 221–26. Publisher: MEDKNOW PUBLICATIONS PVT LTD.; doi:10.4103/0253-7613.44154., PMID: 20040961

> "The results suggest that the methanolic extract of Morbus alba L. possesses antidopaminergic activity. Further neurochemical investigation can explore the mechanism of action of the plant drug with respect to dopaminergic functions and help to establish the plant as an antipsychotic agent."

Yokukansan (Yi-gan san)

Yokukansan is a Potential Adjunctive Treatment Strategy for Treatment-Resistant Schizophrenia

Miyaoka, Tsuyoshi, et al., "Efficacy and Safety of Yokukansan in Treatment-Resistant Schizophrenia: A Randomized, Double-Blind, Placebo-Controlled Trial (a Positive and Negative Syndrome Scale, Five-Factor Analysis)." *Psychopharmacology*, June 13, 2014. Publisher: SPRINGER-VERLAG; doi:10.1007/s00213-014-3645-8., PMID: 24923986

> "The results of the present study indicate YKS to be a potential adjunctive treatment strategy for treatment-resistant schizophrenia, particularly to improve excitement/hostility symptoms."

Provides Highly Significant Improvement in Psychotic Symptoms

Miyaoka, Tsuyoshi, et al., "Yokukansan (TJ-54) for Treatment of Very-Late-Onset Schizophrenia-like Psychosis: An Open-Label Study." *Phytomedicine: International Journal of Phytotherapy and Phytopharmacology* 20, no. 7 (May 15, 2013): 654–58. Publisher: URBAN UND FISCHER; doi:10.1016/j.phymed.2013.01.007., PMID: 23453830

> ➤ A highly significant (p<0.001) improvement on all measures of psychotic symptomology was observed in all patients. TJ-54 was very well tolerated by the patients, and no clinically significant adverse effects were observed. Scores on all abnormal movement scales did not differ significantly prior to and after TJ-54 treatment.

Yi-gan san is Effective for the Treatment of Visual Hallucinations

Miyaoka, Tsuyoshi, et al., "Yi-Gan San for Treatment of Charles Bonnet Syndrome (visual Hallucination due to Vision Loss): An Open-Label Study." *Clinical Neuropharmacology* 34, no. 1 (February 2011): 24–27. Publisher: LIPPINCOTT WILLIAMS & WILKINS doi:10.1097/WNF.0b013e318206785a., PMID: 21164340

> ➤ "Yi-gan san may be effective and safe therapy to control visual hallucinations in patients with CBS and should be further tested in double-blind, placebo controlled trials."

Yi-gan san Decreases Positive and Negative Symptoms in Schizophrenia

Miyaoka, Tsuyoshi, et al., "Yi-Gan San as Adjunctive Therapy for Treatment-Resistant Schizophrenia: An Open-Label Study." *Clinical Neuropharmacology* 32, no. 1 (February 2009): 6–9. Publisher: LIPPINCOTT WILLIAMS & WILKINS doi:10.1097/WNF.0b013e31817e08c3., PMID: 19471183

> ➤ "A significant decrease was observed at 2 weeks and at 4 weeks in each Positive and Negative Syndrome Scale for Schizophrenia subscale score in the YGS group, but not observed in the control group."

Kampo Yokukansan Alkaloid Geissoschizine Methyl Ether May Be a New Set of Candidates for Atypical Antipsychotics

Ueda, Takashi, et al., "Geissoschizine Methyl Ether Has Third-Generation Antipsychotic-like Actions at the Dopamine and Serotonin Receptors." *European Journal of Pharmacology* 671, no. 1–3 (December 5, 2011): 79–86. Publisher: ELSEVIER BV doi:10.1016/j.ejphar.2011.09.007., PMID: 21951966

> ➤ "GM and GM derivatives may compromise a new set of candidates for atypical antipsychotics."

CODEX ALTERNUS

Yokukansan and its Ingredients have Antipsychotic Effects

Yu, Chuan-Hsun, et al., "Yokukansan and Its Ingredients as Possible Treatment Options for Schizophrenia." *Neuropsychiatric Disease and Treatment* 10 (2014): 1629–34. Publisher: DOVE MEDICAL PRESS LTD. doi:10.2147/NDT.S67607., PMID: 25210456

> ➤ Yokukansan (TJ-54), also called yi-gan san in Chinese, is a traditional herbal medicine with evident therapeutic effect for neuropsychiatric disorders. There are several open-label clinical studies upholding the possibility of using yokukansan to treat schizophrenia or schizophrenia-like psychosis. Evidence from animal studies and neurobiology also sheds light on the antipsychotic implications of yokukansan and its ingredients. Nevertheless, correlations between the experimental environment and clinical settings may be complicated by a number of confounders. Clinical trials with more sophisticated designs are required to fill the gap between the experimental environment and clinical settings.

Yokukansan Treatment Improves Cognitive Functions in Patient with Schizophrenia

Sakamoto, Shinji, et al., "Adjunctive Yokukansan Treatment Improved Cognitive Functions in a Patient with Schizophrenia." *The Journal of Neuropsychiatry and Clinical Neurosciences* 25, no. 3 (2013): E39–40. Publisher: AMERICAN PSYCHIATRIC PUBLISHING, INC. doi:10.1176/appi.neuropsych.12070166., PMID: 24026738

> ➤ Yokukansan, a traditional Asian herbal medicine, is reported to be safe and effective for behavioral and psychological symptoms of dementia in randomized, controlled trials, and is widely prescribed for patients with dementia in Japan.1 A recent open- label study indicates that adjunctive yokukansan administration in treatment-resistant schizophrenia improved the positive and negative symptoms of schizophrenia.2 In this report, we present a case of schizophrenia in which adjunctive yokukansan treatment dramatically improved severe cognitive dysfunction.

Yumeiho® Therapy

Yumeiho Therapy is a Japanese Therapy Similar to Chiropractic that Helps Balance the Schizophrenic Patients Natural Condition

Favzia, Rahmi, "Yumeiho Therapy for Schizophrenia." International Conference on Economics and Humanities (ICEH '14) Dec. 10-11, 2014 Bali (Indonesia)

> ➤ "Yumeiho therapy is a therapy that focuses on the treatment of the spine and joints. Based on the research that has been done can be concluded that the therapy Yumeiho able to reduce symptoms of psychological or physiological the patients with schizophrenia."

Drugs

Aspirin

Aspirin Therapy Reduces the Symptoms of Schizophrenia

Laan, Wijnand, et al., "Adjuvant Aspirin Therapy Reduces Symptoms of Schizophrenia Spectrum Disorders: Results from a Randomized, Double-Blind, Placebo-Controlled Trial." *The Journal of Clinical Psychiatry* 71, no. 5 (May 2010): 520–27. Publisher: PHYSICIANS POSTGRADUATE PRESS, INC. doi:10.4088/JCP.09m05117yel., PMID: 20492850

> ➤ "Aspirin given as adjuvant therapy to regular antipsychotic treatment reduces the symptoms of schizophrenia spectrum disorders. The reduction is more pronounced in those with the more altered immune function. Inflammation may constitute a potential new target for antipsychotic drug development."

Aspirin Prevents the Niacin Flush in Schizophrenic and Non Schizophrenic Patients

Richard A. Kunin, M.D, "The Action of Aspirin in Preventing the Niacin Flush and its Relevance to the Antischizophrenic Action of Megadose Niacin." *Journal of Orthomolecular Psychiatry,* 1976
http://www.orthomolecular.org/library/jom/1976/pdf/1976-v05n02-p089.pdf

> ➤ Aspirin has been observed to block or attenuate the flush reaction caused by niacin in 90 percent of a group of schizophrenic and nonschizophrenic outpatients. The patients were not treated with tranquilizers or antiinflammatory agents concurrently. The basis for this phenomenon, the blocking of the niacin flush by aspirin, is probably due to inhibition of prostaglandin synthesis by aspirin. In addition inhibition of bradykinin by aspirin may also suppress the flush. The various components of the inflammatory system are briefly described, and their relationship to the flush response is discussed. It is speculated that continued megadose niacin therapy leads to depletion of bradykinin and histamine and a small increase in prostaglandins, particularly of the E type. These are known to exert an inhibitory

Exercise, Aerobics, and Sports

Aqua Therapy

Aqua-Therapy Proven Successful Rehabilitation for Physically Disabled Schizophrenic Patient

CODEX ALTERNUS

Kacavas, J. J., et al., "The Use of Aqua-Therapy with Geriatric Patients." *American Corrective Therapy Journal* 31, no. 2 (April 1977): 52–59., Publisher: AMERICAN CORRECTIVE THERAPY ASSOCIATION; PMID: 855786

➢ Aqua-Therapy, has proven to be a highly effective means of rehabilitation for physically disabled patient. In the treatment and care of the aged patient, situations occur for which there are no immediate solutions. This indicates the need for carefully planned research followed through by an organized treatment program. As a case in point we would like to consider a patient, who for many years was a supervisory problem for many of our staff members, doctors, and therapists. This particular patient, in his early seventies, had stamina of a much younger person. This schizophrenic patient who not direct his energy in a socially acceptable manner would often physically abuse himself to gain attention. He did this to the point where he was not only causing physical damage, but created great uneasiness among other patients on the ward. Two alternatives the ward staff had were to keep him heavily tranquilized to a point where he would remain quiet for several hours, or to work with this man in some constructive ways to channel his energy. The gymnasium offered a number of outlets, such as bicycling, running, calisthenics, etc., but he still would not tire that easily. The patient also had access to apparatus on which he could injure himself unless carefully supervised. The swimming pool and Aqua-Therapy Program became an ideal means of treatment. While the patient was in the water he had no real means to intentionally harm himself since he was a good swimmer and was kept busy diving off the board and swimming to the shallow end. The water temperature of eighty-five degrees and air temperature of ninety-five degrees Fahrenheit provided resistance to his movements, thus fatiguing him while providing effective means of exercise. The patient would usually enter the pool in a very restless state but after a half-hour program of swimming, diving and underwater exercises, he quieted down to the point where he would actually sit down and converse with the therapist. Through Aqua-Therapy he became more manageable and sociable with other patients.

Jogging

Jogging Showed Significantly Less Posttest Trait Anxiety in Chronic Psychiatric Patients

Lion, Lionel S., et al., "Psychological Effects of Jogging: A Preliminary Study." *Perceptual and Motor Skills* 47, no. 3f (December 1, 1978): 1215–18. doi:10.2466/pms.1978.47.3f.1215.

➢ Three chronic psychiatric patients in a halfway house were enrolled in a program of regular supervised jogging. In comparison with three other chronic patients from the same setting who received the same amount of attention but no jogging, the jogging group showed significantly less posttest trait anxiety. No significant posttest differences in body image were found between groups. The role of multi-process relaxation is discussed.

Sports

Soccer Practice is a very Effective Add-on Treatment for Schizophrenic Patients

Battaglia, Giuseppe, et al., "Soccer Practice as an Add-on Treatment in the Management of Individuals with a Diagnosis of Schizophrenia." *Neuropsychiatric Disease and Treatment* 9 (2013): 595–603. Publisher: DOVE MEDICAL PRESS LTD. doi:10.2147/NDT.S44066., PMID: 23662058

> After the training period, the TG showed a relevant decrease by 4.6% in bodyweight (BW) and body mass index compared to baseline. Conversely, the CG showed an increased BW and body mass index by 1.8% from baseline to posttest. Moreover, after 12 weeks we found that control patients increased their BW significantly when compared to trained patients ($\Delta = 5.4\%$; $P < 0.05$). After the training period, comparing the baseline TG's Short Form-12-scores to posttest results, we found an improvement of 10.5% and 10.8% in physical component summary and mental component summary, respectively. In addition, performances on the 30 meter sprint test and slalom test running with a ball in the TG improved significantly ($P < 0.01$) from baseline to posttest when compared to CG. Soccer practice appears able to improve psychophysical health in individuals with diagnosis of schizophrenia. Indeed, our study demonstrated that programmed soccer physical activity could reduce antipsychotic medication-related weight gain and improve SRHQL and sports performance in psychotic subjects.

Sports are Effective Treatments, Improve Self-esteem, Body Awareness and Increase Overall Physical Activity

Längle, G., et al., "[Role of sports in treatment and rehabilitation of schizophrenic patients]." *Die Rehabilitation* 39, no. 5 (October 2000): 276–82. Publisher: wdv, Ges. für Medien und Kommunikation; doi:10.1055/s-2000-7863., PMID: 11089261

> The literature on the role of sports in the treatment and rehabilitation of schizophrenic patients is meagre and no systematic interdisciplinary review of the subject exists. This article reviews the existing literature and summarizes the relevant research findings. It also discusses practical experiences derived from a model project designed to study the role of sports in the management of chronically ill psychiatric patients, which showed that social interaction as well as the ability to organize time and leisure activities improved as did self-esteem, body awareness, and overall physical activity. Sports activities as part of the care of chronically ill psychiatric patients are effective as well as cost-effective and should receive more attention in both practice and research.

CODEX ALTERNUS

Takahashi, H., et al., "Effects of Sports Participation on Psychiatric Symptoms and Brain Activations during Sports Observation in Schizophrenia." *Translational Psychiatry* 2 (2012): e96. Publisher: Nature Pub. Group; doi:10.1038/tp.2012.22., PMID: 22832861

> Compared with baseline, activation of the body-selective extrastriate body area (EBA) in the posterior temporal-occipital cortex during observation of sports related actions was increased in the program group. In this group, increase in EBA activation was associated with improvement in general psychopathology scale of PANSS. Sports participation had a positive effect not only on weight gain but also on psychiatric symptoms in schizophrenia. EBA might mediate these beneficial effects of sports participation. Our findings merit further investigation of neurobiological mechanisms underlying the therapeutic effect of sports for schizophrenia.

Football Teams are Forms of Therapy for Psychiatric Hospitals

Nolot, Franck, et al., "Football and Psychosis." *The Psychiatrist* 36, no. 8 (August 1, 2012): 307–9. Publisher: Royal College of Psychiatrists; doi:10.1192/pb.bp.112.038570.

> Summary; "After 25 years of promoting football in psychiatric hospitals, the authors highlight the potential benefits of sport and physical activity in treating people diagnosed with psychosis. A number of clinical cases are used to illustrate the benefits to individual people as well as to the collective and the institution."

Exercise

High Aerobic Intensity Training Rehabilitation Improved Physical Capacity and Reduced the Risk of Cardiovascular Disease

Heggelund, Jørn, et al., "Effects of High Aerobic Intensity Training in Patients with Schizophrenia: A Controlled Trial." *Nordic Journal of Psychiatry* 65, no. 4 (September 2011): 269–75. Publisher: TAYLOR & FRANCIS LTD; doi:10.3109/08039488.2011.560278., PMID: 21332297

> "VO(2peak) and net mechanical efficiency of walking improved significantly by 8 weeks of HIT. HIT should be included in rehabilitation in order to improve physical capacity and contribute risk reduction of CVD."

Aerobic Exercise May Help Reduce Psychopathological Symptoms and Improve Cognitive Skills in Depressive and Schizophrenic Patients

Oertel-Knöchel, Viola, et al., "Effects of Aerobic Exercise on Cognitive Performance and Individual Psychopathology in Depressive and Schizophrenia Patients." *European Archives of Psychiatry and Clinical Neuroscience*, February 2, 2014. Publisher: DIETRICH/STEINKOPFF VERLAG; doi:10.1007/s00406-014-0485-9., PMID: 24487666

> In sum, the effects for the combined training were superior to the other forms of treatment. Physical exercise may help to reduce psychopathological symptoms and improve cognitive skills. The intervention routines employed in this study promise to add the current psychopathological and medical treatment options and could aid the transition to a multidisciplinary approach. However, a limitation of the current study is the short time interval for interventions (6 weeks including pre- and post-testing).

Exercise Therapy Can Have Healthful Physical and Mental Effects for Individuals with Schizophrenia

Gorczynski, Paul, et al., "Exercise Therapy for Schizophrenia." *The Cochrane Database of Systematic Reviews*, no. 5 (2010): CD004412. Publisher: WILEY INTERSCIENCE; doi:10.1002/14651858.CD004412.pub2., PMID: 20464730

> "…..results indicated that regular exercise programs are possible in this population, and that they can have healthful effects on both the physical and mental health and well-being of individuals with schizophrenia"

Exergames

Microsoft Kinect® Intervention Promotes Healthier Lifestyles and is an Acceptable Alternative to Perform Physical Activity.

Campos, Carlos, et al., "Feasibility and Acceptability of an Exergame Intervention for Schizophrenia." *Psychology of Sport and Exercise* 19 (July 2015): 50–58. doi:10.1016/j.psychsport.2015.02.005.

> This study established the feasibility and acceptability of an exergame intervention for outpatients with schizophrenia. The feasibility and acceptability findings suggest that this intervention should be more thoroughly studied in people with schizophrenia. Despite the costs associated with equipment purchase and the need for technical support for some of the subjects, exergames could provide a low resource dependent intervention to promote physical activity in this population. Moreover, as familiarity with game consoles increases and the recent generation of young adults grows hand-in-hand with videogames, the opportunity for patients with schizophrenia to use exergames, in a home based approach, will increase.

X-Box Video Games are a way to Promote Physical Activity in Older Adults with Schizophrenia

Leutwyler, Heather, et al., "Videogames to Promote Physical Activity in Older Adults with Schizophrenia." *Games for Health Journal* 1, no. 5 (October 2012): 381–83. Publisher: Mary Ann Liebert, Inc; doi:10.1089/g4h.2012.0051., PMID: 24761318

> Older adults with schizophrenia need physical activity programs that promote well-being, are accessible, and are easily incorporated into their treatment programs. Video-games that use the Kinect for X-Box 360 game system are an ideal way to promote physical activity in this population because it makes physical activity fun, accessible, and social. Preliminary acceptability results from an ongoing pilot physical activity program reveal that older adults with schizophrenia rate bowling as an enjoyable and fun way to be active. In order for participants to stay engaged, participants need to feel they have the necessary skills to play the games. Participants who frequently bowled gutter balls rated the game as less enjoyable, whereas participants who bowled strikes indicated greater satisfaction. Offering a practice session prior to playing the game may improve the overall acceptability.

Mindfulness and Meditation

Imagery

Imagery Techniques are Regarded as a Worthwhile Addendum for Emotional Difficulties

Kosbab, F. P., et al., "Imagery Techniques in Psychiatry." *Archives of General Psychiatry* 31, no. 3 (September 1974): 283–90., PMID: 4137715

> Hypnagogic or "affective" imagery is not an uncommon phenomenon; it is based on preconscious, preverbal "thinking in pictures" and characterized by symbol-content, changing thematic scenes, motion, color perception, relative autonomy, and affective connotations. Integrated with established dynamic principles and competently used, imagery techniques are regarded as a worthwhile addendum to the diagnostic-therapeutic armamentarium of the dynamically trained therapist for exploration and therapy of neurotic conflicts and related emotional difficulties. A brief historical overview and "primer" on the topic is presented along with a concise procedural outline of one established clinical method (Leuner's), a didactic approach used by the author, and a discussion of some theoretical questions implied in these approaches.

Meditation

Loving-Kindness Meditation is Associated with Decreased Negative Symptoms, Increased Positive Emotions and Psychological Recovery

Johnson, David P., et al., "A Pilot Study of Loving-Kindness Meditation for the Negative Symptoms of Schizophrenia." *Schizophrenia Research* 129, no. 2–3 (July 2011): 137–40. Publisher: ELSEVIER BV; doi:10.1016/j.schres.2011.02.015., PMID: 21385664

> "This pilot study examined loving-kindness meditation (LKM) with 18 participants with schizophrenia-spectrum disorders and significant negative symptoms. Findings indicate

that the intervention was feasible and associated with decreased negative symptoms and increased positive emotions and psychological recovery."

Loving-Kindness Meditation May Be an Important Intervention for Schizophrenic Patients with Negative Symptoms

Johnson, David P., et al., "Loving-Kindness Meditation to Enhance Recovery from Negative Symptoms of Schizophrenia." *Journal of Clinical Psychology* 65, no. 5 (May 2009): 499–509. Publisher: American Psychological Association; doi:10.1002/jclp.20591., PMID: 19267396

> In this article, we describe the clinical applicability of loving-kindness meditation (LKM) to individuals suffering from schizophrenia-spectrum disorders with persistent negative symptoms. LKM may have potential for reducing negative symptoms such as anhedonia, avolition, and asociality while enhancing factors consistent with psychological recovery such as hope and purpose in life. Case studies will illustrate how to conduct this group treatment with clients with negative symptoms, the potential benefits to the client, and difficulties that may arise. Although LKM requires further empirical support, it promises to be an important intervention since there are few treatments for clients afflicted with negative symptoms.

Mindfulness

The Use of Mindfulness on Anxiety in Schizophrenia

Davis, Louanne W., et al., "Mindfulness: An Intervention for Anxiety in Schizophrenia." *Journal of Psychosocial Nursing and Mental Health Services* 45, no. 11 (November 2007): 23–29., Publisher: SLACK, INC. PMID: 18041355

> Despite evidence that individuals with schizophrenia spectrum disorders experience significant and persistent symptoms of anxiety, there are few reports of the use of empirically supported treatments for anxiety in this population. This article describes how we have tried to adapt mindfulness interventions to help individuals with schizophrenia who experience significant anxiety symptoms. Although mindfulness has been widely used to help individuals without psychosis, to our knowledge, this is the first study adapting it to help those with schizophrenia manage worry and stress. We provide an overview of the intervention and use an individual example to describe how our treatment development group responded. We also explore directions for future research of mindfulness interventions for schizophrenia.

Mindfulness is effective for Distressing Thoughts and Images

> **Chadwick, Paul,** et al., "Mindfulness Groups for Distressing Voices and Paranoia: A Replication and Randomized Feasibility Trial." *Behavioural and Cognitive Psychotherapy* 37, no. 4 (July 2009): 403–12. Publisher: CAMBRIDGE UNIVERSITY PRESS doi:10.1017/S1352465809990166., PMID: 19545481

> ➤ There were no significant differences between intervention and waiting-list participants. Secondary analyses combining both groups and comparing scores before and after mindfulness training revealed significant improvement in clinical functioning (p = .013) and mindfulness of distressing thoughts and images (p = .037). Findings on feasibility are encouraging and secondary analyses replicated earlier clinical benefits and showed improved mindfulness of thoughts and images, but not voices.

Mindfulness Has Beneficial Impact on Cognition and Voices

> **Newman Taylor, Katherine**, et al.,"Impact of Mindfulness on Cognition and Affect in Voice Hearing: Evidence from Two Case Studies." *Behavioural and Cognitive Psychotherapy* 37, no. 4 (July 2009): 397–402. Publisher: CAMBRIDGE UNIVERSITY PRESS doi:10.1017/S135246580999018X., PMID: 19580696

> ➤ "Findings show that mindfulness training has an impact on cognition and affect specifically associated with voices, and thereby beneficially alters relationship with voices."

Mindfulness Can Impact Cognition and Paranoid Beliefs

> **Ellett, Lyn,** et al., "Mindfulness for Paranoid Beliefs: Evidence from Two Case Studies." *Behavioural and Cognitive Psychotherapy* 41, no. 2 (March 2013): 238–42. Publisher: CAMBRIDGE UNIVERSITY PRESS; doi:10.1017/S1352465812000586., PMID: 22974494

> ➤ "Findings suggest that mindfulness training can impact on cognition and affect specifically associated with paranoid beliefs, and is potentially relevant to both Poor Me and Bad Me paranoia."

Autogenic Training

Application of Autogenic Training to Schizophrenic Patients Proves Favorable

> **Shibata J.,** et al., "The Application of Autogenic Training to a Group of Schizophrenic Patients." *The American Journal of Clinical Hypnosis*, Volume X, Number 1, July 1967 Publisher: THE SOCIETY

> The progress of the Standard Exercises of the Autogenic Training program in 65 schizophrenic patients was favorable, being the same as for normal persons, the patients learning them in about two months and being able to proceed on to the Meditation Exercises. All patients progressed favorably during the Standard Exercises, but after proceeding on to the Meditation Exercises there were several patients whose symptoms aggravated.

Shibata J., et al., "Clinical Evaluation with Psychological Tests of Schizophrenic Patients Treated with Autogenic Training." *The American Journal of Clinical Hypnosis*, Volume X, Number 1, July 1967, Publisher: THE SOCIETY

> "What we can say from the results of the psychological tests alone, is that evidently we can obtain good results in some recuperating schizophrenic patients who take up AT as a medium for rehabilitation."

Mind-Body Therapies

Basic Body Awareness Therapy

Schizophrenic Patients Report Positive Effects with Basic Body Awareness Therapy (BBAT) for Increasing Body Awareness and Self-Esteem

Hedlund, Lena, et al., "The Experiences of Basic Body Awareness Therapy in Patients with Schizophrenia." *Journal of Bodywork and Movement Therapies* 14, no. 3 (July 2010): 245–54. Publisher: CHURCHILL LIVINGSTONE; doi:10.1016/j.jbmt.2009.03.002., PMID: 20538222

> Patients with schizophrenia report positive treatment effects of physiotherapy with BBAT. Four main categories were identified: affect regulation, body awareness and self-esteem, effects described in a social context and effects on the ability to think. These should be targeted in a future randomized and controlled study.

Body-ego Technique

Body-ego Technique Focuses on Body Posture and Movement and Improves General Functioning of Schizophrenic Patients

Goertzel, V., et al., "Body-Ego Technique: An Approach to the Schizophrenic Patient." *The Journal of Nervous and Mental Disease* 141, no. 1 (July 1965): 53–60., Publisher: LIPPINCOTT WILLIAMS & WILKINS; PMID: 5841637

> Body-ego technique (BET) is a predominantly nonverbal approach to the psychotic patient that has a theoretic basis in ego psychology. As described in detail in a previous communication by May, Wexler, Salkin and Schoop, this approach focuses attention on

body posture and movement as they relate to body image; on the patients sense of time as experienced and expressed in different speeds of movement; on body-ego boundaries; and on reality contact and experience in movement. There is a deliberate attempt to recreate for the patient the physical experience of the posture and movements associated with a wide range of emotions and attitudes, and by this route to rebuild ego structure. Thus this approach is primarily concerned with the process of recathexis of ego function.

> In this first controlled clinical trial of its use with chronic regressed schizophrenic patients, the therapists felt that they could establish contact and elicit cooperation in a high proportion of cases. Those treated with BET did significantly better than the controls in terms of independent psychiatric ratings of overall improvement and affective contact and nursing ratings of motility and general functioning. On other ratings there were no significant differences between the groups. These results and the results that BET has some promise for further research study and clinical exploration. It is not proposed as a therapeutic cure-all for schizophrenic patients, but rather it is suggested that it may have value in making contact and establishing a relationship and as an adjunct to, or in preparing the way for, the more verbal forms of therapy such as psychotherapy and the social therapies.

Body-oriented Psychotherapy

Body-Oriented Psychological Therapy Significantly Lowers Negative Symptoms after Treatment

---

Röhricht, Frank, et al., "Effect of Body-Oriented Psychological Therapy on Negative Symptoms in Schizophrenia: A Randomized Controlled Trial." *Psychological Medicine* 36, no. 5 (May 2006): 669–78. Publisher: CAMBRIDGE UNIVERSITY PRESS doi:10.1017/S0033291706007161., PMID: 16608559

> Patients receiving BPT attended more sessions and had significantly lower negative symptom scores after treatment (PANSS negative, blunted affect, motor retardation). The differences held true at 4-month follow-up. Other aspects of psychopathology and subjective quality of life did not change significantly in either group. Treatment satisfaction and ratings of the therapeutic relationship were similar in both groups. BPT may be an effective treatment for negative symptoms in patients with chronic schizophrenia. The findings should merit further trials with larger sample sizes and detailed studies to explore the therapeutic mechanisms involved.

Röhricht, Frank, et al., "Ego-Pathology, Body Experience, and Body Psychotherapy in Chronic Schizophrenia." *Psychology and Psychotherapy* 82, no. Pt 1 (March 2009): 19–30. Publisher: JOHN WILEY & SONS LTD. doi:10.1348/147608308X342932., PMID: 18789189

> "In patients with chronic schizophrenia, body oriented psychological interventions may be effective for both positive therapeutic changes in ego-pathology and negative symptoms..."

Massage

Physically Oriented Massage Therapy Give Schizophrenic Patients an Increase in Awareness in Their Body Limits

> **Andres, K.,** et al., "[Empirical study of a physically oriented therapy with schizophrenic patients]." *Zeitschrift Für Klinische Psychologie, Psychopathologie Und Psychotherapie / Im Auftrag Der Görres-Gesellschaft* 41, no. 2 (1993): 159–69., PMID: 8511959

> ➤ Ten predominantly chronic schizophrenics were given body therapy, including massage to the feet, back and neck. The aim of the therapy was to increase patients' awareness of their own bodily limits. This objective is based on the view that schizophrenia is a problem of delimitation, that psychic problems have their physical embodiment, and that problems of delimitation can therefore be tackled at the physical level by enhancing the patients' ability to experience their own bodily limits. The relaxing effect of the therapy is indicated in physiological measurements of skin conductance and heart rate, plus patients' self-perceptions. The close physical presence of the therapist did not trigger any anxiety conditions. The study shows that this body-oriented therapy is worthy of consideration as a method for giving schizophrenic patients a greater awareness of their own bodily limits.

Progressive Muscle Relaxation

Progressive Muscle Relaxation May Be a Cost Effective Way to Treat Persecutory Ideation

> **Ben-Zeev, Dror,** et al., "A Possible Role for Progressive Muscle Relaxation in the Treatment of Persecutory Ideation." *Medical Hypotheses* 75, no. 6 (December 2010): 568–71. Publisher: CHURCHILL LIVINGSTONE; doi:10.1016/j.mehy.2010.07.033., PMID: 20709459

> ➤ We hypothesize that PMR could be used to help ameliorate anxiety in patients who are at risk or already experiencing persecutory ideation, subsequently reducing the frequency, level of conviction, and distress associated with persecutory thoughts. Our hypothesis could be tested through feasibility and randomized control trials of PMR for treatment of persecutory ideation in individuals with schizophrenia. We expect the relationship between PMR and persecutory ideation will be mediated by reduction in anxiety. Potential advantages of examining our hypothesis include identifying a viable, efficacious, cost-effective novel intervention for paranoia in patients with psychosis. In addition, PMR could be easily facilitated by practitioners with varying levels of training and integrated with other existing interventions for persecutory ideation.

Progressive Muscle Relaxation Might Be a Useful Add-on Treatment to Reduce Anxiety in Schizophrenia

> **Vancampfort, Davy,** et al., "Progressive Muscle Relaxation in Persons with Schizophrenia: A Systematic Review of Randomized Controlled Trials." *Clinical Rehabilitation* 27, no. 4 (April 2013): 291–98. Publisher: HODDER ARNOLD JOURNALS doi:10.1177/0269215512455531., PMID: 22843353

  ➢ "Progressive muscle relaxation might be a useful add-on treatment to reduce state anxiety and psychological distress and improve subjective well-being in persons with schizophrenia."

Progressive Muscle Relaxation Can Effectively Alleviate Anxiety in Schizophrenia

> **Chen, Wen-Chun,** et al., "Efficacy of Progressive Muscle Relaxation Training in Reducing Anxiety in Patients with Acute Schizophrenia." *Journal of Clinical Nursing* 18, no. 15 (August 2009): 2187–96. Publisher: BLACKWELL PUBLISHING LTD. doi:10.1111/j.1365-2702.2008.02773.x., PMID: 19583651

  ➢ "This study demonstrated that progressive muscle relaxation can effectively alleviate anxiety in patients with schizophrenia"

Relaxation Exercises Reduce Anxiety Levels in Psychiatric Inpatients

> **Weber, S.,** et al., "The Effects of Relaxation Exercises on Anxiety Levels in Psychiatric Inpatients." *Journal of Holistic Nursing: Official Journal of the American Holistic Nurses' Association* 14, no. 3 (September 1996): 196–205., Publisher: SAGE PUBLICATIONS INC. PMID: 8900613

  ➢ The purpose of this study was to investigate the effects of relaxation exercises on anxiety levels in an inpatient general psychiatric unit. The conceptual framework used was holism. A convenience sample of 39 subjects was studied. Anxiety levels were measured prior to and post interventions with the state portion of the State-Trait Anxiety Inventory. Progressive muscle relaxation, meditative breathing, guided imagery, and soft music were employed to promote relaxation. A significant reduction in anxiety level was obtained on the post-test. The findings of this study can be incorporated by holistic nurses to help reduce anxiety levels of general psychiatric inpatients by using relaxation interventions.

Qigong

Qigong is a Mindful Exercise that Assists with Recovery for the Mentally Ill

Lloyd C., et al., "Qigong as a mindful exercise intervention for people living with mental ill health." *International Journal of Therapy and Rehabilitation,* 16 (7), 393-399, Publisher: MA Healthcare Ltd.

> "It is suggested that mindful exercise may be used as an intervention to assist people living with mental ill health to improve their community functioning and hence their recovery."

Shiatsu Therapy

Shiatsu Therapy Provides Substantial Improvement for Schizophrenia

Lichtenberg, Pesach, et al., "Shiatsu as an Adjuvant Therapy for Schizophrenia: An Open-Label Pilot Study." *Alternative Therapies in Health and Medicine* 15, no. 5 (October 2009): 44–46., Publisher: INNOVISION HEALTH MEDIA; PMID: 19771930

> "On the scales of psychopathology and side effects, the subjects showed a statistically and clinically significant improvement by the end of treatment. This improvement was maintained at the 12 week follow-up."

Tai-Chi

Tai-Chi is Beneficial for Movement Coordination and Interpersonal Functioning in Schizophrenia

Ho, Rainbow TH., et al., "Tai-Chi for Residential Patients with Schizophrenia on Movement Coordination, Negative Symptoms, and Functioning: A Pilot Randomized Controlled Trial." *Evidence-Based Complementary and Alternative Medicine,* Volume 2012. Publisher: OXFORD UNIVERSITY PRESS (UK)

> Tai-Chi buffered from deteriorations in movement coordination and interpersonal functioning, the latter with sustained effectiveness 6 weeks after the class was ended. Controls showed marked deteriorations in those areas, The Tai-chi group also experienced fewer disruptions to life activities at the 6-week maintenance. There was no significant improvement in negative symptoms after Tai-chi. The study demonstrated encouraging benefits of Tai-chi in preventing deteriorations in movement coordination and interpersonal functioning for residential patients with schizophrenia. The ease of implementation facilitates promotion at institutional psychiatric services.

Yoga

Yoga is a Feasible Add-on Intervention for the Treatment of Psychotic Disorder

Manjunath, R. B., et al., "Efficacy of Yoga as an Add-on Treatment for in-Patients with Functional Psychotic Disorder." *Indian Journal of Psychiatry* 55, no. Suppl 3 (July 2013): S374–378. Publisher: Indian Psychiatric Society; doi:10.4103/0019-5545.116314., PMID: 24049202

> "Adding yoga intervention to standard pharmacological treatment is feasible and may be beneficial even in the early and acute stage of psychosis."

Yoga Therapy Can Help Improve Basic Living Skills of Persons with Schizophrenia

Paikkatt, Babu, et al., "Efficacy of Yoga Therapy on Subjective Well-Being and Basic Living Skills of Patients Having Chronic Schizophrenia." *Industrial Psychiatry* Journal 21, no. 2 (July 2012): 109–14. Publisher: Association of Industrial Psychiatry of India doi:10.4103/0972-6748.119598., PMID: 24250042

> "Yoga could improve patients' subjective well-being, their daily basic living functioning, personal hygiene, self-care, interpersonal activities and communication, and prompted more involvement in routine work."

Yoga Provides Better Clinical Outcome in Schizophrenia

Vancampfort, Davy, et al., "State Anxiety, Psychological Stress and Positive Well-Being Responses to Yoga and Aerobic Exercise in People with Schizophrenia: A Pilot Study." *Disability and Rehabilitation* 33, no. 8 (2011): 684–89. Publisher: TAYLOR & FRANCIS LTD doi:10.3109/09638288.2010.509458., PMID: 20718623

> "After single sessions of yoga and aerobic exercises individuals with schizophrenia or schizoaffective disorder showed significantly decreased state anxiety, decreased psychological stress and increased subjective well-being compared to no exercise control."

Visceglia, Elizabeth, et al., "Yoga Therapy as an Adjunctive Treatment for Schizophrenia: A Randomized, Controlled Pilot Study." *Journal of Alternative and Complementary Medicine* (New York, N.Y.) 17, no. 7 (July 2011): 601–7. Publisher: REASONHOLD LTD doi:10.1089/acm.2010.0075., PMID: 21711202

> The YT group obtained significant improvements in positive and negative symptoms of schizophrenia symptoms compared to WL, including PANSS scores on positive syndrome, negative syndrome, general psychopathology. Activation, paranoia, and depression subscales. YT had improved perceived quality of life in physical and psychological domains.

Duraiswamy, G., et al., "Yoga Therapy as an Add-on Treatment in the Management of Patients with Schizophrenia--a Randomized Controlled Trial." *Acta Psychiatrica Scandinavica* 116, no. 3 (September 2007): 226–32. Publisher: BLACKWELL MUNKSGAARD doi:10.1111/j.1600-0447.2007.01032.x., PMID: 17655565

> "Subjects in the YT group had significantly less psychopathology than those in the PT group at the end of four months"

Yoga Therapy Improves Cognitive Function in Schizophrenia

Bhatia, Triptish, et al., "Adjunctive Cognitive Remediation for Schizophrenia Using Yoga: An Open, Non-Randomized Trial." *Acta Neuropsychiatrica* 24, no. 2 (April 1, 2012): 91–100. Publisher: BLACKWELL PUBLISHING; doi:10.1111/j.1601-5215.2011.00587.x., PMID: 22661830

> ➤ Compared with the SZ/TAU group, the SZ/YT group showed significantly greater improvement with regard to measures of attention following corrections for multiple comparisons; the changes were more prominent among the men. In the other diagnostic groups, differing patterns of improvements were noted with small to medium effect sizes. Our initial analyses suggest nominally significant improvement in cognitive function in schizophrenia with adjunctive therapies such as YT. The magnitude of the change varies by cognitive domain and may also vary by diagnostic group.

Sensory Therapies

Color Therapy

Color Therapy May Play a Role in Hospital Wards Recovery of Patients

Ajayi, O. O., et al. "An Appraisal of the Colour of Hospital Wards on the Recovery Attitudes of Psychiatric Patients." *Global Journal of Environmental Sciences* 4, no. 2 (March 8, 2006): 165–70. doi:10.4314/gjes.v4i2.2460.

> ➤ The environment where psychiatric patients are kept has been identified as an aid to their recovery attitudes. Based on the fact that the patients were being treated by qualified hands, an attempt is made to examine the significance of colour of the psychiatry ward environment as relating to the patients' rehabilitation in this paper. Number of patients admitted for psychiatric problem and those recovered (from the illness) and discharged in five psychiatric hospitals randomly selected from the western part of Nigeria were collected for a period five years (1995–2000). Among other things collected was the colour of the ward where the patients were kept for treatments. The data were analyzed using Statistical Package for Social Sciences (SPSS 10.0). Results showed that out 3125 patients admitted 73.3% of them recovered, of which 26.3% came from green, 37.6% from blue, 5.1% from neutralized yellow and the remaining 4.3% from white colour. Furthermore, it was observed that 93.8% of the patients kept under green, 93.9% under blue, 29.1% under neutralized yellow and 30.1% under white colour recovered from the illness. There is association between the recovery attitudes of patients and the different colours (P-value < 0.001). The strength of the relationship is also significant (P-value < 0.001). When the colours were gouped in two, namely dull (green

and blue) and bright (neutralized yellow and white), out of the 73.3% that recovered 63.9% came from dull and the remaining 9.4% from bright colour. In addition, we observed that 93.9% of the patients kept under dull and 29.5% under bright colour recovered from the illness. The association between recovery attitudes and the different colours is still evident (P-value < 0.001); and that the strength of the relationship is also significant (P-value < 0.001). Consequently, the dull colours have a better positive influence on the recovery attitudes of psychiatric patients.

Eye Movement Desensitization and Reprocessing (EMDR)

EMDR is Effective Therapy for PTSD Patients with Psychosis

Van den Berg, DP, et al., "Treating Trauma in Psychosis with EMDR: A Pilot Study." *Journal of Behavior Therapy and Experimental Psychiatry* 43, no. 1 (March 2012): 664–71. doi:10.1016/j.jbtep.2011.09.011., PMID: 21963888

> ➤ This pilot study shows that a short EMDR therapy is effective and safe in the treatment of PTSD in subjects with a psychotic disorder. Treatment of PTSD has a positive effect on auditory verbal hallucinations, delusions, anxiety symptoms, depression symptoms, and self-esteem. EMDR can be applied to this group of patients without adapting the treatment protocol or delaying treatment by preceding it with stabilizing interventions.

Hydrotherapy

Hydrotherapy Works as a Neuroleptic and Sedative Treatment

Shevchuk, Nikolai A., et al., "Hydrotherapy as a Possible Neuroleptic and Sedative Treatment." *Medical Hypotheses* 70, no. 2 (2008): 230–38. Publisher: CHURCHILL LIVINGSTONE; doi:10.1016/j.mehy.2007.05.028., PMID: 17640827

> ➤ As described previously, an adapted cold shower could work as a mild electroshock applied to the sensory and therefore, it might have an antipsychotic effect similar to that of electroconvulsive therapy. Additionally, a cold shower is a vivid example of stress-induced analgesia and would also be expected to "crowd out" or suppress psychosis related neurotransmission with-in the mesolimbic system.

Harmon, Rebecca Bouterie, et al., "Hydrotherapy in State Mental Hospitals in the Mid-Twentieth Century." *Issues in Mental Health Nursing* 30, no. 8 (August 2009): 491–94. Publisher: TAYLOR & FRANCIS INC. doi:10.1080/01612840802509460., PMID: 19591022

> ➤ "Student and graduate nurses were required to demonstrate competence in hydrotherapy treatments used to calm agitated or manic patients in the era before

neuroleptics. The nurses interviewed for this study indicated that, although labor intensive, hydrotherapy worked, at least temporarily......."

Heliotherapy

Sun Bathing has a Therauetic Effect on Psychotic Patients

Jackson, Allen J., et al. ""Heliotherapy in the Treatment of Mental Patients" *Medical Journal and Record*, 126, 731-734, 1927

> ➤ Although our studies are restricted to forty-four cases, we are convinced : 1, that heliotherapy has its usefulness in treatment of mental patients; 2, that the expense incurred in the physical appurtenance is nil; 3, that it has a sedative, relaxing and pleasing effect on the patient with a tendency to encourage metabolism; 4, that it will continue a rout! ne procedure at' this hospital; 5, that it is worth recommending to all institutions treating; the mentally ill.

Bright Light and Dark Therapy

Bright Light Therapy is Safe and Effective for Schizophrenia

Aichhorn, Wolfgang, et al., "Bright Light Therapy for Negative Symptoms in Schizophrenia: A Pilot Study." *The Journal of Clinical Psychiatry* 68, no. 7 (July 2007): 1146., Publisher: PHYSICIANS POSTGRADUATE PRESS, INC. PMID: 17685757

> ➤ "Bright light therapy was safe in our patients and did not result in psychotic exacerbation, as seen in unchanged positive scores on the PANSS. The subjective improvement in drive was statistically significant after 4 weeks, but did not persist after discontinuation of bright light therapy."

Heim, M., et al., "[Bright light therapy in schizophrenic diseases]." *Psychiatrie, Neurologie, Und Medizinische Psychologie* 42, no. 3 (March 1990): 146–50., PMID: 1972581

> ➤ 20 patients with schizophrenic disorders, displaying a depressive syndrome, were given bright-light therapy, and compared with 11 patients treated by means of partial deprivation of sleep. Against a figure of 27% in the case of sleep-deprivation, syndrome remittance was 55% in the case of bright-light therapy. As depressive syndromes improve under bright-light therapy, schizophrenic syndromes also recede, which suggests close syndromatologic links....

Bright Light Therapy Proves Superior to Previous Medications for Depression in Schizoaffective Patient

Oren, D. A., et al., "Bright Light Therapy for Schizoaffective Disorder." *The American Journal of Psychiatry* 158, no. 12 (December 2001): 2086–87., Publisher: AM PSYCHIATRIC ASSN PMID: 11729035

> "Bright light therapy proved comparable or superior to treatment with previous medications for depression for this patient."

Early Morning Sunlight Reduces Length of Hospitalization

Benedetti, F., et al., "Morning Sunlight Reduces Length of Hospitalization in Bipolar Depression." *Journal of Affective Disorders* 62, no. 3 (February 2001): 221–23, Publisher: ELSEVIER BV; PMID: 11223110

> *"Natural sunlight can be an underestimated and controlled light therapy for bipolar depression."*

Dark Therapy: The Use of Amber Tinted Safety Glasses for Creating Virtual Darkness in the Treatment of Schizoaffective Disorder

Gómez-Bernal, Germán, et al., "Dark Therapy for Schizoaffective Disorder. A Case Report." *Medical Hypotheses* 72, no. 1 (January 2009): 105–6. Publisher: CHURCHILL LIVINGSTONE; doi:10.1016/j.mehy.2008.08.008., PMID: 18812254

> James Phelps describes how amber-tinted safety glasses, could be useful for patients with rapid cycling bipolar disorder. These lens could block more than 90% wavelengths around 450mm (blue to blue-green) of light spectrum creating "virtual darkness" which could has a physiologic effect equivalent to true darkness, at least at the level of melatonin synthesis. I report a case that could support Phelps hypotheses.

Neurofeedback and Biofeedback

Neurofeedback has Been Found Effective for the Treatment of Schizophrenia

Surmeli, Tanju, et al., "Schizophrenia and the Efficacy of qEEG-Guided Neurofeedback Treatment: A Clinical Case Series." *Clinical EEG and Neuroscience* 43, no. 2 (April 2012): 133–44. Publisher: ELECTROENCEPHALOGRAPHY AND CLINICAL NEUROSCIENCE SOCIETY ; doi:10.1177/1550059411429531., PMID: 22715481

> Changes in PANSS, MMPI, and TOVA were analyzed to evaluate the effectiveness of NF treatment. The mean number of sessions completed by the participants was 58.5 sessions within 24 to 91 days. Three dropped out of treatment between 30 and 40 sessions on NF, and one did not show any response. Of the remaining 48 participating 47 showed clinical improvement after NF treatment, based on changes in their PANSS scores. The participants who were able to take the MMPI ant the TOVA showed significant improvements in these measures as well. Forty were followed up for more than 22 months, 2 for 1 year, 1 for 9 months, and 3 for between 1 and 3 months after completion of NF. Overall NF was shown to be effective.

CODEX ALTERNUS

Bolea AS., et al., "Neurofeedback Treatment of Chronic Inpatient Schizophrenia." *Journal of Neurotherapy: Investigations in Neuromodulation, Neurofeedback and Applied Neuroscience,* Volume 14, Issue 1, 2010, Publisher: THE/HAWORTH MEDICAL PRESS

> ➤ This is a study on the effect of neurofeedback on chronic inpatient complex paranoid schizophrenics. The purpose of this research was twofold: first, to determine the effects of the application of neurofeedback to very chronic cases of schizophrenia that had been resistant to years of inpatient medical and psychological treatment and second, to propose a connection paradigm of schizophrenia. The author obtained progress using affective neurofeedback with more than 70 hospitals in patients with chronic schizophrenia. Improvements were seen in the EEG patterns and in cognitive, affective and behavioral patterns that often resulted in successful release from the hospital to live in the community. A 2-year follow up found that positive changes were sustained. It is the author's impression that reinforcement of right parietal alpha and inhibiting frontal delta and fast beta activity obtained the best results.

Neurofeedback Treatments Enhance Cognitive Performance in Schizophrenia

Rocha N., et al., "Neurofeedback Treatment to Enhance Cognitive Performance in Schizophrenia". *Porto* 17-18, June 2011

> ➤ Following treatment, patients showed evidence of improved performance in different cognitive measures. The most important and consistent increases were observed in attention/vigilance, working memory and processing speed. We also observed changes in
> EEG patterns during the treatment, suggesting a learning effect. Patients were very collaborative during the treatment sessions and showed increased interest in their performance. Results from this exploratory study support the feasibility of using neurofeedback to enhance cognition in schizophrenia, but this method should not be considered alone for this purpose.

Biofeedback Improves Social Competence and Interest Factors for Schizophrenics

Pharr, O. M., et al., "The Use and Utility of EMG Biofeedback with Chronic Schizophrenic Patients." *Biofeedback and Self-Regulation* 14, no. 3 (September 1989): 229–45., Publisher: PLENUM PRESS. PMID: 2597713

> ➤ "On the nurses observation scale for inpatient evaluation the biofeedback group significantly improved on the Social Competence and Social Interest factors"

CODEX ALTERNUS

Biofeedback Induces Neuroleptic-like EEG Changes

> **Schneider, S. J.,** et al., "Neuroleptic-like Electroencephalographic Changes in Schizophrenics through Biofeedback." *Biofeedback and Self-Regulation* 7, no. 4 (December 1982): 479–90., Publisher: PLENUM PRESS. PMID: 6131700

> ➢ "The results suggest that the EEG of schizophrenics can be temporarily altered, using feedback techniques, in a way that mimics the EEG changes that have been shown to occur with neuroleptic induced clinical improvement."

Anxiety Reduction in Schizophrenia through Thermal Biofeedback and Relaxation Training

> **Hawkins, R. C.,** et al., "Anxiety Reduction in Hospitalized Schizophrenics through Thermal Biofeedback and Relaxation Training." *Perceptual and Motor Skills* 51, no. 2 (October 1980): 475–82. Publisher: AMMONS SCIENTIFIC LTD. doi:10.2466/pms.1980.51.2.475., PMID: 7443365

> ➢ The present study investigated the efficacy of thermal biofeedback and relaxation as adjunctive treatments to antipsychotic medication for reduction of anxiety in 40 hospitalized schizophrenics who were randomly assigned to four groups: biofeedback, relaxation, biofeedback and relaxation, and minimal treatment control. Significant reduction in anxiety followed treatment, but there were no between-group differences. One year follow-up and post boc analyses indicated a subgroup of "anxious" schizophrenics who showed substantial reduction in anxiety following treatment with biofeedback and relaxation.

Sound Therapy

Masking Techniques for Tinnitus Work Well for Auditory Hallucinations in Schizophrenia

> **Musiek, Frank,** et al., "Auditory Hallucinations: An Audiological Perspective." *The Hearing Journal* 60, no. 9 (September 2007): 32–52. Publisher: LIPPINCOTT WILLIAMS & WILKINS; doi:10.1097/01.HJ.0000295756.39258.41.

> ➢ Using one earplug and distracting oneself with external sounds or self-vocalization has been reported to help patients with Ahs. In one study of 20 patients with AHs, 14 reported that listening to an external acoustic stimulus was helpful, while 8 found the earplug useful. Collins et al., had mixed results when they used an earplug in one ear and had the subjects listen to music, the news, and discussions. It is difficult from an auditory stand-point to understand how an earplug in one ear influences the perception of AHs. It might allow the patient to hear his or her own voice better through the occlusion effect, but it is difficult to envision any other advantage in regard to AHs. Shergill et al. relates that acoustic stimuli serve primarily as a distraction, which prevents the patient from focusing on the hallucinations. Auditory distractions seem to work reasonably well. We would submit that, in addition to distraction, there is another

phenomenon known as "auditory masking" that plays a role in helping these patients. Auditory masking is defined as one sound (the masker) interfering with or even obliterating the perception of another sound. In the first author's experience, use of a white noise masker and appropriate masking protocols easily masked AHs, much to the patient's surprise. Wearable maskers have been used for many years to treat patients with tinnitus. Masking techniques may also hold much promise for helping patients with auditory hallucinations.

White Noise Therapy Might Decrease Auditory Hallucinations, Behavioral and Psychological Symptoms of Dementia in Schizophrenic Patients

> **Kaneko, Yutaka,** et al., "Efficacy of White Noise Therapy for Dementia Patients with Schizophrenia." *Geriatrics & Gerontology International* 13, no. 3 (July 2013): 808–10. Publisher: BLACKWELL PUBLISHING ASIA ; doi:10.1111/ggi.12028., PMID: 231819634

➤ We suggest that white noise therapy might decrease BPSD in dementia patients with schizophrenia. The mechanisms of white noise decreasing BPSD are not known. We note that BPSD in dementia patients without schizophrenia is often associated with confusion as to why they cannot live their lives as before; they might express anger if they perceive they are not being treated properly relative to their expectations, even when these might be unrealistic. However, patients with dementia coupled with schizophrenia often lash out without a reason and are difficult to comfort. These are completely different from those patients with BPSD, but without schizophrenia. White noise might mask these auditory hallucinations in patients with schizophrenia, and lead at least transiently to some level of relaxation for the patients. This is consistent with previous case reports, which also support the idea that white noise might soften or mitigate some aspects of auditory hallucination in patients with schizophrenia. The present study suggests that white noise therapy is a candidate of non-medical care to decrease BPSD in dementia patients with schizophrenia.

Humming My Help Reduce Auditory Hallucinations

> **Green, M. F.,** et al., "Auditory Hallucinations in Schizophrenia: Does Humming Help?" *Biological Psychiatry* 25, no. 5 (March 1, 1989): 633–35., Publisher: ELSEVIER INC.; PMID: 2920196

➤ "Though Falloon and Talbot (1981) did not list humming as a spontaneously used coping strategy, we found that it reduced reported hallucinations in our subjects. The present study demonstrates the value of using behavioral techniques (with a hypothesis-driven approach) to control auditory hallucinations."

CODEX ALTERNUS

Ear Plug Reduces Auditory Hallucinations in Schizophrenic Patient

Done, D. J., et al., "Reducing Persistent Auditory Hallucinations by Wearing an Ear-Plug." *The British Journal of Clinical Psychology / the British Psychological Society* 25 (Pt 2) (May 1986): 151–52., Publisher: BRITISH PSYCHOLOGICAL SOCIETY; PMID: 3730653

> ➤ "A case study is presented of the effects of wearing an ear-plug in a single patient with persistent auditory hallucinations. Beneficial effects were detected when the plug was in the dominant ear only."

Personal Stereo to Treat Auditory Hallucinations Leads to Decrease in Psychopathology

Johnston, Olwyn, et al., "The Efficacy of Using a Personal Stereo to Treat Auditory Hallucinations. Preliminary Findings." *Behavior Modification* 26, no. 4 (September 2002): 537–49., Publisher: SAGE PUBLICATIONS, INC.; PMID: 12205826

> ➤ This article presents preliminary findings from the first participant to complete an experiment assessing the efficacy of the personal stereo in treating auditory hallucinations. O.C., a 50-year-old woman, took part in a controlled treatment trial in which 1-week baseline, personal stereo, and control treatment (nonfunctioning hearing aid) stages were alternated for 7 weeks. The Positive and Negative Syndrome Scale, Clinical Global Impression Scales, Beliefs About Voices Questionnaire, Rosenberg Self-Esteem Scale, and Topography of Voices Rating Scale were used. The personal stereo led to a decrease in the severity of O.C.'s auditory hallucinations. For example, she rated her voices as being fairly distressing during baseline and control treatment stages but neutral during personal stereo stages. A slight decrease in other psychopathology also occurred during personal stereo stages. Use of the personal stereo did not lead to a decrease in self-esteem, contradicting suggestions that counter stimulation treatments for auditory hallucinations may be disempowering.

Reading Out Loud Reduces Levels of Auditory Hallucinations

Gallagher, A. G., et al., "The Effects of Varying Auditory Input on Schizophrenic Hallucinations: A Replication." *The British Journal of Medical Psychology* 67 (Pt 1) (March 1994): 67–75., Publisher: CAMBRIDGE UNIVERSITY PRESS, PMID: 8204543

> ➤ The aim of this study was to investigate the effects of different types of auditory stimulation on reports of auditory hallucinations at the time of the experiment. The results showed that self-reports by seven schizophrenic patients of auditory hallucinations were reduced by different types of auditory stimulation, particularly by listening to pop music. Requiring the subject to read a passage aloud also reduced the levels reported. This study was a replication of one by Margo, Hemsley & Slade (1981) who reported similar findings.

CODEX ALTERNUS

Sound Therapy with a Tinnitus Sound Generators Successfully Treats Auditory Hallucinations in Treatment Resistant Schizophrenia

Kaneko, Yutaka, et al., "Two Cases of Intractable Auditory Hallucination Successfully Treated with Sound Therapy." *The International Tinnitus Journal* 16, no. 1 (2010): 29–31., Publisher: STATE UNIV OF NEW YORK, HEALTH SCI CTR; PMID: 21609910

> ➤ We report two cases of AVHs successfully treated with sound therapy safely using a tinnitus control instrument (sound generator). The present study showed that sound therapy induced a complete remission of AVHs safely in two patients 2 years 7 months and 1 year 6 months. These results imply that the neuromechanism of AVHs is sensitive to sound therapy.

Audio Hallucinations Eliminated with Radio Headphones

Feder, R., et al., "Auditory Hallucinations Treated by Radio Headphones." *The American Journal of Psychiatry* 139, no. 9 (September 1982): 1188–90., Publisher: AM PSYCHIATRIC ASSN; PMID: 7114315

> ➤ "Listening to a radio through stereo headphones in conditions of low auditory stimulation eliminated the patient's hallucinations."

Auditory Hallucinations Decreased with Personal Stereo

Johnston, Olwyn, et al., "The Efficacy of Using a Personal Stereo to Treat Auditory Hallucinations. Preliminary Findings." *Behavior Modification* 26, no. 4 (September 2002): 537–49., Publisher: SAGE PUBLICATIONS, INC; PMID: 12205826

> ➤ "The personal stereo led to a decrease in severity of O.C.'s auditory hallucinations. A slight decrease in other psychopathology also occurred during personal stereo stages."

Sony Walkman Eliminates Auditory Hallucinations in Patient

Mallya, A. R., et al., "Radio in the Treatment of Auditory Hallucinations." *The American Journal of Psychiatry* 140, no. 9 (September 1983): 1264–65., Publisher: AM PSYCHIATRIC ASSN; PMID: 6614254

> ➤ From 1976 to 1981 he did well receiving 40mg/day of fluphenazine hydrochloride and 6 mg/day of trihexyphenityl. In 1981 his disability benefit was terminated and the financial stress increased his hallucinations, but the neurologist warned against the increase of neuroleptics for fear of worsening his parkinsonism. The patient was advised to buy a pair of headphones to control his hallucinations. The relief was so dramatic that the patient bought a Sony Walkman. However, when he takes off the headphones, auditory hallucinations recur immediately.

Audiotape Therapy Decreased Persistent Auditory Hallucinations in Patient

> **McInnis, M.,** et al., "Audiotape Therapy for Persistent Auditory Hallucinations." *The British Journal of Psychiatry: The Journal of Mental Science* 157 (December 1990): 913–14., Publisher: ROYAL MEDICO-PSYCHOLOGICAL ASSOCIATION; PMID: 2289102

  ➢ We report a case of a man with recurrent depression and persistent second-person auditory hallucinations telling him to kill himself. Using and audiotape cassette and headphones the duration of the hallucinations decreased significantly. Helpfulness of the audiotape continued at 15 months follow-up.

Vestibular Stimulation

Vestibular Stimulation for the Treatment of Schizophrenia

> **Baker, G.,** et al., "Vestibular Stimulation with Autistic and Schizophrenic Children." *The Alabama Journal of Medical Sciences* 14, no. 4 (October 1977): 434–35., Publisher: UNIVERSITY OF ALABAMA MEDICAL CENTER, PMID: 305727

  ➢ Behavior changes such as increased awareness, increased eye contact and verbalization, and decrease of self-destructive behaviors were also observed in the experimental group. The hypothesis was supported that vestibular stimulation can lower the threshold for vestibular activation to improve system functioning.

Psychosocial Therapies

Befriending

Befriending Patients with Medication Resistant Schizophrenia Can Predict a Good Response for those that are Delusional and Not for those Who Have Hallucinations

> **Samarasekera, N.,** et al., "Befriending Patients with Medication-Resistant Schizophrenia: Can Psychotic Symptoms Predict Treatment Response?" *Psychology and Psychotherapy* 80, no. Pt 1 (March 2007): 97–106. Publisher: JOHN WILEY & SONS LTD. doi:10.1348/147608306X108998., PMID: 17346383

  ➢ "Baseline delusions predicted a good response and auditory hallucinations predicted a poor response at 9 months."

Bibliotherapy

Bibliotherapy is Important for Rehabilitation of Schizophrenics

CODEX ALTERNUS

Alexander, R. H., et al., "Bibliotherapy with Chronic Schizophrenics." *Journal of Rehabilitation* 33, no. 6 (December 1967): 26–27 passim., Publisher: NATIONAL REHABILITATION ASSOCIATION; PMID: 6073694

> ➤ Bibliotherapy should continue to play an increasingly important function in the rehabilitation of chronic schizophrenics. Schizophrenic persons have shown ready response to the reality approach of bibliotherapy when it is presented in an interesting and challenging manner by a skilled therapist. With careful professional guidance bibliotherapy can provide a significant "first step" in the rehabilitation of mental patients to become interacting members of society. A significant finding of the study of which the above is a resume and one which the study was not aimed at, is that with the application of bibliotherapy, a group of chronic schizophrenic patients undergoing drug therapy can learn to consistently perform tasks heretofore considered beyond their ability.

Exposure Control

Exposure approach could help patients gain more control over persistent auditory hallucinations.

Persaud, R., et al., "A Pilot Study of Exposure Control of Chronic Auditory Hallucinations in Schizophrenia." *The British Journal of Psychiatry: The Journal of Mental Science* 167, no. 1 (July 1995): 45–50., Publisher: ROYAL MEDICO-PSYCHOLOGICAL ASSOCIATION; PMID: 7551607

> ➤ Many patients complain less of their auditory hallucinations per se than of lack of control of the experiences. There is reason to believe that a non-distraction (exposure) approach could help patients gain more control over persistent auditory hallucinations and teach them that their experience is a form of thinking and has no external source. This study is a pilot test of that idea. Five DSM-III-R schizophrenic outpatients with medication-resistant auditory hallucinations improved with a mean of 31 hour-long sessions over 3 months of therapist-guided exposure to their hallucinations and situations likely to evoke them. Improvement was the greatest in the patient's anxiety and sense of control over their hallucinations, less in social use of leisure and hallucinating time. These mildly encouraging pilot results warrant a controlled study of exposure for drug-resistant chronic auditory hallucinations and other psychotic experiences which are associated with anxious avoidance.

Hypnosis

Hypnosis Shows Positive Effects in Schizophrenic Patients

Scagnelli, J., et al., "Hypnotherapy with Schizophrenic and Borderline Patients: Summary of Therapy with Eight Patients." *The American Journal of Clinical Hypnosis* 19, no. 1 (July 1976): 33–38., Publisher: THE SOCIETY; PMID: 937214

> ➤ As a result of this program of traditional insight-oriented, dynamic therapy and hypnotherapy using the techniques described above, all eight patients discussed in this

paper have shown progress. They were generally able to reduce their medication requirements and to achieve partial or full time status as functioning members of society as students or job holders. All the patients achieved varying levels of reintegration of personalities. Although the growth and development of two of the patients appear to be subject to some of the inevitable schizophrenic setbacks, the general overall results of hypnotherapy appear to be positive and progressive.

Hypnosis May Be a Highly Successful Technique for Schizophrenia

> **Izquierdo, Santiago A.,** et al., "Hypnosis for Schizophrenia." *The Cochrane Database of Systematic Reviews,* no. 3 (2004): CD004160. Publisher: WILEY INTERSCIENCE doi:10.1002/14651858.CD004160.pub2., PMID: 15266520

> ➤ "Hypnosis could be helpful for people with schizophrenia"

> **Abrams, S.** "Short-Term Hypnotherapy of a Schizophrenic Patient." *The American Journal of Clinical Hypnosis* 5 (April 1963): 237–47., Publisher: THE SOCIETY ; PMID: 14010779

> ➤ "The only generalization that can be made from this study is that hypnotherapy may be a highly successful technique with some schizophrenic patients; but whether this is a method that might be of value for schizophrenia in general remains inconclusive. "

> **Abrams, S.,** et al., "THE USE OF HYPNOTIC TECHNIQUES WITH PSYCHOTICS; A CRITICAL REVIEW." *American Journal of Psychotherapy* 18 (January 1964): 79–94., Publisher: ASSOCIATION FOR THE ADVANCEMENT OF PSYCHOTHERAPY ; PMID: 14104802

> ➤ The case histories of psychotics treated by hypnotic methods point up the value of this treatment modality. Some patients improved with hypnotherapy after other therapeutic techniques had failed, and other patients with long-term illness dramatically recovered when hypnosis was employed. This would strongly suggest that hypnotherapeutic methods may be valuable tool for the treatment of specific psychotic disorders.

Language Therapy

Significant Reductions in Auditory Hallucinations from Language Therapy for Schizophrenic Patients

> **Hoffman, R. E.,** et al., "Language Therapy for Schizophrenic Patients with Persistent 'Voices.'" *The British Journal of Psychiatry: The Journal of Mental Science* 162 (June 1993): 755–58., Publisher: ROYAL MEDICO-PSYCHOLOGICAL ASSOCIATION; PMID: 8330107

> ➤ One of us has hypothesized that the 'voices' of schizophrenic patients reflect altered preconscious planning of discourse that can produce involuntary 'inner speech' as well as incoherent overt speech. Some schizophrenic patients reporting voices do not,

however, have disorganized speech. We hypothesize that these 'counterexample' patients compensate for impairments of discourse planning by reducing language complexity and relying on highly rehearsed topics. A 'language therapy' designed to challenge and enhance novel discourse planning was administered to four such patients; three had significant albeit temporary reductions in the severity of their voices. These clinical findings provide further evidence that alterations of discourse planning may underlie hallucinated voices.

Maudsley Review

The Maudsley Review Computerized Training Program Targets Reasoning Biases in Delusions

Waller, Helen, et al., "Targeting Reasoning Biases in Delusions: A Pilot Study of the Maudsley Review Training Programme for Individuals with Persistent, High Conviction Delusions." *Journal of Behavior Therapy and Experimental Psychiatry* 42, no. 3 (September 2011): 414–21. Publisher: PERGAMON; doi:10.1016/j.jbtep.2011.03.001., PMID: 21481815

> ➤ The computerized programme was developed on Microsoft PowerPoint and then transferred to a Real BASIC programme to incorporate the interactive elements. It comprised a general introduction to JTC and five training tasks (see below). It was designed to be completed together with a therapist, who emphasized key messages and provided together with a therapist, who emphasized key messages and provided feedback on participants' comments, for example by reinforcing useful insights and normalizing JTC. This was summarized, with participants' permission, in a handout to be taken away at the end of the session. No explicit mention of psychosis or direct challenging of beliefs was included. However, in order to increase relevance to delusional experience, video clips and scenarios, with the potential for paranoid interpretation, were used.

> ➤ Overall, the results suggest that the programme holds promise in changing, over a single session, outcomes which are typically resistant to standard treatments. Additionally, the programme is relatively easy to administer and may hold potential to be delivered by 'non-expert' staff following brief training.

Morita Therapy

Morita Therapy for Schizophrenia May Have Some Positive Effects

Li, Chunbo, et al., "Morita Therapy for Schizophrenia." *Schizophrenia Bulletin* 34, no. 6 (November 2008): 1021–23. Publisher: OXFORD UNIVERSITY PRESS doi:10.1093/schbul/sbn124., PMID: 18852234

> "Morita therapy may have some positive effects, but there are no data to assess whether this sustained. For schizophrenia, therefore, Morita therapy remains and experimental intervention."

Nidotherapy

Nidotherapy is a Novel Therapy Distinctly Different form Standard Treatment

Chamberlain, Ian J., et al., "Nidotherapy for People with Schizophrenia." *The Cochrane Database of Systematic Reviews* 3 (2013): CD009929. Publisher: WILEY INTERSCIENCE doi:10.1002/14651858.CD009929.pub2., PMID: 23543583

> "Further research is needed into the possible benefits or harms of this newly-formulated therapy. Until such research is available, patients, clinicians, managers and policymakers should consider it an experimental approach."

Personal Therapy

Personal Therapy A Disorder-Relevant Psychotherapy for Schizophrenia

Hogarty, G. E., et al., "Personal Therapy: A Disorder-Relevant Psychotherapy for Schizophrenia." *Schizophrenia Bulletin* 21, no. 3 (1995): 379–93., Publisher: OXFORD UNIVERSITY PRESS; PMID: 741569

> While the long-term care of ambulatory schizophrenia patients requires highly effective interpersonal treatment skills among clinicians, there is little evidence to support an empirically validated individual psychotherapy of schizophrenia. Personal therapy (PT) attempts to address the apparent limitations of traditional psychotherapy by modifying the "model of the person" to accommodate an underlying pathophysiology, minimizing potential iatrogenic effects of maintenance antipsychotic medication, controlling sources of environmental provocation, and extending therapy to a time when crisis management has lessened and stabilization is better ensured. By means of graduated, internal coping strategies, PT attempts to provide a growing awareness of personal vulnerability, including the "internal cues" of affect dysregulation. The goals are to increase foresight through the accurate appraisal of emotional states, their appropriate expression, and assessment of the reciprocal response of others. The strategies are supplemented by phase-specific psychoeducation and behavior therapy techniques. Practical issues in the application of this new intervention are discussed. Preliminary observations from two samples of patients, one living with and the other living independent of family, suggest differential improvement over time among PT recipients.

CODEX ALTERNUS

Creative Engagement Therapies

Agrotherapy

Agrotherapy is a Way to Keep Patients Occupied in a Rural Agriculture Setting with Structured Activities.

Javed, M. A., et al., "Agrotherapy--New Concept of Rehabilitation for Chronic Schizophrenics in Pakistan." *JPMA. The Journal of the Pakistan Medical Association* 43, no. 12 (December 1993): 251–53., PMID: 8133634

> ➢ The provision of comprehensive programme for mental health in the community setting has achieved an important place in the field of psychiatric rehabilitation. The concept of agrotherapy which is based on the philosophy of keeping patients occupied in a rural and agricultural setting with more structured activities has been found to be a promising innovation for the rehabilitation of chronic schizophrenics in this regard. This paper describes the results of a three years follow-up study conducted at Fountain House Farm, Farooqabad to evaluate the effectiveness of agrotherapy. The findings are discussed in terms of practical implications of this innovative approach in the rehabilitation of chronic schizophrenic patients.

Animal Assisted Therapy

Therapeutic Riding Sessions Improve Negative Symptoms and Reduce Rate of Hospitalization

Cerino, Stefania, et al., "Non-Conventional Psychiatric Rehabilitation in Schizophrenia Using Therapeutic Riding: The FISE Multicentre Pindar Project." *Annali dell'Istituto Superiore Di Sanità* 47, no. 4 (2011): 409–14. doi:DOI: 10.4415/ANN_11_04_13., PMID: 22194076

> ➢ The FISE (Federazione Italiana Sport Equestri) Pindar is a multicentre research project aimed at testing the potential effects of therapeutic riding on schizophrenic patients. Twenty-four subjects with a diagnosis of schizophrenia were enrolled for a 1 year-treatment involving therapeutic riding sessions. All subjects were tested at the beginning and at the end of treatment with a series of validated test batteries (BPRS and 8 items-PANSS). The results discussed in this paper point out an improvement in negative symptoms, a constant disease remission in both early onset and chronic disease subjects, as well as a reduced rate of hospitalization.

CODEX ALTERNUS

Therapeutic Horseback Riding Benefits Individuals with Schizophrenia

Corring, Deborah, et al., "Therapeutic Horseback Riding for ACT Patients with Schizophrenia." *Community Mental Health Journal* 49, no. 1 (February 2013): 121–26. Publisher: SPRINGER NEW YORK LLC; doi:10.1007/s10597-011-9457-y., PMID: 22015959

> ➤ One form of psychiatric leisure rehabilitation which has only recently been explored for individuals with schizophrenia is Therapeutic Horseback Riding (THBR). This study is the first to examine THBR for Assertive Community Treatment (ACT) patients with schizophrenia. A sample of· 6 ACT patients with schizophrenia or schizoaffective disorder who reside in the community and 6 mental health care staff participated in 10 weeks of weekly horseback riding sessions with an experienced THBR instructor. Participating patients, staff and the THBR instructor were qualitatively interviewed at the start, during and at the end of the THBR program and these semi-structured interviews were analyzed for recurrent themes. We found that THBR benefitted this group of patients. In spite of our study's limitations, such as its exploratory nature and the small sample size, it demonstrates that THBR has promise and should be further developed and studied for individuals with schizophrenia.

Farm-based Interventions Can Alleviate Psychiatric Symptoms in Patients with Persistent Mental Disorders

Iancu, Sorana C., et al., "Farm-Based Interventions for People with Mental Disorders: A Systematic Review of Literature." *Disability and Rehabilitation,* June 25, 2014, 1–10. Publisher: TAYLOR & FRANCIS LTD; doi:10.3109/09638288.2014.932441., PMID: 24963943

> ➤ Our results suggest that the farm environment should be considered, especially for patients with mental disorders who do not achieve an adequate response with other treatment options. Further research is needed to clarify potential social and occupational benefits. Implications for Rehabilitation Despite the developments in mental healthcare, in many countries farms still play a role in the provision of psychiatric rehabilitation services. Farm-based interventions can alleviate psychiatric symptoms in patients with persistent mental disorders and can facilitate mental health recovery. The social and occupational aspects of the farm-based interventions are central to the experiences of mental health recovery.

Animal Assisted Therapy is Associated with Reduced Anxiety Levels for Hospitalized Patients

Barker, S. B., et al., "The Effects of Animal-Assisted Therapy on Anxiety Ratings of Hospitalized Psychiatric Patients." *Psychiatric Services (Washington, D.C.)* 49, no. 6 (June 1998): 797–801., Publisher: Stm Editores; PMID: 9634160

> "Animal-assisted therapy was associated with reduced state anxiety levels for hospitalized patients with a variety of psychiatric diagnoses, while a routine therapeutic recreation session was associated with reduced levels only for patients with mood disorders."

Animal-assisted Therapy May Contribute to Psychosocial Rehabilitation for Schizophrenia Patients

Nathans-Barel, Inbar, et al., "Animal-Assisted Therapy Ameliorates Anhedonia in Schizophrenia Patients. A Controlled Pilot Study." *Psychotherapy and Psychosomatics* 74, no. 1 (2005): 31–35. Publisher: S./KARGER AG; doi:10.1159/000082024., PMID: 15627854

> The AAT group showed a significant improvement in the hedonic tone compared to controls. They also showed an improvement in the use of leisure time and a trend towards improvement in motivation. AAT may contribute to the psychosocial rehabilitation and quality of life of chronic schizophrenia patients.

Animal-assisted Therapy Improves Non-verbal Communication in Schizophrenic Patients

Kovacs Z., et al., "An Exploratory Study of the Effect of Animal-assisted Therapy on Nonverbal Communication in Three Schizophrenic Patients." *A Multidisciplinary Journal of the Interactions of People & Animals*, 1 December 2006, vol.19, no.4, pp353-364(12)

> The therapy was oriented toward improving non-specific (i.e., general well-being) and specific (i.e., communication patterns) areas of the patient's daily activities. The outcome measure was the change in the patient's nonverbal communication, as measured by analysis of standardized, video-recorded scenarios registered at the beginning of the therapy, and six months later, and the end of it. Because two patients completed less than half of the sessions, we analyzed the data of only three parameters. All three patients improved in the usage of space during communication, while partial improvement in other domains of nonverbal communication (anatomy of movements, dynamics of gestures, regulator gestures) was also observed. Animal-assisted therapy can improve certain aspects of nonverbal communication in schizophrenic patients.

Animal-assisted Therapy Improves Socialization, ADL's and General Well-being in Elderly Schizophrenic Patients

Barak, Y., et al., "Animal-Assisted Therapy for Elderly Schizophrenic Patients: A One-Year Controlled Trial." *The American Journal of Geriatric Psychiatry: Official Journal of the American Association for Geriatric Psychiatry* 9, no. 4 (2001): 439–42., Publisher: AMERICAN PSYCHIATRIC PUBLISHING, INC. PMID: 11739071

> The authors evaluated, in a blinded, controlled manner, the effects of AAT in a closed psychogeriatric ward over 12 months. Subjects were 10 elderly schizophrenic patients

and 10 matched patients (mean age: 79.1 +/-6.7 years). The outcome measure was the Scale for Social Adaptive Functioning Evaluation (SAFE). AAT was conducted in weekly 4-hour sessions. Treatment encouraged mobility, interpersonal contact, and communication and reinforced activities of daily living (ADLs), including personal hygiene and independent self-care, through the use of cats and dogs as "modeling companions." The SAFE scores at termination showed significant improvement compared with baseline scores and on the Social Functions subscale. AAT proved a successful tool for enhancing socialization, ADLs, and general well-being.

Animal-assisted Therapy with Farm Animals May Have Positive Influences on Self-Efficiency for Persons with Schizophrenia

> **Berget B.,** et al., "Animal-assisted Therapy with Farm Animals for Persons with Psychiatric Disorders: Effects on Self-efficiency, Coping Ability and Quality of Life, a Randomized Controlled Trial." *Clinical Practice and Epidemiology in Mental Health* 2008, 4:9, Publisher: BIOMED CENTRAL LTD.

> ➤ "AAT with farm animals may have positive influences on self-efficiency and coping ability among psychiatric patients with long lasting psychiatric symptoms."

Art Therapy

Art Therapy Can Help Alter Psychotic Projections and Aid in Psychotherapeutic Rehabilitation

> **Honig, Sylvia,** et al., "Art Therapy Used in Treatment of Schizophrenia." *Art Psychotherapy* 4, no. 2 (1977): 99–104. Publisher: PERGAMON. doi:10.1016/0090-9092(77)90007-2.

> ➤ "I have found that art therapy, used in a positive, realistic, structured and supportive way, such as displayed in contour drawing sessions, can help alter psychotic projections and aid in overall psychotherapeutic rehabilitation of schizophrenia."

Computer-based Art Therapy Helps Decrease Fear and Let Patients Transfer Feelings to Drawings

> **Hartwich, Peter,** et al., "Computer-Based Art Therapy with Inpatients: Acute and Chronic Schizophrenics and Borderline Cases." *The Arts in Psychotherapy* 24, no. 4 (1997): 367–73. Publisher: PERGAMON; doi:10.1016/S0197-4556(97)00042-7.

> ➤ Many people feel inhibited when they are asked to paint in a traditional way. They do not feel able to transfer their feelings and experiences onto paper. They argue that they are not artists. With computer based painting this threshold of fear is decreased. After a little training they are able to express at least some intrapsychic experiences. The stimulating nature of colors, shapes and tools is great and seems to be like a box of toys for the patients. The second important difference between traditional and computer-

based painting is that one can save the painting in its various steps of development. The whole process of events in drawing a picture can be fixed and saved step by step. The painting can be brought back to the screen whenever wanted or any aspect of the painting can be accessed at will. Also, the whole process of the painting can be put on a videotape electronically without using a camera. One then has two different opportunities to mirror the patient's creative drawing process. The finished picture is the goal in the traditional way of painting. The process is over when the picture is completed. Painting by computer enables us to store the process and to recall it. The patient gets into an "interaction" with the computer and the painting process becomes a mirror of the relationship. The outer expression of an intrapsychic process can be recorded with the help of technology. The reproduction of the unfolding intrapsychic events becomes possible.* Our computer painting therapy is not to be regarded as exclusive psychotherapeutic method. We hope it becomes a helpful part in the concerted action of all our therapeutic efforts. Schizophrenic patients' treatment should always be a combination of different pharmacotherapeutic and psychotherapeutic methods adapted to individual needs.

Art Therapies Improve Mental Health and Negative Symptoms of Schizophrenia

> **Crawford, Mike J.**, et al., "Arts Therapies for People with Schizophrenia: An Emerging Evidence Base." *Evidence-Based Mental Health* 10, no. 3 (August 2007): 69–70., Publisher: B M J PUBLISHING GROUP; PMID: 17652554

> ➤ An evidence base for the effectiveness of arts therapies in the treatment of people with schizophrenia is beginning to emerge. Arts therapies combine the use of art materials with psychotherapeutic techniques that aim to encourage self-expression and promote self-awareness. They appear to be popular with patients and may result in improved mental health, especially reductions in negative and general symptoms of schizophrenia, which are those least responsive to pharmacological interventions. Further research is needed to establish the effects and cost effectiveness of arts therapies for people with schizophrenia outside of specialist centres.

Group Art Therapy for Psychosis may have a Positive Effect

> **Montag, Christiane,** et al., "A Pilot RCT of Psychodynamic Group Art Therapy for Patients in Acute Psychotic Episodes: Feasibility, Impact on Symptoms and Mentalising Capacity." *PloS One* 9, no. 11 (2014): e112348. Publisher: PUBLIC LIBRARY OF SCIENCE doi:10.1371/journal.pone.0112348., PMID: 25393414

> ➤ Evidence on the efficacy and effectiveness of AT in patients with schizophrenia is far from being conclusive and benefits might be limited to a subgroup of patients. Results of this pilot study suggest that RCTs of AT can be implemented in routine hospital settings for patients experiencing acute psychotic states. With all due caution, findings from this first European pilot RCT of psychodynamic AT in acutely psychotic inpatients prove the feasibility of similar projects and point to a possible positive effect of the intervention on psychotic symptoms, psychosocial functioning and the ability to mentalise emotions. These preliminary results must be substantiated by further independent research.

CODEX ALTERNUS

Art Therapy Strengthens the Sense of Self in Schizophrenic Patients

Teglbjaerg, Hanne Stubbe, et al., "Art Therapy May Reduce Psychopathology in Schizophrenia by Strengthening the Patients' Sense of Self: A Qualitative Extended Case Report." *Psychopathology* 44, no. 5 (2011): 314–18. Publisher: S./KARGER AG doi:10.1159/000325025.

> ➤ "The most important benefit of the art therapy was a strengthening of the patients' sense of self. All patients reported a good outcome, and qualitative analysis showed that the positive effect of art therapy is mainly due to a strengthening of patients' minimal sense of self."

Art as a Therapeutic Tool Help Clients Communicate and Express Themselves

Noronha, Konrad J., et al., "Working with Art in a Case of Schizophrenia." *Indian Journal of Psychological Medicine* 35, no. 1 (January 2013): 89–92. doi:10.4103/0253-7176.112215., Publisher: Indian Psychiatric Society, South Zone; PMID: 23833350

> ➤ This study used art as a therapeutic tool in therapy with a client diagnosed with schizophrenia, along with medical management. The purpose of using art was to enable the non-communicative client to communicate. The client's drawings were used as a process medium. Progress was seen in changes in social behaviors and communication evidenced by him speaking more, expressing feelings and gaining better insight.

Games

The Card Game "Michael's Game" is Feasible for Treatment of Delusional Behaviors

Khazaal, Yasser, et al., "A Card Game for the Treatment of Delusional Ideas: A Naturalistic Pilot Trial." *BMC Psychiatry* 6 (2006): 48. doi:10.1186/1471-244X-6-48., Publisher: BIOMED CENTRAL LTD. PMID: 17074084

> ➤ Michael's Game", a training module for hypothetical reasoning is a treatment inspired by CBTs of psychotic symptoms. It was conceived by the first two authors as a tool to promote the dissemination of CBTs in natural clinical settings. Principles of the game are founded on cognitive therapy of psychotic symptoms and use their techniques such as: developing a therapeutic alliance based on the patients perspective, normalizing psychotic symptoms, cognitive restructuring techniques aiming to develop alternative explanations to their delusions, reality testing and connecting belief to emotion and behavior. It could be used as a preliminary or complement of individual CBTs. "Michael's Game" is a program aiming at training hypothetical reasoning. Participants have to help Michael to find alternatives to the erroneous conclusions that Michael draws from situations described on each card. It was conceived as a group card game in order to allow patients to become partners of fictive character (Michael) interacting

together with cards containing impersonal information which may however reflect their own problems.

> ➤ This pilot study supports the feasibility of this therapeutic approach and the ease of its diffusion in various clinical settings. "Michael's game" has been used easily after a short training, in different sites that were not specialized in CBTs.

A Card Game Helps Those Preoccupied with Psychotic Symptoms

Khazaal, Yasser, et al., "'Michael's Game,' a Card Game for the Treatment of Psychotic Symptoms." *Patient Education and Counseling* 83, no. 2 (May 2011): 210–16. Publisher: ELSEVIER IRELAND LTD; doi:10.1016/j.pec.2010.05.017., PMID: 20646892

> ➤ Data about 107 patients were included in the entire analyses. Significant improvements were observed on BCIS subscales as well as a reduction of severity of conviction and preoccupation scores on the PDI-21. The intervention has a moderate effect on the PDI-21 preoccupation and conviction as well as the BCIS subscales. Patients who benefit the most from the program are patients who have a low degree of self-reflectiveness and patients who are concomitantly preoccupied by their symptoms. The present study supports the feasibility and effectiveness of "Michael's Game" in naturalistic settings. The game seems to be a useful tool for patients with psychotic disorders.

Playing Chess Can Easily Restore Executive Functions in Schizophrenics

Demily, Caroline, et al., "The Game of Chess Enhances Cognitive Abilities in Schizophrenia." *Schizophrenia Research* 107, no. 1 (January 2009): 112–13. doi:10.1016/j.schres.2008.09.024., Publisher: ELSEVIER BV; PMID: 18995990

> ➤ When considered together, our results suggest that playing chess for mere 10 h can restore (at least partially) executive functions of patients with schizophrenia. It may be interesting to note that chess can be proposed easily –at almost no cost—to all psychotic patients. Most of the patients kept playing chess on their own, after the completion of the study.

Cognitive Training via a Laptop Computer Games is a Promising Treatment for Schizophrenia

Fisher, Melissa, et al., "Neuroplasticity-Based Auditory Training Via Laptop Computer Improves Cognition in Young Individuals With Recent Onset Schizophrenia." *Schizophrenia Bulletin,* January 20, 2014. Publisher: OXFORD UNIVERSITY PRESS doi:10.1093/schbul/sbt232., PMID: 24444862

> ➤ Neuroscience-informed cognitive training via laptop computer represents a promising treatment approach for cognitive dysfunction in early schizophrenia. An individual's baseline motivational system functioning (reward anticipation), and ability to engage in

auditory processing speed improvement, may represent important predictors of treatment outcome. Future studies must investigate whether cognitive training improves functioning and how best to integrate it into critical psychosocial interventions.

Creative Writing

Evidence that Creative Writing Forms an Important Recovery Experience

> **King, Robert,** et al., "Creative Writing in Recovery from Severe Mental Illness." *International Journal of Mental Health Nursing* 22, no. 5 (October 2013): 444–52. Publisher: BLACKWELL PUBLISHING ASIA; doi:10.1111/j.1447-0349.2012.00891.x. , PMID: 23211053

➢ There is evidence that creative writing forms an important part of the recovery experience of people affected by severe mental illness. In this paper, we consider theoretical models that explain how creative writing might contribute to recovery, and we discuss the potential for creative writing in psychosocial rehabilitation. We argue that the rehabilitation benefits of creative writing might be optimized through focus on process and technique in writing, rather than content, and that consequently, the involvement of professional writers might be important. We describe a pilot workshop that deployed these principles and was well-received by participants. Finally, we make recommendations regarding the role of creative writing in psychosocial rehabilitation for people recovering from severe mental illness and suggest that the development of an evidence base regarding the effectiveness of creative writing is a priority.

Camping

Camping Allows Patients to Be More Assertive and a Better View of Their Peers

> **Shearer, R. M.** "Camping as a Therapeutic Experience for Depressed and Schizophrenic Patients." *Hospital & Community Psychiatry* 26, no. 8 (August 1975): 494–97., PMID: 1165083

➢ The experience in living gave staff and patients from each group a view of the total person in a variety of situations and circumstances not usually evident in group sessions and in-house programs at the hospital. The dynamics of personality and behavior take a more realistic perspective when related to an extended experience in living. Patients indicate they feel much freer to assert themselves in groups, whether the assertion is directed toward the leader or others.

Dance

Traditional Dancing Improves Functional Capacity and Quality of Life in Patients with Schizophrenia

CODEX ALTERNUS

Kaltsatou, A., et al., "Effects of Exercise Training with Traditional Dancing on Functional Capacity and Quality of Life in Patients with Schizophrenia: A Randomized Controlled Study." *Clinical Rehabilitation*, December 18, 2014, Publisher: HODDER ARNOLD JOURNALS; doi:10.1177/0269215514564085.

> After the eight months, Group A increased walking distance in the 6-minute walk test (328.4 ± 35.9 vs. 238.0 ± 47.6 m), sit-to-stand test (19.1 ± 1.8 vs. 25.1 ± 1.4 seconds), Berg Balance Scale score (53.1 ± 2.1 vs. 43.2 ± 6.7), lower limbs maximal isometric force (77.7 ± 25.7 vs. 51.0 ± 29.8 lb.), Positive and Negative Syndrome Scale total score (77.0 ± 23.1 vs. 82.0 ± 24.4), Global Assessment of Functioning Scale total score (51.3 ± 15.5 vs. 47.7 ± 13.3) and Quality of Life total score (34.9 ± 5.2 vs. 28 ± 4.5), compared with Group B. Our results demonstrate that Greek traditional dances improve functional capacity and quality of life in patients with schizophrenia.

Dance Group for Psychotic Patients is used as a Therapeutic Tool for Recovery

Tavormina, Romina, et al., "The Advantages of 'Dance-Group' for Psychotic Patients." *Psychiatria Danubina* 26 Suppl 1 (November 2014): 162–66., Publisher: FACULTAS UNIVERSITATIS [I.E. FACULTAS MEDICA UNIVE; PMID: 25413534

> Psychosocial rehabilitation and in particular group dances allow the recovery of lost or compromised ability of patients with mental illness, and they facilitate their reintegration into the social context. The dance group has enabled users of the Day Centre of the Unit of Mental Health Torre del Greco ASL NA 3 south to achieve the objectives of rehabilitation such as: taking care of themselves, of their bodies and their interests, improving self-esteem, the management of pathological emotions, socialization and integration, overcoming the psychotic closing and relational isolation. In particular, patients with schizophrenia, psychotic and mood disorders had a concrete benefit from such rehabilitation activities, facilitating interpersonal relationships, therapy compliance and significantly improved mood, quality of life, providing them with the rhythm and the security in their relationship with each other. The dance group and for some individuals, also psychotherapy and drug therapy, have facilitated social inclusion, improved the quality of life and cured their diseases. The work is carrying out in a group with patients, practitioners, family members, volunteers, social community workers, following the operating departmental protocols. Using the chorus group "Sing that you go" as an operational tool for psychosocial rehabilitation and therapeutic element we promote the psychological well-being and the enhancement of mood.

CODEX ALTERNUS

Dance Therapy is a Non-verbal Variant of Psychotherapy that Explores the Unconscious Process in Schizophrenic Patients

> **Romero, Emilio F.,** et al., "Dance Therapy on a Therapeutic Community for Schizophrenic Patients." *The Arts in Psychotherapy* 10, no. 2 (1983): 85–92. Publisher: PERGAMON doi:10.1016/0197-4556(83)90034-5.

> ➤ We have discussed dance therapy as a nonverbal variant of psychotherapy. This experience allowed many patients to explore their own creativity and to experiment with new behaviors. After several weeks, some patients and staff became more and more creative, selecting new records, steps, movements, and themes. We have not found dance therapy to differ from or to oppose reconstructive psychotherapy; rather, it coadunates it. Dance is an additional way to explore unconscious processes in the schizophrenic patient.

Dance Therapy is a Communication Activating Non-verbal Psychotherapy

> **Natalia Oganesian,** et al., "Dance therapy as form of communication activating psychotherapy for schizophrenic patients" *Body, Movement and Dance in Psychotherapy* Vol. 3, No. 2, September 2008, 97–106, Publisher: ROUTLEDGE DOI:10.1080/17432970802080057

> ➤ Before dance therapy, the patients were characterized by certain fencing off, instability in their mood, communication problems, and psycho-motoric inhibition. After dance therapy, their cooperation with the doctors improved, their stigmatization phenomena became less evident, their psycho-motoric inhibition decreased, and the patients became more accessible to contact and more active. As for medication therapy, in most cases it did not change. In conclusion, it may be said that dance therapy is a communication activating non-verbal psychotherapy. Introduction of dance therapy into the complex of clinical psychological interferences enables us to intensify the rehabilitation process for schizophrenic patients.

Application of the Primitive Expression Form of Dance Therapy in Psychotic Patients Leads to Increased Happiness and Positive Attitude

> **Margariti A., et al.,** "An Application of the Primitive Expression Form of Dance Therapy in a Psychiatric Population." *The Arts in Psychotherapy* 39 (2012) 95-101, Publisher: PERGAMON

> ➤ In this paper we present preliminary results of PE-based protocol with a small group of psychiatric patients (psychotic and depressive disorders). It is shown that a relatively short duration of PE treatment led to observable changes in psychological state, behavior, and brain physiology. It was found that the patients (1) experienced an increase in their happiness level, (2) expressed a positive attitude to the PE process by utilizing appropriate word associations, and (3) exhibited (a patient subset) an increase in EEG activity related to relaxed awake state. The study presents encouraging results related to the application of PE therapy with psychiatric patients. PE can be added to other dance

therapy methodologies which have been shown to be promising therapeutic approaches in psychiatric populations.

Social Partnered Dance May Benefit those with Serious and Persistent Mental Illness

Hackney, Madeleine E., et al., "Social Partnered Dance for People with Serious and Persistent Mental Illness: A Pilot Study." *The Journal of Nervous and Mental Disease* 198, no. 1 (January 2010): 76–78. Publisher: LIPPINCOTT WILLIAMS & WILKINS doi:10.1097/NMD.0b013e3181c81f7c., PMID: 20061874

> Individuals with serious mental illness (SMI) often experience isolation and poor health, but normalized social opportunities aid recovery. This study aimed to determine social dance's feasibility and effects on mood, functional mobility, and balance confidence in 12 people with SMI. Participants danced once per week in 1-hour lessons for 10 weeks. Before and after lessons, participants were evaluated for gait velocity and with one-leg stance, Timed Up and Go, and 6-minute walk tests. Participants self-completed Beck Depression II and Beck Anxiety Inventories and the Activities-specific Balance Confidence Scale. Posttesting included an exit questionnaire assessing participant experiences. Participants significantly improved on the Timed Up and Go, (p = 0.012, effect size = 0.68), and demonstrated nonsignificant improvements in anxiety, depression, and balance confidence (effect sizes of 0.41, 0.54, and 0.64, respectively). Participants reported enjoying classes, and interest to continue. Social dance is feasible and may benefit mobility for those with SMI.

Drama

Improvisational Drama Groups are Beneficial for Psychiatric Inpatients

Sheppard, J., et al., "Improvisational Drama Groups in an Inpatient Setting." *Hospital & Community Psychiatry* 41, no. 9 (September 1990): 1019–21., Publisher: THE ASSOCIATION; PMID: 2210698

> Many descriptive case studies have been written about psychodrama, drama therapy, and related therapies. However, few studies have used experimental techniques to demonstrate the positive effects of these therapies. This study found nearly a 100 percent increase in the frequency of appropriate verbalization for a group of ten inpatients in a psychiatric rehabilitation program. Quantitative procedures were useful for measuring changes in verbalization. Nineteen of the initial 29 participants chose not to continue in the drama groups. Many of these people were restless or incapable of concentrating. The drop-out group differed from those who completed in that they were slightly older, included a higher percentage of women, and included two people with a diagnosis of mental retardation. Subjects' creativity flourished in the improvisational drama sessions. Some presented soliloquies they had memorized. Others sang or read their own poetry. They were fascinated to watch themselves on videotape. Participants interacted in an increasingly cooperative manner. After scheduled drama group sessions, subjects began to use role playing, role reversal and charades in ward meetings, creating a relaxed

atmosphere and breaking down role and communication barriers in the hospital environment. These effects continued for months after the sessions had ended.

Drama Therapy May Be an Adjunctive Therapy for Schizophrenia

> **Ruddy, R. A.,** et al., "Drama Therapy for Schizophrenia or Schizophrenia-like Illnesses." *The Cochrane Database of Systematic Reviews,* no. 1 (2007): CD005378. doi:10.1002/14651858.CD005378.pub2., Publisher: WILEY INTERSCIENCE; PMID: 17253555

> ➢ Drama therapy is one of the creative therapies suggested to be of value as an adjunctive treatment for people with schizophrenia or schizophrenia-like illnesses. Randomised studies have been successfully conducted in this area but poor study reporting meant that no conclusions could be drawn from them. The benefits or harms of the use of drama therapy in schizophrenia are therefore unclear and further large, high quality studies are required to determine the true value of drama therapy for schizophrenia or schizophrenia-like illnesses.

Flower Workshop

Flower Workshop Helps Schizophrenics with Cognitive Coordination and Promotes New Ways of Psychosocial Rehabilitation

> **Pereira, Alfredo**, et al. "The Flower Workshop in Psychosocial Rehabilitation: A Pilot Study." *Issues in Mental Health Nursing* 30, no. 1 (January 2009): 47–50. doi:10.1080/01612840802555216. PMID: 19148821

> ➢ We believe that the Workshop was successful in providing an adequate context with facilitations that compensate a putative biological vulnerability (defective synchronization of neuronal oscillations) of the participants, and in collaborating with the emergence of new ways to promote psychosocial rehabilitation. It helps the cognitive coordination of the participants in the task of dynamical grouping of objects (flowers, materials for the vase), and creates a social environment that promotes the development of affective bonds. It can be used in a variety of conditions in mental health assistance for persons with and without schizophrenia.

Humor

Humor Skills Training Can Improve Rehabilitation Outcomes for Schizophrenic Patients

> **Cai, Chunfeng,** et al., "Effectiveness of Humor Intervention for Patients with Schizophrenia: A Randomized Controlled Trial." *Journal of Psychiatric Research* 59 (December 2014): 174–78. Publisher: PERGAMON; doi:10.1016/j.jpsychires.2014.09.010., PMID: 25266473

> "The implementation of humor skill training in a mental health service can improve rehabilitative outcomes and sense of humor for schizophrenia patients who were in the rehabilitation stage."

Humor has Positive Effect on Hospitalized Schizophrenic Patients

Gelkopf, M. "Laughter in a Psychiatric Ward. Somatic, Emotional, Social, and Clinical Influences on Schizophrenic Patients." *The Journal of Nervous and Mental Disease* 181, no. 5 (May 1993): 283–89., Publisher: LIPPINCOTT WILLIAMS & WILKINS; PMID: 8501443

> The study was designed to explore the potential therapeutic effects of humor on hospitalized schizophrenics. For this purpose, in the first stage, we conducted a review of findings in regard to physical health, emotions, psychiatric state, and social behavior. In the second stage, we carried out an experiment with 34 resident patients in two chronic schizophrenic wards who were exposed to 70 movies during 3 months. The experimental group was exposed to humorous movies only, and the control group to different kinds of movies. Before and after the exposure to films for 3 months, both groups were tested on different health, emotional, social, and clinical measures using the Cognitive Orientation of Health Questionnaire, the Shalvata Symptom Rating Scale, blood pressure, heart rate, Perceived Verbal and Motor Aggression (rated by nurses), the Multiple Affect Adjective Check List, the Social Support Questionnaire 6, and the Brief Psychiatric Rating Scale (BPRS; rated by psychiatrists). Covariance analyses yielded significant reductions in Perceived Verbal Hostility, BPRS scales (total score, anxiety/depression), and significant increases in BPRS (activation) and degree of staff support experienced by the patients. The results indicate that the effects of exposure to humor may be mediated by the effects on the staff of the incidental exposure to humorous films.

Humorous Movies Reduce Levels of Psychopathology of Schizophrenics

Gelkopf, M., et al., "Therapeutic Use of Humor to Improve Social Support in an Institutionalized Schizophrenic Inpatient Community." *The Journal of Social Psychology* 134, no. 2 (April 1994): 175–82. Publisher: American Psychological Association doi:10.1080/00224545.1994.9711380., PMID: 17102716

> "Reduced levels of psychopathology, anger, anxiety, and depression symptoms and improvement in social competence were reveled in the study group."

The Use of Humor with Chronic Schizophrenic Patients Raises Patient Self-esteem

Witztum E., et al., "The Use of Humor with Chronic Schizophrenic Patients." *Journal of Contemporary Psychotherapy*, Volume 29, Number 3, 1999, pp 223-234 (12), Publisher: SPRINGER NEW YORK LLC

> The use of humorous therapeutic approach combined with drug therapy in the treatment of chronic schizophrenia patients institutionalized for prorated periods of time led to positive changes in their symptoms. The majority of the patients responded well to humorous interpretations. The patients felt that they had the option of adopting the doctor's humorous manner. This approach appealed to them and raised self-esteem; they likewise gained confidence in their own ability to form judgments. They cooperated better with the doctor in issues pertaining to treatment. The fact that humor made an impact on the patient's cognition was evaluated according to the BPRS scale, before the treatment, on a monthly basis during the treatment, and three months upon the completion of the experiment. In the course of the experiment, pharmacological treatment remained unchanged. On average, a perceptible reduction in the BPRS value (p<.05) was detected as a result of humor therapy. Amusing representations of affective external stimuli were incorporated into the patient's cognition and, along with a newly gained awareness of the possibility of relating to them with humor, were retained long after the termination of the project.

Music Therapy

Karaoke Therapy is Effective at Improving Social Interaction in Mental Patients

Leung, C. M., et al., "Karaoke Therapy in the Rehabilitation of Mental Patients." *Singapore Medical Journal* 39, no. 4 (April 1998): 166–68., Publisher: SINGAPORE MEDICAL ASSOCIATION; PMID: 9676147

> Karaoke therapy may be more effective than simple singing in improving social interaction. There is preliminary evidence that it may be anxiety-provoking for unstable schizophrenic patients. More research is required for further elucidation of the characteristics of favourable candidates, optimal schedule and active components of the therapy.

Music Improvisation Improves Schizophrenics Self-assessment Scores

Pfeiffer, H., et al., "Music improvisation with schizophrenic patients--a controlled study in the assessment of therapeutic effects]." *Die Rehabilitation* 26, no. 4 (November 1987): 184–92., Publisher: wdv, Ges. für Medien und Kommunikation; PMID: 3423420

> The effects of a course of music therapy with free improvisation, consisting of 27 sessions over a period of 6 months, were examined in a controlled study of matched therapy and waiting group, each comprising 7 patients with a diagnosis of schizophrenia or schizoaffective psychosis. The psychopathologic picture having essentially remained unaltered on the measuring instrument used (Lorr scales), significant positive changes were found in the self-assessment questionnaires completed by the participants. Improvements in recreational and social behaviours could not be shown. The disease and reintegration processes took similarly positive courses in both groups, supported by the

extensive range of psychiatric/psychotherapeutic services available in the Munich area. The improvising orientation of the music therapy course had mostly been approved of by the patients, it however also gave rise to a desire for more structuring and a more goal-directed therapeutic approach. A tendency towards the initial values, i.e. a deterioration, was stated in the therapy group at follow-up six months post-therapy.

Music Therapy May Diminish Schizophrenic Symptoms

Na, Hyun-Joo, et al., "[Effects of listening to music on auditory hallucination and psychiatric symptoms in people with schizophrenia]." *Journal of Korean Academy of Nursing* 39, no. 1 (February 2009): 62–71. Publisher: Korean Society of Nursing Science doi:10.4040/jkan.2009.39.1.62., PMID: 19265313

> ➤ "....listening to music may be useful for managing auditory hallucinations in schizophrenic inpatients.

Ulrich, G. "The Additional Therapeutic Effect of Group Music Therapy for Schizophrenic Patients: A Randomized Study." *Acta Psychiatrica Scandinavica* 116, no. 5 (November 2007): 362–70. Publisher: BLACKWELL MUNKSGAARD; doi:10.1111/j.1600-0447.2007.01073.x., PMID: 17919155

> ➤ "Musical activity diminishes negative symptoms and improves interpersonal contact."

Tang, W., et al., "Rehabilitative Effect of Music Therapy for Residual Schizophrenia. A One-Month Randomised Controlled Trial in Shanghai." *The British Journal of Psychiatry. Supplement,* no. 24 (August 1994): 38–44., Publisher: ROYAL MEDICO-PSYCHOLOGICAL ASSOCIATION; PMID: 7946230

> ➤ "Music therapy significantly diminished patient's negative symptoms, increasing their ability to converse with one another."

Mössler, Karin, et al., "Music Therapy for People with Schizophrenia and Schizophrenia-like Disorders." *The Cochrane Database of Systematic Reviews,* no. 12 (2011): CD004025. doi:10.1002/14651858.CD004025.pub3., Publisher: WILEY INTERSCIENCE ;PMID: 22161383

> ➤ Music therapy as an addition to standard care helps people with schizophrenia to improve their global state, mental state (including negative symptoms) and social functioning if a sufficient number of music therapy sessions are provided by qualified music therapists. Further research should especially address the long-term effects of music therapy, dose-response relationships, as well as the relevance of outcomes measures in relation to music therapy.

CODEX ALTERNUS

Music Therapy Could Be a Useful Adjunct to Pharmacotherapy during In-Patient Hospital Stay

---

Morgan, K., et al., "A Controlled Trial Investigating the Effect of Music Therapy during an Acute Psychotic Episode." *Acta Psychiatrica Scandinavica* 124, no. 5 (November 2011): 363–71. Publisher: BLACKWELL MUNKSGAARD; doi:10.1111/j.1600-0447.2011.01739.x, PMID: 21740403

> Statistically significant changes in BPRS scores were seen in the treatment group (n = 25) compared with the control group (n = 24). No significant differences were seen in the results of the Calgary, NOSIE-30 or DASS21 scores. Despite the treatment group, having a 9.3% decrease in their length of stay in hospital as opposed to the control group, this did not reach statistical significance. No significant differences were found when comparing the two groups in their doses of antipsychotic, benzodiazepine, mood stabilising or antidepressant medication or at the 1-month follow-up assessment.

Music Alleviates Cognitive Dysfunction in Schizophrenia

Glicksohn, J., et al., "Can Music Alleviate Cognitive Dysfunction in Schizophrenia?" *Psychopathology* 33, no. 1 (February 2000): 43–47. Publisher: S./KARGER AG ; doi:29118., PMID: 10601827

> It has recently been reported that students performed relatively better on cognitive tasks after listening to music. Conceivably, music might reduce the level of arousal in subjects who are tense, thereby improving their performance. A test case would be schizophrenic subjects, noted for poor performance on tasks demanding attention, who have been characterized as suffering from hyperarousal, which mediates these attentional deficits. We investigated whether cognitive task performance could be facilitated by music in schizophrenics and report a beneficial effect.

Nature Therapy

Horticulture Therapy May Be an Effective Treatment for Schizophrenia

---

Kamioka, Hiroharu, et al., "Effectiveness of Horticultural Therapy: A Systematic Review of Randomized Controlled Trials." *Complementary Therapies in Medicine* 22, no. 5 (October 2014): 930–43. Publisher: CHURCHILL LIVINGSTONE; doi:10.1016/j.ctim.2014.08.009., PMID: 25440385

> Although there was insufficient evidence in the studies of HT due to poor methodological and reporting quality and heterogeneity, HT may be an effective treatment for mental and behavioral disorders such as dementia, schizophrenia, depression, and terminal-care for cancer.

Reliable Evidence Supports the Effectiveness of Nature-assisted Therapy for Psychiatric Illness

> **Annerstedt, Matilda,** et al., "Nature-Assisted Therapy: Systematic Review of Controlled and Observational Studies." *Scandinavian Journal of Public Health* 39, no. 4 (June 2011): 371–88. Publisher: TAYLOR & FRANCIS A S; doi:10.1177/1403494810396400., PMID: 21273226

> ➤ This review gives at hand that a rather small but reliable evidence base supports the effectiveness and appropriateness of NAT as a relevant resource for public health. Significant improvements were found for varied outcomes in diverse diagnoses, spanning from obesity to schizophrenia. Recommendations for specific areas of future research of the subject are provided.

Adventure and Recreation Based Group Intervention Promotes Well Being and Weight Loss in Schizophrenia

> **Voruganti, Lakshmi N. P.,** et al., "Going beyond: An Adventure- and Recreation-Based Group Intervention Promotes Well-Being and Weight Loss in Schizophrenia." *Canadian Journal of Psychiatry. Revue Canadienne De Psychiatrie* 51, no. 9 (August 2006): 575–80., Publisher: CANADIAN PSYCHIATRIC ASSOCIATION. PMID: 17007224

> ➤ Treatment adherence was 97%, and there were no dropouts. Patients in the study group showed marginal improvement in perceived cognitive abilities and on domain-specific functioning measures but experienced a significant improvement in their self-esteem and global functioning ($P < 0.05$), as well as a weight loss of over 12 lb. Improvement was sustained over 1 year with further occupational and social gains. In the context of overcoming barriers to providing early intervention for youth and preventing metabolic problems among older adults with schizophrenia, adventure and recreation-based interventions could play a useful complementary role.

Outdoor Adventure Camp for People with Mental illness Demonstrates Significant Improvements in Mastery, Self-esteem, and Social Connectedness

> **Cotton, Sue,** et al., "Outdoor Adventure Camps for People with Mental Illness." *Australasian Psychiatry: Bulletin of Royal Australian and New Zealand College of Psychiatrists* 21, no. 4 (August 2013): 352–58. Publisher: BLACKWELL PUBLISHING ASIA doi:10.1177/1039856213492351., PMID: 23828947

> ➤ "Participants demonstrated significant improvements in mastery, self-esteem and social connectedness from baseline to end of the camp; however, these improvements were not sustained by the four-week follow-up."

CODEX ALTERNUS

Gardening May Be a Therapeutic Form of Exercise for Schizophrenia

Sullivan, M. E., et al., "Horticultural Therapy--the Role Gardening Plays in Healing." *Journal - American Health Care Association* 5, no. 3 (May 1979): 3, 5–6, 8., Publisher: AMERICAN HEALTH CARE ASSOCIATION. PMID: 10316809

> ➤ Horticultural therapy is an adjunct therapy--to be used in addition to occupational and physical therapies, and combining means used by both. It is meant to increase the motivation of the physically and/or mentally handicapped, while at the same time stimulating the five senses and furnishing a means of self-gratification and self-esteem. Now that neurologically orientated psychologists are identifying schizophrenia as being biologically based and capable of being reversed with exercise, it is time to study the many benefits of gardening as a therapy method.

Community Coping Skills Enhanced by an Adventure Camp for Chronic Adult Psychiatric Patients

Banaka, W. H., et al., "Community Coping Skills Enhanced by an Adventure Camp for Adult Chronic Psychiatric Patients." *Hospital & Community Psychiatry* 36, no. 7 (July 1985): 746–48., Publisher: THE ASSOCIATION; PMID: 4018750

> ➤ The effect of a two-week wilderness camp on ten skill areas related to community survival of the chronic mentally ill was assessed both by participants, who were adult chronic psychiatric patients from two Oregon state mental hospitals, and by camp and hospital staff. Compared with 30 controls, the 48 participants improved on seven of the ten areas by the end of camp and maintained their improvements in four of the seven areas for several weeks following their return to the hospital. Although discharge and recidivism rates for participants and controls did not differ at six-month follow-up, participants spent a greater proportion of time in the community than did controls. The authors discuss the specific skills improved by the program and those that contributed to duration of community survival, as well as the program's cost-effectiveness.

Sailing Can Improve Quality of Life of People with Severe Mental Disorders

Carta, Mauro Giovanni, et al., "Sailing Can Improve Quality of Life of People with Severe Mental Disorders: Results of a Cross over Randomized Controlled Trial." *Clinical Practice and Epidemiology in Mental Health: CP & EMH* 10 (2014): 80–86. Publisher: BIOMED CENTRAL LTD.doi:10.2174/1745017901410010080., PMID: 25191521

> ➤ The aim of this study was to evaluate the impact of a sailing rehabilitation program on the quality of life (QoL) in a sample of patients with severe mental disorders. The study adopted a randomized, crossover, waiting-list controlled design. The participants enrolled in the study were outpatients diagnosed with severe chronic mental disorders.

The participants (N=40) exposed to rehabilitation with sailing took part in a series of supervised cruises near the gulf of Cagliari, South Sardinia, and showed a statistically significant improvement of their quality of life compared to the control group. This improvement was comparable to the improvement in psychopathologic status and social functioning as shown in a previous report of the same research project. The improvement was maintained at follow-up only during the trial and for a few months later: after 12 months, patients returned to their baseline values and their quality of life showed a worsening trend. This is the first study to show that rehabilitation with sailing may improve the quality of life of people with severe chronic mental disorders. In all likelihood, a program grounded on learning how to manage a sailing vessel - during which patients perform cruises that emphasize the exploration of the marine environment by sailing - might be interesting enough and capture the attention of the patients so as to favour greater effectiveness of standard rehabilitation protocols, but this should be specifically tested.

Photography

Article Demonstrates How Real Life Photo Stories Can Help Patients Reformulate Meaning and Clinicians Can Broaden Their Understanding of Practice

Sitvast, J. E., et al., "Photo Stories, Ricoeur, and Experiences from Practice: A Hermeneutic Dialogue." *ANS. Advances in Nursing Science* 31, no. 3 (September 2008): 268–79. doi:10.1097/01.ANS.0000334290.04225.be., PMID: 18724116

> The purpose of this article is to demonstrate how a particular narrative approach in nursing, namely the photo instrument can be connected with Ricoeur's hermeneutic philosophy. Ricoeur's concept of mimesis, when supplemented with the concept of performance, is shown relevant for understanding how patients construct and reformulate meaning in illness experiences. A single-case study is presented for a tentative exploration of how the key concepts of mimesis and performance can broaden our understanding of practice. More specifically it concerned the use of photographs in a group with psychiatric patients.

Photography is a Way to Capture and Reflect on the World of a Persons Life with Mental Illness

Erdner, Anette, et al., "Photography as a Method of Data Collection: Helping People with Long-Term Mental Illness to Convey Their Life World." *Perspectives in Psychiatric Care* 47, no. 3 (July 2011): 145–50. doi:10.1111/j.1744-6163.2010.00283.x. , PMID: 21707630

> When auto photography is used, the world inhabited by the participants is captured while, at the same time, they seek to reflect the worlds they live in. These life worlds are the patients' source of material and what is reflected in their narratives and pictures.

There is a need for more studies to investigate photography as a qualitative research tool in mental health. Nurses can use this tool to discover the life worlds of the patients they treat and study.

Play Therapy

Play Therapy can be used in Treatment of Hebephrenia Schizophrenia

> **Hudson, W. C.,** et al., "Play Therapy in the Treatment of Hebephrenia." *Psychotherapy and Psychosomatics* 26, no. 5 (1975): 286–93., Publisher: S./KARGER AG; PMID: 1234663

> ➢ This paper has attempted to outline a multiple technique therapy designed for the treatment of hebephrenia. The first phase of the technique utilizes play therapy, followed by an interchange of therapist and patient's drawings, and finally, analytic psychotherapy. These three phases may be characterized, respectively, as expressive, expressive-communicative, and communicative.

Television Therapy

Television Therapy with Closed Circuit and Commercial Television Combined Improved Behavior 16.2%

> **Lewis, R. B.,** et al., "Television Therapy; Effectiveness of Closed-Circuit Television as a Medium for Therapy in Treatment of the Mentally Ill." *A.M.A. Archives of Neurology and Psychiatry* 77, no. 1 (January 1957): 57–69., PMID: 13381217

> ➢ Comparisons were made for the control group (no television and commercial television), and the experimental group (commercial television and closed-circuit television); the results of these comparisons were based on scores computed from the rating/rerating for each group on the Hospital Adjustment Scale (Table 3). These data revealed that the addition of a commercial television set on the control ward improved group behavior patterns 5.1% in three months, and the addition of closed circuit television to the experimental ward, following 20 months of commercial television, improved group behavior patterns 9.4%. The use of closed-circuit television plus commercial television resulted in an average improvement in behavior for the experimental group of 16.2%.

Electric Brain Stimulation Therapies

Cranial Electrotherapy

Cranial Electrotherapy Stimulation Reduces Aggression in Violent Schizophrenic Patient

CODEX ALTERNUS

Childs, Allen, et al., "Cranial Electrotherapy Stimulation Reduces Aggression in a Violent Retarded Population: A Preliminary Report." *The Journal of Neuropsychiatry and Clinical Neurosciences* 17, no. 4 (2005): 548–51. Publisher: AMERICAN PSYCHIATRIC PUBLISHING, INC. doi:10.1176/appi.neuropsych.17.4.548., PMID: 16387997

> ➤ Nine aggressive, retarded patients refractory to conventional care at a maximum security hospital were given a 3-month course of cranial electrotherapy stimulation. Aggressive episodes declined 59% from baseline; seclusions were down 72%; restraints were down 58%; and use of prescribedas needed sedative medications decreased 53%. The most dramatic change was that of a disorganized, schizophrenic patient whose aggressive episodes declined from 62 to 9, seclusions from 53 to 8, restraints from 9 to 1 and PRNs from 25 to 1. No patients discontinued cranial electrotherapy stimulation (CES) because of side effects. This preliminary report indicates that CES appears to be an efficacious, safe, and cost-effective addition to the treatment regimen in this patient population.

Neuro-electric Therapy

Neuro-electric Therapy is an Effective Treatment for Schizophrenia and Affective Psychosis

Klimke, A., et al., "[Effectiveness of neuro-electric therapy in drug resistant endogenous psychoses]." *Fortschritte Der Neurologie-Psychiatrie* 59, no. 2 (February 1991): 53–59. Publisher: Thieme; doi:10.1055/s-2007-1000679., PMID: 1673954

> ➤ A retrospective chart review of 50 pharmacotherapeutically resistant patients was performed after treatment with NET in 1986-1988. 28 patients suffered from schizophrenia and 22 from affective psychosis. In contrast to literature where NET as therapy of first choice has favourable results in depression in this study 60.7% of the treatment resistant acute schizophrenics responded well to NET. 3 months after discharge from hospital 9 schizophrenics (32.1%) but only 3 patients with affective psychosis (13.6%) presented a 'good' outcome (full remission). A longer duration of schizophrenia (more than 5 years since first manifestation) and a good response to neuroleptics in history was predictive for a good actual NET response (14 of 17 patients), whereas 7 of 11 patients suffering from schizophrenia less than 3 years without any period of full remission on neuroleptics were also non-responders to NET.

Transcranial Direct Current Stimulation

Transcranial Direct Current Stimulation May Be Effective for Treatment Catatonic Schizophrenia

Shiozawa, Pedro, et al., "Transcranial Direct Current Stimulation (tDCS) for Catatonic Schizophrenia: A Case Study." *Schizophrenia Research* 146, no. 1–3 (May 2013): 374–75. Publisher: ELSEVIER BV; doi:10.1016/j.schres.2013.01.030., PMID: 23434501

➢ The intervention protocol consisted in 10 consecutive daily tDCS sessions (including the weekend). The cathode was positioned over the right and the anode over the left dorsolateral prefrontal cortex. We used a direct current of 2.0 mA for 20 mn. The 35 cm_2-rubber electrodes were wrapped in cotton material, which was moistened with saline to reduce impedance. For, assessment of catatonic symptoms we used the Bush-Francis catatonic scale, a widely used assessment tool in clinical practice that account for the main symptoms of schizophrenia. As shown in Fig. 1, catatonic symptoms substantially improved during the treatment course. After one month of treatment, she progressively started to perform eye and verbal contact with the medical team and engaged in daily activities such as eating, walking and showering without help. After four months, the patients remain without catatonic symptoms.

Transcranial Direct Current Stimulation May be a Promising Tool for the Treatment of Negative Symptoms in Schizophrenia

Palm, Ulrich, et al., "Prefrontal Transcranial Direct Current Stimulation (tDCS) Changes Negative Symptoms and Functional Connectivity MRI (fcMRI) in a Single Case of Treatment-Resistant Schizophrenia." *Schizophrenia Research* 150, no. 2–3 (November 2013): 583–85. Publisher: ELSEVIER BV; doi:10.1016/j.schres.2013.08.043., PMID: 24060570

➢ In conclusion, anodal tDCS of the left DLPFC seems to be a promising tool for the treatment of negative symptoms in schizophrenia and may even alter positive symptoms. However, randomized controlled trials are needed for investigating the specific action of tDCS on the symptom spectrum in schizophrenia, using different electrode placements and stimulation protocols.

Once to Twice Daily Transcranial Direct Current Stimulation is Effective for Severe Clozapine Refractory Continuous Auditory Hallucinations in Schizophrenia

Andrade, Chittaranjan, et al., "Once- to Twice-Daily, 3-Year Domiciliary Maintenance Transcranial Direct Current Stimulation for Severe, Disabling, Clozapine-Refractory Continuous Auditory Hallucinations in Schizophrenia." *The Journal of ECT* 29, no. 3 (September 2013): 239–42. Publisher: International Society for ECT and Neurostimulation; doi:10.1097/YCT.0b013e3182843866., PMID: 23377748

➢ Once daily, 20-minute tDCS sessions at 1-mA intensity produced noticeable improvement within a week: cognitive and psychosocial functioning improved, followed by attenuation in the experience of hallucinations. There was greater than 90% self-reported improvement within 2 months. Benefits accelerated when the current was raised to 3 mA; treatment duration was increased to 30-minute sessions, and session frequency was increased to twice daily. The patient improved from a psychosocially vegetative state to near-normal functioning. Once- to twice-daily domiciliary tDCS was continued across nearly 3 years and is still ongoing. Benefits attenuated or were even lost when alternate day session spacing was attempted, or when electrode positioning was changed; benefits were regained when the original stimulation protocol was reintroduced. There was confirmation of benefit in 2 separate on-off-on situations, which occurred inadvertently and under blinded conditions. There were no adverse events attributable to tDCS.

Add-on Transcranial Direct Current Stimulation is Effective for Rapid Amelioration of Auditory Hallucinations in Schizophrenics

Shivakumar, Venkataram, et al., "Rapid Improvement of Auditory Verbal Hallucinations in Schizophrenia after Add-on Treatment with Transcranial Direct-Current Stimulation." *The Journal of ECT* 29, no. 3 (September 2013): e43–44. Publisher: International Society for ECT and Neurostimulation; doi:10.1097/YCT.0b013e318290fa4d., PMID: 23965609

➢ Treatment of nonresponsive auditory hallucinations in schizophrenia have been reported to improve with transcranial direct-current stimulation. This case description illustrates the use of add-on transcranial direct-current stimulation for rapid amelioration of auditory hallucinations in schizophrenia during the acute phase. Because transcranial direct-current stimulation is safe, largely well tolerated, and relatively inexpensive, this add-on treatment option is worth exploring through further rigorous studies.

Transcranial Direct Current Stimulation Improves Treatment-resistant Auditory Hallucinations in Schizophrenic Patient

Nawani, Hema, et al., "Neural Basis of tDCS Effects on Auditory Verbal Hallucinations in Schizophrenia: A Case Report Evidence for Cortical Neuroplasticity Modulation." *The Journal of ECT* 30, no. 1 (March 2014): e2–4. doi:10.1097/YCT.0b013e3182a35492., Publisher: International Society for ECT and Neurostimulation; PMID: 24080544

➢ Transcranial direct current stimulation (tDCS) has been reported to ameliorate auditory hallucinations that are nonresponsive/minimally responsive to antipsychotic treatment in schizophrenia. The neurobiological basis of the tDCS effects in ameliorating auditory hallucinations is yet to be explored. In this case report, for the first time, using the novel method for noninvasive assessment of cortical plasticity, we demonstrate potential neuroplasticity effect of tDCS in improving treatment-resistant auditory hallucinations in a schizophrenic patient.

Transcranial Random Noise Stimulation

Transcranial Random Noise Stimulation is a Sustainable Treatment in Drug-free Schizophrenic Patients

CODEX ALTERNUS

Haesebaert, Frederic, et al., "Efficacy and Safety of Fronto-Temporal Transcranial Random Noise Stimulation (tRNS) in Drug-Free Patients with Schizophrenia: A Case Study." *Schizophrenia Research* 159, no. 1 (October 2014): 251–52. Publisher: ELSEVIER BV doi:10.1016/j.schres.2014.07.043., PMID: 25129852

➤ "This case illustrates for the first time that fronto-temporal high frequency tRNS seems to be a sustainable treatment in drug-free patients with schizophrenia, alleviating delusions and enhancing insight of the illness."

Modest Clinical Improvement was shown with Transcranial Random Noise Stimulation for the Treatment of Schizophrenia

Palm, Ulrich, et al., "Transcranial Random Noise Stimulation for the Treatment of Negative Symptoms in Schizophrenia." *Schizophrenia Research* 146, no. 1–3 (May 2013): 372–73. Publisher: ELSEVIER BV; doi:10.1016/j.schres.2013.03.003., PMID: 23517664

➤ At baseline, the patient presented with a Positive and Negative Symptom Scale (PANSS) score of 102 (subscales: positive 9, negative 34, cognition 32, excitement/hostility 4, depression/anxiety 23), a Scale for the Assessment of Negative Symptoms (SANS) score of 73, and a Calgary Depression Scale in Schizophrenia (CDSS) score of 6. For the Trail Making Test (TMT), he needed 19 s (TMT-A) and 55 s (TMT-B). After 20 stimulations he showed a modest clinical improvement in the domain of negative symptoms (i.e. emotional withdrawal, poor rapport, lack of spontaneity), cognition (i.e. disorganization, difficulties in abstract thinking, and disturbance of volition) and depression/anxiety: PANSS score 68 (subscales: positive 5, negative 21, cognition 25, excitement/hostility 4, depression/anxiety 13), SANS score 48, CDSS score 5, TMT-A 17 s, TMT-B 38 s. tRNS was well tolerated and there were no adverse effects. However, there are some limitations: clinical improvement could also be due to non-specific effects of the treatment or a delayed onset of medication effects. Furthermore, information processing (TMT-A) and executive functioning (TMT-B) were intact at baseline and the modest improvement could be due to learning effects. There also may be several factors limiting the efficacy of tRNS, e.g. chronicity of the disease, short duration of treatment and concomitant medication (Fertonani et al.,2011). For example, lamotrigine and pregabaline may potentially decrease the neuromodulatory effects of tRNS by blocking the opening of voltage-gated sodium channels (lamotrigine) or voltage-gated calcium channels (pregabaline) (Nitsche et al., 2012). However, this case report supports the findings of cognitive enhancement by excitatory noninvasive electrical brain stimulation (Kuo and Nitsche, 2012; Nitsche et al., 2012). Thus, therapeutic effects of tRNS in psychiatric disorders merit systematic investigation.

Alternative Reality

Avatar Therapy

Avatar Therapy is Effective for Persecutory Auditory Hallucinations

CODEX ALTERNUS

Leff, Julian, et al., "Avatar Therapy for Persecutory Auditory Hallucinations: What Is It and How Does It Work?" *Psychosis* 6, no. 2 (June 2014): 166–76. Publisher: Routledge doi:10.1080/17522439.2013.773457., PMID: 24999369

> We have developed a novel therapy based on a computer program, which enables the patient to create an avatar of the entity, human or non-human, which they believe is persecuting them. The therapist encourages the patient to enter into a dialogue with their avatar, and is able to use the program to change the avatar so that it comes under the patient's control over the course of six 30-min sessions and alters from being abusive to becoming friendly and supportive. The therapy was evaluated in a randomised controlled trial with a partial crossover design. One group went straight into the therapy arm: "immediate therapy". The other continued with standard clinical care for 7 weeks then crossed over into Avatar therapy: "delayed therapy". There was a significant reduction in the frequency and intensity of the voices and in their omnipotence and malevolence. Several individuals had a dramatic response, their voices ceasing completely after a few sessions of the therapy. The average effect size of the therapy was 0.8. We discuss the possible psychological mechanisms for the success of Avatar therapy and the implications for the origins of persecutory voices.

Computer-assisted Therapy for Medication-resistant Auditory Hallucinations

Leff, Julian, et al., "Computer-Assisted Therapy for Medication-Resistant Auditory Hallucinations: Proof-of-Concept Study." *The British Journal of Psychiatry: The Journal of Mental Science* 202 (June 2013): 428–33. Publisher: ROYAL MEDICO-PSYCHOLOGICAL ASSOCIATION; doi:10.1192/bjp.bp.112.124883., PMID: 23429202

> Avatar therapy was evaluated by a randomized, single blind, partial crossover trial comparing the novel therapy with treatment as usual (TAU). We used three main outcome measures: (a) the Psychotic Symptom Rating Scale (PSYRATS), hallucination section; (b) the Omnipotence and Malevolence subscales of Revised Beliefs About Voices Questionnaire (BAVQ-R); and (c) the Calgary Depression Scale (CDS). The control group showed no change over time in their scores on three assessments, whereas the novel therapy group showed mean reductions in total PSYRATS score (auditory hallucinations) of 8.75 (P=0.003) and in the BAVQ-R combined score of omnipotence and malevolence of the voices of 5.88 (P=0.004). There was no significant reduction in the CDS total score for depression. For the crossover group, comparison of the period of the TAU with the period of avatar therapy confirmed the findings of the previous analysis. The effect size of therapy was 0.8. Avatar therapy represents a promising treatment for medication resistant auditory hallucinations.

Video Games

Videogames as Game Therapy are Attractive, Safe, and Easy to Monitor

CODEX ALTERNUS

Samoilovich, S., et al., "Attitude of Schizophrenics to Computer Videogames." *Psychopathology* 25, no. 3 (1992): 117–19., Publisher: S./KARGER AG; PMID: 1448536

> ➤ "Considered as labor or game therapy, the games are attractive, safe and easy to monitor, even in defected patients. The value of continued use of videogames in individual or group sessions merits to be investigated."

Video Game Training could be Used to Counteract Risk Factors Such as Smaller Hippocampus and Prefrontal Cortex in Schizophrenia

Kühn, S., et al., "Playing Super Mario Induces Structural Brain Plasticity: Gray Matter Changes Resulting from Training with a Commercial Video Game." *Molecular Psychiatry* 19, no. 2 (February 2014): 265–71. Publisher: NATURE PUBLISHING GROUP doi:10.1038/mp.2013.120., PMID: 24166407

> ➤ Video gaming is a highly pervasive activity, providing a multitude of complex cognitive and motor demands. Gaming can be seen as an intense training of several skills. Associated cerebral structural plasticity induced has not been investigated so far. Comparing a control with a video gaming training group that was trained for 2 months for at least 30 min per day with a platformer game, we found significant gray matter (GM) increase in right hippocampal formation (HC), right dorsolateral prefrontal cortex (DLPFC) and bilateral cerebellum in the training group. The HC increase correlated with changes from egocentric to allocentric navigation strategy. GM increases in HC and DLPFC correlated with participants' desire for video gaming, evidence suggesting a predictive role of desire in volume change. Video game training augments GM in brain areas crucial for spatial navigation, strategic planning, working memory and motor performance going along with evidence for behavioral changes of navigation strategy. The presented video game training could therefore be used to counteract known risk factors for mental disease such as smaller hippocampus and prefrontal cortex volume in, for example, post-traumatic stress disorder, schizophrenia and neurodegenerative disease.

Video Games Used to Treat Mental Disorders Including Schizophrenia

Fernández-Aranda, et al., "Video Games as a Complementary Therapy Tool in Mental Disorders: PlayMancer, a European Multicentre Study." *Journal of Mental Health (Abingdon, England)* 21, no. 4 (August 2012): 364–74. Publisher: ROUTLEDGE doi:10.3109/09638237.2012.664302., PMID: 22548300

> ➤ The video game was created and developed within the European research project PlayMancer. It aims to prove potential capacity to change underlying attitudinal, behavioural and emotional processes of patients with impulse-related disorders. New interaction modes were provided by newly developed components, such as emotion

recognition from speech, face and physiological reactions, while specific impulsive reactions were elicited. The video game uses biofeedback for helping patients to learn relaxation skills, acquire better self-control strategies and develop new emotional regulation strategies. In this article, we present a description of the video game used, rationale, user requirements, usability and preliminary data, in several mental disorders.

Internet Video Game Play was found to Have Clinical Improvement and Could Be an Adjunctive Treatment for Rehabilitation of Schizophrenic Patients

> **Han, Doug Hyun,** et al., "The Effect of Internet Video Game Play on Clinical and Extrapyramidal Symptoms in Patients with Schizophrenia." *Schizophrenia Research* 103, no. 1–3 (August 2008): 338–40. Publisher: ELSEVIER BV; doi:10.1016/j.schres.2008.01.026., PMID: 18304782

> ➤ To the best of our knowledge, this is the first clinical study to assess psychiatric symptoms and EPS in schizophrenic patients who engage in internet videogame play. In addition, the current study also showed that EPS in IVP-SCZ was improved, as compared to nIVP-SCZ. Based on the current findings of improvement in clinical symptoms and EPS, we suggest that limited internet video game play could be considered as an adjunctive treatment and rehabilitation modality for patients with schizophrenia.

Virtual Reality

Virtual Reality-Integrated Program May Be Effective for Improving Social Skills

> **Rus-Calafell, Mar,** et al., "A Virtual Reality-Integrated Program for Improving Social Skills in Patients with Schizophrenia: A Pilot Study." *Journal of Behavior Therapy and Experimental Psychiatry* 45, no. 1 (March 2014): 81–89. Publisher: PERGAMON doi:10.1016/j.jbtep.2013.09.002., PMID: 24063993

> ➤ The results of a series of repeated measures ANOVA revealed significant improvement in negative symptoms, psychopathology, social anxiety and discomfort, avoidance and social functioning. Objective scores obtained through the use of the VR program showed a pattern of learning in emotion perception, assertive behaviours and time spent in a conversation. Most of these gains were maintained at four-month follow-up. The results showed that the intervention may be effective for improving social dysfunction. The use of the VR program contributed to the generalisation of new skills into the patient's everyday functioning.

Virtual Reality for Treatment of Schizophrenia

> **Da Costa, Rosa Maria,** et al., "The Acceptance of Virtual Reality Devices for Cognitive Rehabilitation: A Report of Positive Results with Schizophrenia." *Computer Methods and Programs in Biomedicine* 73, no. 3 (March 2004): 173–82. Publisher: ELSEVIER IRELAND LTD; doi:10.1016/S0169-2607(03)00066-X., PMID: 14980398

> ➢ "The subjects that participated in this experiment accepted to work with computers and immersive glasses and demonstrated a high level of interest in the proposed tasks. No problems of illness have been observed."

Virtual Reality for Paranoia

> **Fornells-Ambrojo, Miriam,** et al., "Virtual Reality and Persecutory Delusions: Safety and Feasibility." *Schizophrenia Research* 104, no. 1–3 (September 2008): 228–36. Publisher: ELSEVIER BV; doi:10.1016/j.schres.2008.05.013., PMID: 18571899

> ➢ "Exposure to social situations using VR has the potential to be incorporated into cognitive behavioral interventions for paranoia."

Virtual Reality Cognitive Training Program Offers Potential for Significant Gains in Cognitive Function in Older Adults with Schizophrenia

> **Chan, Christopher L. F.,** et al., "Effect of the Adapted Virtual Reality Cognitive Training Program among Chinese Older Adults with Chronic Schizophrenia: A Pilot Study." *International Journal of Geriatric Psychiatry* 25, no. 6 (June 2010): 643–49. Publisher: JOHN/WILEY & SONS LTD. doi:10.1002/gps.2403., PMID: 19806599

> ➢ After the 10-session intervention, older adults with chronic schizophrenia preformed significantly better than control in overall cognitive function (p .000), and in two cognitive subscales: repetition (p .001) and memory (p .040). These participants engaged in the VR activities volitionally. No problem of cybersickness was observed. The results of the current study indicate that engaging in the adapted virtual reality cognitive training program offers the potential for significant gains in cognitive function of the older adults with chronic schizophrenia.

Energy & Spiritual Healing

Exorcism

Exorcism used by Traditional Healer Cures Bedouin Patient

CODEX ALTERNUS

Al-Krenawi, Alean, "Spirit Possession and Exorcism in the Treatment of Bedouin Psychiatric Patient" *Clinical Social Work Journal,* Vol.25, No. 2, Summer 1997

A male Bedouin psychiatric patient was initially misdiagnosed and treated as a paranoid schizophrenic. The modern mental health care system correctly understood the "form" of the patient's symptoms, auditory and visual hallucinations. It did not however at first appreciate their "content", or cultural significance. The patient had unresolved anger toward his family which was manifested in an angry exchange with his mother. This exchange created guilt and the belief that the patient had sinned against God and was possessed by demons. A psychiatric social worker was able to reconcile the patient with his mother and to incorporate a traditional Bedouin healer, the Dervish, to exorcise the patient. The patient was cured by the Dervish, re-diagnosed as a neurotic by the modern system, and continued successfully with both systems for several months in follow-up treatment before being discharged.

Personal Belief System

Sound Spiritual, Religious or Personal Belief System is Associated with Adaptive Coping Skills in Schizophrenia

Shah, Ruchita, et al., "Relationship between Spirituality/religiousness and Coping in Patients with Residual Schizophrenia." *Quality of Life Research: An International Journal of Quality of Life Aspects of Treatment, Care and Rehabilitation* 20, no. 7 (September 2011): 1053–60. Publisher: SPRINGER-VERLAG DORDRECHT; doi:10.1007/s11136-010-9839-6., PMID: 21222165

> ➤ "A sound spiritual, religious, or personal belief system is associated with active and adaptive coping skills in subjects with residual schizophrenia. Understanding and assessing the spirituality and religiousness of subjects with schizophrenia can help in better management of the disorder."

Religion Has a Clinical Significance in the Care of Patients with Schizophrenia

Mohr, Sylvia, et al., "Toward an Integration of Spirituality and Religiousness into the Psychosocial Dimension of Schizophrenia." *The American Journal of Psychiatry* 163, no. 11 (November 2006): 1952–59. Publisher: AM PSYCHIATRIC ASSN doi:10.1176/appi.ajp.163.11.1952., PMID: 17074947

> ➤ Our results highlight the clinical significance of religion in the care of patients with schizophrenia. Religion is neither a strictly personal matter nor a strictly cultural one. Spirituality should be integrated into the psychosocial dimension of care. Our results suggest that the complexity of the relationship between religion and illness requires a highly sensitive approach to each unique story.

Prayer

Prayer May Offer Good Health and Contribute to the Healing of Trauma and Psychosis

Luhrmann, Tanya Marie, "Making God Real and Making God Good: Some Mechanisms through Which Prayer May Contribute to Healing." *Transcultural Psychiatry* 50, no. 5 (October 2013): 707–25. doi:10.1177/1363461513487670., PMID: 23793786

> ➢ This paper argues that another mechanism may be a positive relationship with the supernatural, a proposal that builds upon anthropological accounts of symbolic healing. Such a mechanism depends upon the learned cultivation of the imagination and the capacity to make what is imagined more real and more good. This paper offers a theory of the way that prayer enables this process and provides some evidence, drawn from experimental and ethnographic work, for the claim that a relationship with a loving God, cultivated through the imagination in prayer, may contribute to good health and may contribute to healing in trauma and psychosis.

Religious Support

Religious Support and Enduring with Faith Were Positively Associated with Recovery from Severe Mental Illness

Webb, Marcia, et al., "Struggling and Enduring with God, Religious Support, and Recovery from Severe Mental Illness." *Journal of Clinical Psychology* 67, no. 12 (December 2011): 1161–76. Publisher: American Psychological Association; doi:10.1002/jclp.20838., PMID: 22072528

> ➢ "Religious support and enduring with faith were positively associated with recovery. Struggling was negatively associated with recovery, and that relationship was mediated by religious support."

Spiritual Emotional Freedom Technique

Spiritual Emotional Freedom Technique (SEFT) is Effective in Schizophrenia

Puspitaningrum Ike, et al., "Effectiveness of Spiritual Emotional Freedom Technique (SEFT) Intervention in Schizophrenia with Depression, Anxiety, Stress." *Nursing Intervention, Complementary and Alternative Therapy, In JAVA International Nursing Conference* 2012 October 6-7, Semarang

> ➢ "The results of statistical tests concluded that the variables had a significant result (0.017). It can be concluded that SEFT intervention was effective to reduce depression anxiety stress levels in patients with schizophrenia."

Spiritual Healer

Help of a Spiritual Healer Led to Recovery in a Homeless Hispanic Man

Tsemberis, Sam et al., "The Role of an Espiritista in the Treatment of a Homeless, Mentally Ill Hispanic Man." *Psychiatric Services* 51: 1572-1574, 2000, PMID: 11097657

> This paper presents a case study from an emergency psychiatric outreach team that serves homeless and mentally ill persons in New York City. Mr. V was homeless and believed that he was possessed by evil spirits who were causing his physical and mental problems. He was hospitalized involuntarily twice for medical reasons, but he refused to cooperate in his treatment and returned to the streets after his first hospitalization. After one visit by a spiritual healer during his second hospitalization, Mr. V began to participate in his treatment. He was discharged to a nursing home, and after three years he had not returned to the streets.

Spiritually Oriented Group Therapy

Spiritually Oriented Group Therapy as a Tool for Healing Mental Illness

Sageman, Sharon, et al., "Breaking through the Despair: Spiritually Oriented Group Therapy as a Means of Healing Women with Severe Mental Illness." *The Journal of the American Academy of Psychoanalysis and Dynamic Psychiatry* 32, no. 1 (2004): 125–41., Publisher: GUILFORD PUBLICATIONS INC; PMID: 15132194

> ➢ Studies have shown that 96% of Americans believe in God and over 90% pray yet there is relatively little education available for clinicians on how to use spirituality as a tool for healing mental illness, particularly when treating very sick patients. This article illustrates how spiritually oriented group therapy with severely ill women can help to improve mood, affect, motivation, interpersonal bonding, and sense of self, and can succeed in reaching patients and promoting recovery in ways that traditional therapy cannot. Specific modalities including group prayer, yoga breathing, and spiritual readings are described. Breaking Through the Despair offers both a psychodynamic and a neurophysiologic perspective for understanding how this type of treatment helps patients transcend their mental illness and be able to grasp abstract spiritual concepts, develop a sense of belonging to a caring community, and integrate a new sense of themselves as productive and valued individuals.

Reiki & Pranic Healing

Energy Healing Shows Promise as a Complementary Treatment for Paranoid Schizophrenia

CODEX ALTERNUS

Chibber K., et al.,"Energy Healing as a Complementary Treatment for Paranoid Schizophrenia: A Case Report." *141st APHA Annual Meeting* (November 2-November 6, 2013) APHA 2013

> ➢ Energy Healing Treatments: The subject received 4 energy healing treatments daily for a period of 16 weeks, consisting of both Pranic healing and Reiki. Additional treatments were administered as necessary, when hallucinations or abnormal behavior persisted. Results: Subject noted feelings of lightness, with sustained periods of calmness and coherence. The subjects mother/father also observed changes in mood and behavior, including increased responsiveness and social proclivity. Hallucinations and erratic behavior diminished in frequency and magnitude. Physician recommended lowering lowering dosage of main antipsychotic based on observations. The subject continues to exhibit improvement. These results indicate Energy healing to be a potent and effective method of complementary therapy for schizophrenia.

Combination Therapies

Alpha Lipoic Acid and Niacinamide

Alpha Lipoic Acid and Niacinamide Help Preserve Mitrochondrial Integrity and Protect from Oxidative Stress which Contributes to the Pathophysiology of Schizophrenia

Seybolt, Sheila E. J., et al., "Is It Time to Reassess Alpha Lipoic Acid and Niacinamide Therapy in Schizophrenia?" *Medical Hypotheses* 75, no. 6 (December 2010): 572–75. Publisher: CHURCHILL LIVINGSTONE; doi:10.1016/j.mehy.2010.07.034., PMID: 20708342

> ➢ As sulfur containing thiols, alpha lipoic acid (ALA) and its reduced form dihydrolipoic acid (DHLA) are powerful antioxidants and free radical scavengers capable of performing many of the same functions as glutathione (GSH). ALA supplementation may help protect mitochondria from oxidative stress, a possible mechanism contributing to certain forms of brain diseases called schizophrenia. Shortly before the advent of antipsychotic medications, two small studies found ALA relieved psychiatric symptoms in schizophrenia. More recently, animal studies have shown ALA augmentation improves mitochondrial function. At pharmaceutical levels, niacinamide helps preserve mitochondrial membrane integrity and acts as an antioxidant. ALA is a precursor for lipoamide, an essential mitochondrial coenzyme and niacinamide is a component of niacinamide adenine dinucleotide (NAD). NADH, the reduced form of NAD, is involved in the reduction of ALA to DHLA within the mitochondria. This is relevant to contemporary research because DHLA increases GSH and low GSH levels contribute to mitochondrial dysfunction and oxidative stress which have been implicated in the pathophysiology of schizophrenia.

CODEX ALTERNUS

Antioxidants

Adjunctive Treatment with Antioxidants May Prevent Further Oxidative Injury and Deterioration Associated with Schizophrenia

Mahadik, S. P., et al., "Oxidative Injury and Potential Use of Antioxidants in Schizophrenia." *Prostaglandins, Leukotrienes, and Essential Fatty Acids* 55, no. 1–2 (August 1996): 45–54., Publisher: CHURCHILL LIVINGSTONE; PMID: 8888122

> ➤ "Adjunctive treatment with antioxidants (e.g. vitamins E and C, beta-carotene and quinones) at the initial stages of illness may prevent further oxidative injury and thereby ameliorate and prevent further possible deterioration of associated neurological and behavioral deficits in schizophrenia."

Antioxidants and Omega-3 fatty acids

Prevention of Oxidative Stress Neuropathology in Schizophrenia

Mahadik, Sahebarao P., et al., "Prevention of Oxidative Stress-Mediated Neuropathology and Improved Clinical Outcome by Adjunctive Use of a Combination of Antioxidants and Omega-3 Fatty Acids in Schizophrenia." *International Review of Psychiatry (Abingdon, England)* 18, no. 2 (April 2006): 119–31. Publisher: ROUTLEDGE doi:10.1080/09540260600581993., PMID:16777666

> ➤ In summary, oxidative stress and cell damage likely exist at very early stages of schizophrenia and if not treated early, it can trigger progressive deterioration of neuropathology and thereby symptomology; dietary antioxidants and omega-3 fatty acids are found to effectively prevent and restore the oxidative neuropathology and improve the outcome under a variety of situations. Moreover, these supplements are also found to prevent and cure important medical morbidities such as obesity, hypertension, diabetes, and cardiovascular abnormalities that are often associated with illness and treatment.

Bodywork and Psychotherapy

Combination of Bodywork and Psychotherapy can Enhance, Accelerate and Improve Therapy

Ventegodt, Søren, et al., "Clinical Holistic Medicine (mindful Short-Term Psychodynamic Psychotherapy Complimented with Bodywork) in the Treatment of Schizophrenia (ICD10-F20/DSM-IV Code 295) and Other Psychotic Mental Diseases." *TheScientificWorldJournal* (2007): 1987–2008. Publisher: Corpus Alienum Oy doi:10.1100/tsw.2007.298., PMID: 18167614

> Clinical holistic medicine (CHM) has developed into a system that can also be helpful with mentally ill patients. CHM therapy supports the patient through a series of emotionally challenging, existential, and healing crises. The patient's sense of coherence and mental health can be recovered through the process of feeling old repressed emotions, understanding life and self, and finally letting go of negative beliefs and delusions. The Bleuler's triple condition of autism, disturbed thoughts, and disturbed emotions that characterizes the schizophrenic patient can be understood as arising from the early defense of splitting, caused by negative learning from painful childhood traumas that made the patient lose sense of coherence and withdraw from social contact. Self-insight gained through the therapy can allow the patients to take their bodily, mental, and spiritual talents into use. At the end of therapy, the patients are once again living a life of quality centered on their life mission and they relate to other people in a way that systematically creates value. There are a number of challenges meeting the therapist who works with schizophrenic and psychotic patients, from the potential risk of experiencing a patient's violence, to the obligation to contain the most difficult and embarrassing of feelings when the emotional and often also sexual content of the patient's unconsciousness becomes explicit. There is a long, well-established tradition for treating schizophrenia with psychodynamic therapy, and we have found that the combination of bodywork and psychotherapy can enhance and accelerate the therapy and might improve the treatment rate further.

Cranial Electric Stimulation with Thermal Biomedical Feedback

Cranial Electric Stimulation with Thermal Biofeedback is Effective in Schizophrenics with Depression, Anxiety, Sleep Loss, Low Back Pain, Migraines, Obsessive Symptoms, Headaches, and Loss of Libido

Kelley, J. W., et al. "Cerebral Electric Stimulation with Thermal Biomedical Feedback." *The Nebraska Medical Journal* 62, no. 9 (September 1977): 322–27., PMID: 895932

> With over 50 cases in which cerebral electric stimulation, thermal biomedical feedback and psychotherapeutical phrases have been used concurrently there is a large enough statistical sample to allow us to infer some trends. Each of the three modalities have therapeutic values individually. Together they seem to synergize each other. The time necessary to reach therapeutic response seems to be markedly shortened, and the persistence of results appear to be lengthened over the results achieved by either of the modalities alone. Tis method is pleasant to the patient, has practically no risk, has none of the bad side effects and is far less expensive to the patient. Hospitalization generally can be averted.

Exercise and Glucose

Exercise and Glucose Supplement My Effectively Treat Cognitive Impairment in Schizophrenia

CODEX ALTERNUS

Li, Yuet-Keung, et al., "Coupling Physical Exercise with Dietary Glucose Supplement for Treating Cognitive Impairment in Schizophrenia: A Theoretical Model and Future Directions." *Early Intervention in Psychiatry* 8, no. 3 (August 2014): 209–20. Publisher: BLACKWELL PUBLISHING INC; doi:10.1111/eip.12109., PMID: 24224943

> ➢ The paper represents a first step in providing a theoretical model of how coupling of exercise with glucose supplement may help to alleviate cognitive impairment in schizophrenia patients. Exercise and glucose supplement work in concert to enhance glucose transport and insulin into the brain, and at the same time augment IGF-1 and BNDF output. Indeed, most research on cognitive benefits of glucose supplement and exercise and their underlying mechanisms is conducted in the general population. Research should first confirm the benefits and their mechanisms of action in schizophrenia patients, and then to elucidate the right dose of physical exercise and glucose to effectively treat cognitive impairment in schizophrenia.

Insulin and D-ribose

High Doses of Insulin and D-ribose for the Treatment of Frontal Lobe Dysfunction in Schizophrenia

Lichtigfeld, F., et al., "New Vistas in Chronic Schizophrenia." *The International Journal of Neuroscience* 38, no. 3–4 (February 1988): 355–67., Publisher: TAYLOR & FRANCIS INC. PMID: 3286558

> ➢ In view of the distinct possibility that the disturbed glucose regulation in the frontal area and basal ganglia of chronic schizophrenia is very germane to the successful treatment of this condition, a survey is given of the many factors that have to be considered in developing a therapy that takes into account this new information. The suggestion is made that the balance between cAMP and cGMP in the cells affected are dysregulated so that there is an excessive activity of the cAMP generating system which eventually leads to the pathological picture found in this condition. To restore the normal metabolic balance, use will have to be made of the various substances that are known to enhance the cGMP generating system in the cell, thereby restoring a more normal metabolic integrity. In this connection, the use of high doses of insulin under cover of hyperglycaemia and also the addition of D-ribose could become the cornerstone of a series of treatments to enhance the action of currently used medications in this often intractable illness.

Leucine and Genistein

Leucine and Genistein Combined Have Potential Antipsychotic Activity

CODEX ALTERNUS

Suresh, Palle, et al., "Antidopaminergic Effects of Leucine and Genistein on Schizophrenic Rat Models." *Neurosciences* (Riyadh, Saudi Arabia) 18, no. 3 (July 2013): 235–41., Publisher: Elsevier BV; PMID: 23887213

> ➤ "The individual administration of leucine and genistein had less anti dopaminergic activity when compared with their combined administration. These results suggest that leucine and genistein may have a potential clinical application in the management of psychiatric disorders."

Pregnenolone with L-theanine

Pregnenolone and L-theanine were Found to Reduce Negative Symptoms and Anxiety in Schizophrenic Pateints

---

Kardashev, Adasa, et al. "Add-on Pregnenolone with L-Theanine to Antipsychotic Therapy Relieves Negative and Anxiety Symptoms of Schizophrenia: An 8-Week, Randomized, Double-Blind, Placebo-Controlled Trial." *Clinical Schizophrenia & Related Psychoses*, July 28, 2015. doi:10.3371/CSRP.KARA.070415.

> ➤ Negative symptoms such as blunted affect, alogia, and anhedonia (SANS) were found to be significantly improved, with moderate effect sizes among patients who received PREG-LT, in comparison with the placebo group. Add-on PREG-LT also significantly associated with a reduction of anxiety scores such as anxious mood, tension, and cardiovascular symptoms (HAM-A), and elevation of general functioning (GAF). Positive symptoms, antipsychotic agents, concomitant drugs, and illness duration did not associate significantly with effect of PREG-LT augmentation. PREG-LT was well-tolerated.

Transcranial Direct Current Stimulation and Exercise

tDCS Combined with Exercise May Improve Cogntive Function

Moreau, David, et al. "Blending Transcranial Direct Current Stimulations and Physical Exercise to Maximize Cognitive Improvement." *Frontiers in Psychology* 6 (2015): 678. doi:10.3389/fpsyg.2015.00678., PMID: 26052301

> ➤ Given the promising results of non-invasive brain stimulation in the laboratory, one might ask whether there is any way to further maximize the size and the durability of improvements. We argue that one possible approach is tocombine brain Stimulation with physical exercise. Cognitive enhancement has Recently been associated with sport and exercise experience There is increasing evidence that physical exercise can improve brain health and plasticity via a variety of mechanisms from cellular to system levels,

such as brain-derived neurotrophic factor (BDNF) andinsulin-like growth factor (IGF-1) concentrations, brainvolume,complexity of neuronalactivity,and white matter integrity. Beyond aerobic fitness, studies have also shown that skill sets that are associated with a specific sport can also modulate cognitive e performance.For example,tennis players possess better temporal processing than fitness-matched athlete controls, bad mintonplayers have superior visuo- spatial skills and great ermodulationson neural oscillations than naïve controls, and wrestlers are better at solving mental rotation problems than runners.These findings suggest that beyond the general effect of aerobic fitness s on cognition, there also is an additional domain-specific benefit to begained from sports training.Thus, sport can be one type of cognitive training that, over a reasonable amount of time, results in more efficient brain functioning. Given the known effects of tDCS on motor learning, it appears that, if appropriately utilized (e.g.,timingofstimulation), tDCS could maximize the effectiveness of sports interventions, either by aiding cognitive or motor learning.

Vitamins and Fatty Acids

Omega-3 Fatty Acids, Vitamin C and E Supplementation have a Beneficial Effect on Positive and Negative Symptoms in Schizophrenia

> **Sivrioglu, E. Y.,** et al., "The Impact of Omega-3 Fatty Acids, Vitamins E and C Supplementation on Treatment Outcome and Side Effects in Schizophrenia Patients Treated with Haloperidol: An Open-Label Pilot Study." *Progress in Neuro-Psychopharmacology & Biological Psychiatry* 31, no. 7 (October 1, 2007): 1493–99. Publisher: ELSEVIER INC. doi:10.1016/j.pnpbp.2007.07.004., PMID: 17688987

> ➤ Our results support the beneficial effect of the supplementation on positive and negative symptoms of schizophrenia as well as the severity of side effects induced by haloperidol. The effect of supplementation on akathisia is especially noteworthy and it has not been investigated in previous studies.

Supplementation with Omega-3 Fatty Acids and Vitamin E and C Significantly Reduces Psychopathology in Schizophrenia

> **Arvindakshan, Meena,** et al., "Supplementation with a Combination of Omega-3 Fatty Acids and Antioxidants (vitamins E and C) Improves the Outcome of Schizophrenia." *Schizophrenia Research* 62, no. 3 (August 1, 2003): 195–204., Publisher: ELSEVIER BV; PMID: 12837515

> ➤ Concomitantly, there was significant reduction in psychopathology based on reduction in individual total scores for brief psychiatric rating scale (BPRS) and positive and negative syndrome scale (PANSS), general psychopathology-PANSS and increase in Henrich's Quality of Life (QOL) scale.

CODEX ALTERNUS

Vitamin E and Polyunsaturated Fatty Acids Supplementation Improves Antioxidant Defense in Schizophrenic Patients

> **Bošković, Marija,** et al., "Vitamin E and Essential Polyunsaturated Fatty Acids Supplementation in Schizophrenia Patients Treated with Haloperidol." *Nutritional Neuroscience*, July 24, 2014. Publisher: Maney Publishing doi:10.1179/1476830514Y.0000000139., PMID: 25056532

> ➤ Discussion Our study indicates that supplementation with vitamin E and EPUFAs may improve the antioxidative defense, especially glutathione system, while there is no major effect on symptoms severity. Supplemental treatment with EPUFAs and vitamin E in schizophrenia patients treated with haloperidol is potentially beneficial and a larger independent study appears warranted.

Vitamins and Beta-carotene

Vitamin E, Vitamin C, and Beta Carotene May Prevent Oxidative Injury and Deterioration Associated with Schizophrenia

> **D'Souza, Benedicta,** et al., "Oxidative Injury and Antioxidant Vitamins E and C in Schizophrenia." *Indian Journal of Clinical Biochemistry: IJCB* 18, no. 1 (January 2003): 87–90. Publisher: ASSOCIATION OF CLINICAL BIOCHEMISTS OF INDIA doi:10.1007/BF02867671., PMID: 23105377

> ➤ "Impaired antioxidant defense and increased lipid peroxidation suggests that treatment with antioxidants (Vitamin E, Vitamin C, beta carotene) at the initial stages of illness may prevent further oxidative injury and deterioration of associated neurological deficits in Schizophrenia."

Citicoline and Galantamine

Citicoline and Galantamine Combined Showed a Reduction in Positive and Negative Symptoms

> **Deutsch, Stephen I.,** et al., "First Administration of Cytidine Diphosphocholine and Galantamine in Schizophrenia: A Sustained alpha7 Nicotinic Agonist Strategy." *Clinical Neuropharmacology* 31, no. 1 (February 2008): 34–39. Publisher: LIPPINCOTT WILLIAMS & WILKINS; doi:10.1097/wnf.0b013e31806462ba., PMID: 18303489

> ➤ The combination of CDP-choline and galantamine was administered to 6 schizophrenic patients with residual symptoms in a 12-week, open-label trial. Patients were maintained on stable dose regimens of antipsychotic medications for 4 weeks before study entry and for the trial duration. All reached target doses of both agents and completed the trial. Transient side effects resolved without slowing of dose titration. Gastrointestinal adverse effects were most common. Of the 6 patients, 5 showed

reduction in Clinical Global Impressions severity scores and Positive and Negative Syndrome Scale total scores. Three patients requested continuation of the adjunctive combination at the end of the trial. These results suggest further investigation of the combination of CDP-choline and galantamine as an alpha7 nAChR agonist intervention.

Enterosorption and Antioxidants

Entersorption and Antioxidants Has a Significant Effect on a Majority of Schizophrenics Tested

Rachkauskas, G. S., et al., "[The efficacy of enterosorption and a combination of antioxidants in schizophrenics]." *Likars'ka Sprava / Ministerstvo Okhorony Zdorov'ia Ukraïny,* no. 4 (June 1998): 122–24., PMID: 9784725

> A total of 143 patients with schizophrenia, who ranged from 28 to 42 years old, were studied. Of these, 68 patients were running a continuously progredient course, 75 were in the phase of exacerbation of the attack-like progredient course of schizophrenia. Group I (n = 76) of patients received the enterosorbent polysorb and a complex of antioxidants (tocoferolum acetatum, ascorbic acid, quercetin) as a supplement to the conventional therapy, group II (n = 67) was placed on the conventional therapy only. A complex of the antioxidants as well as the enterosorbent had a positive effect on the clinical course of the condition in 63.2% of group I patients who managed, among other therapeutic benefits, to achieve a stable remission. They have also demonstrated a concomitant improvement or normalization of indices for lipid peroxidation.

Blood Detoxification Treatments

Dialysis

Dialysis Treatment is Effective for Schizophrenia

Splendiani, G., et al., "Dialysis Treatment in Schizophrenia: Two Years Experience." *Artificial Organs* 5, no. 2 (May 1981): 175–77., Publisher: BLACKWELL PUBLISHING, INC. PMID: 7271531

> The authors summarize two years trial of dialysis treatment of schizophrenia. Twenty-five schizophrenic patients were treated with hemodialysis using PAN membranes. The dialysis schedule was: dialyzer; RP 610; blood flow: 250 ml/min; dialysate flow: 500 ml/min; time: 3 hr; vascular access: arteriovenous fistula, femoral vein, antebrachial veins. Dialysis was first performed for three days, repeated after one week, two weeks, three weeks, and one month, and then performed once a month. The drug regimen was never modified or interrupted. The results were evaluated with the Overall and Lorr scale. Nine patients interrupted the treatment early and were not considered; nine patients showed disappearance of psychiatric symptomatology (Overall and Lorr index

decreased to 21.8 at 2); non-significant modifications of the main schizophrenic symptoms were observed in seven patients. According to our trial, dialysis with polyacrylonitrile membranes can modify the psychotic attitude in a group of schizophrenic "dialysis responders.

Dialysis is Effective for Treatment of Schizophrenia

> **Splendiani, G.,** et al., "Five-Year Trial of Dialytic Treatment for Schizophrenia." *Artificial Organs* 7, no. 3 (August 1983): 322–25., Publisher: BLACKWELL PUBLISHING, INC. PMID: 6625961

> ➢ Thirty schizophrenic patients were treated with hemodialysis for 4-36 months. The clinical results were evaluated using two psychiatric scales: the Brief Psychiatric Rating Scale and the Inpatient Multidimensional Psychiatric Scale. In 13 schizophrenic patients psychiatric symptoms disappeared completely, and complete social reintegration followed. Eight patients showed no significant modification of schizophrenic disease after more than 30 dialysis sessions. Nine patients were not considered because their treatment was interrupted during the first month. Dialysis improved the psychotic attitude in one group of schizophrenic patients. The best results were obtained using polyacrylonitrile membranes.

Hemodialysis Puts Auditory Hallucinations in Remission

> **Malek-Ahmadi, P.,** et al., "Effect of Hemodialysis on Hallucinations." *Southern Medical Journal* 73, no. 4 (April 1980): 520–21., Publisher: SOUTHERN MEDICAL ASSOCIATION; PMID: 7367947

> ➢ A patient with chronic schizophrenia had two hemodialyses and two sham dialyses in a single-blind design. There was no change in the patient's affect after either procedure, but her auditory hallucinations disappeared after both hemodialysis and sham dialysis, with hemodialysis inducing a much longer partial remission.

Dialysis May Be Effective for Treatment of Schizophrenia

> **Fogelson, D. L.,** et al., "Dialysis for Schizophrenia: Review of Clinical Trials and Implications for Further Research." *The American Journal of Psychiatry* 137, no. 5 (May 1980): 605–7., Publisher: AM PSYCHIATRIC ASSN; PMID: 7369409

> ➢ At least 67 schizophrenic patients have undergone dialysis for renal failure, without improvement in schizophrenic symptoms. Ninety-two nonuremic schizophrenic patients have received dialysis in nonblind studies; 22 improved, 21 improved partially, 47 showed no change, and 2 became worse. The authors point out factors other than dialysis that may affect outcome, including family respones and reduction in drug dose.

They believe that until the results of current double-blind, sham-controlled trials are known, dialysis should not be prescribed as a treatment for schizophrenia.

Hemodialysis Improves Schizophrenic Symptoms

Malek-Ahmadi, P., et al., "Hemodialysis and Schizophrenia: A Double-Blind Study." *Southern Medical Journal* 73, no. 7 (July 1980): 873–74., Publisher: SOUTHERN MEDICAL ASSOCIATION. PMID: 6992283

> ➢ Partial or total remission of schizophrenic symptoms after exchange transfusion or hemodialysis have been reported in the literature. Although the results of these reports are encouraging, they have not been confirmed by controlled studies. We have conducted a double-blind placebo-controlled study to evaluate the effect of hemodialysis on chronic schizophrenia. Our data seem to indicate that some schizophrenic symptoms improve after hemodialyses.

Dialysis Pretreatment Improved Depression and Anxiety in Schizophrenic Patients

Scheiber, S. C., et al., "Dialysis for Schizophrenia: An Uncontrolled Study of 11 Patients." *The American Journal of Psychiatry* 138, no. 5 (May 1981): 662–65., Publisher: AM PSYCHIATRIC ASSN; PMID: 7235065

> ➢ The authors evaluated hemodialysis as a treatment for schizophrenia in an uncontrolled study of 11 patients. Eight men and two women with chronic schizophrenia who had responded poorly to conventional treatments or who had sought alternate treatments received three dialyses weekly for 3 weeks; 1 additional subject dropped out after eight treatments. MMPI, Psychiatric Status Scale, and Inpatient Multidimensional Psychiatric Scale scores were obtained before, immediately following, and at intervals after the nine treatments. Preliminary results, including 1-month follow-up, suggest that subjects with pretreatment anxiety and depression improved. No endorphins were discovered in the dialysate.

Haemodialysis Removes Some Endogenous Dialysable Substance in the Pathogenesis of Mood Disturbances in Schizophrenia

Vanherweghem, J. L., et al., "Haemodialysis in Schizophrenia: A Double Blind Study - Preliminary Report." *Proceedings of the European Dialysis and Transplant Association. European Dialysis and Transplant Association* 16 (1979): 148–54., Publisher: PITMAN; PMID: 548976

> ➢ Nine of the 12 patients were improved by both extracorporeal procedures with or without active dialysis. No significant difference appeared however between both groups in the rate and degree of improvement of nuclear symptoms of schizophrenia. Nevertheless, AD was significantly more efficient in relieving affective symptomatology,

suggesting the potential involvement of some endogenous dialysable substance (s) in the pathogenesis of mood disturbances in schizophrenia.

Blood Detoxification

Blood Detoxification Treatment in Schizophrenia Proves to Be Therapeutic

> **Nedopil, N.,** et al., "Detoxification Treatment for Chronic Schizophrenic Patients: Experimental Results and Data from a Survey." *Artificial Organs* 7, no. 3 (August 1983): 304–9., Publisher: BLACKWELL PUBLISHING, INC. PMID: 6625959

> ➤ Blood detoxification as a treatment of schizophrenia has been studied intensively since 1977 by a number of research centers. Results of an open study on 10 chronic schizophrenic patients--two showing improvement--were less favorable than those reported in the initial publications. In order to possibly identify a subgroup of responders to this treatment, a survey was undertaken in which 95 centers were invited to participate. Of the 95 centers which originally treated schizophrenic patients with detoxification and which were asked to send data on these patients to the Registry of the European Dialysis and Transplant Association, 39 centers replied (35 from Europe and four from the United States). From the 100 patients reported on in Europe, 17 were reported to be very much improved and 22 to be improved. Of the patients from the United States, 86% were reported as improved. No subgroup of responders could be identified, and differences between centers concerning nosological subgroups, treatment methods, and results were so great that no real comparison was possible. Although data from this survey are not totally conclusive, in connection with the updated literature they do not encourage further research in this treatment of schizophrenia.

Hallucination Reduction Treatments

Autohemotherapy

Autohemotherapy is the Reinjecting of Patients Blood from the Arm to Buttock and Has Incredible Results in Improving Psychotic Symptoms

> **Reddick, R. H.** "Autohemotherapy in Chronic Mental Disorders; a Preliminary Report." *Journal of the American Institute of Homeopathy* 43, no. 10 (December 1950): 263–69., PMID: 14803231

> ➤ Twenty-five chronically ill state hospital patients were treated by hemotherapy during a period of six months. The group consisted of 13 schizophrenics, 6 involutionals, 3 paranoid conditions, and one each of manic depressive psychosis, psychosis with cerebral arteriosclerosis, and psychosis due to alcohol. Nineteen patients or 76 percent of

those treated displayed a social recovery, inasmuch as they were able to leave the hospital and resume their former activities. Of the six patients still requiring hospitalization at the conclusion of the treatment period, three were much better ; two were somewhat better ; and one remained unchanged. Eleven out of thirteen or 85 percent of the schizophrenics improved sufficiently to no longer require hospitalization, while 66-2/3 percent of the involutionals and paranoid conditions also displayed social recovery. Three cases and their progress are individually described in some detail. The theories of numerous investigators concerning the modus operandi of autohemotherapy are listed; and various somato-therapeutic and psychotherapeutic aspects of autohemotherapy are discussed. The use of autohemotherapy in the treatment of chronic mental disorders presents a new application of an old method of treatment; beneficial effects from the use of autohemotherapy have been reported in a wide variety of clinical conditions (50 or more); but I have yet to find any prior report indicating that it has ever been used before in the therapy of psychoses.

Continuous Positive Air Pressure (CPAP)

CPAP led to Complete Remission of Hallucinations in Schizophrenic Patient

Karanti, Alina, et al., "Treatment Refractory Psychosis Remitted upon Treatment with Continuous Positive Airway Pressure: A Case Report." *Psychopharmacology Bulletin* 40, no. 1 (2007): 113–17., Publisher: MEDWORKS MEDIA GLOBAL; PMID: 17285102

> ➤ A 63-year-old women previously diagnosed with hebephrenic schizophrenia developed treatment resistant auditory hallucinations along with extreme daytime fatigue and obesity. She was eventually diagnosed with Pickwickian syndrome or OHS and received treatment with continuous positive airway pressure (CPAP). Restoring the patient's alveolar hypoventilation with nocturnal CPAP led to the complete remission of hallucinations.

CPAP Treatment of Obstructive Sleep Apnea Should Be More Highly Acknowledged in Clinical Psychiatry

Hiraoka, Toshiaki, et al., "[Treatment of psychiatric symptoms in schizophrenia spectrum disorders with comorbid sleep apnea syndrome: a case report]." *Seishin Shinkeigaku Zasshi = Psychiatria Et Neurologia Japonica* 115, no. 2 (2013): 139–46., Publisher: JAPAN PUBLICATIONS TRADING CO. LTD., PMID: 23691802

> ➤ Sleep apnea syndrome (SAS) is characterized by apnea and hypopnea during sleep. SAS manifests various symptoms, and can become a risk factor for a variety of diseases. Typical psychiatric presentations of SAS are depressive symptoms, and those resembling negative symptoms in schizophrenia. We report two patients with schizophrenia spectrum disorders. Both patients showed the partial improvement of

psychiatric symptoms with pharmacotherapy. After diagnosing comorbid SAS and subsequent treatment with continuous positive airway pressure (CPAP), the psychiatric symptoms improved. The first case was a 54-year-old woman, who presented with auditory hallucinations and delusions and was diagnosed with schizophrenia at 32 years of age. Her positive symptoms responded immediately to medication; however, her negative symptoms persisted despite switching to atypical antipsychotics. We diagnosed her with SAS using pulse oximetry and portable polysomnography (PSG), and, after treatment with CPAP, her fatigue and shallow sleep improved, as well as her quality of life (QOL). The second case was is a 61-year-old man, who presented with delusions of persecution and was diagnosed with delusional disorder at 49 years of age. His delusional symptoms fluctuated under medication, and repeatedly worsened under stressful situations. We suspected SAS as a Complicating factor, and diagnosed him with severe SAS using PSG. After treatment with CPAP, his hypertension and delusions of persecution improved. Screening for SAS is available in psychiatric hospitals and outpatient clinics. We believe that the possibility of comorbid SAS in psychiatric patients should be more widely acknowledged in clinical psychiatry.

CPAP can be Effective for Negative Symptoms and Remission of Auditory Hallucination in Schizophrenia

> **Sugishita, Kazuyuki,** et al., "Continuous Positive Airway Pressure for Obstructive Sleep Apnea Improved Negative Symptoms in a Patient with Schizophrenia." *Psychiatry and Clinical Neurosciences* 64, no. 6 (December 2010): 665. Publisher: BLACKWELL PUBLISHING ASIA; doi:10.1111/j.1440-1819.2010.02146.x., PMID: 21105956

> ➢ "The present case report is in line with previous reports, including a patient with delusional schizophrenia showing improvement of negative symptoms and a case of hebephrenic schizophrenia showing complete remission of auditory hallucinations after successful treatments of OSA with CPAP."

Endovascular Laser Therapy

Endovascular Laser Therapy is Effective for Treatment of Viruses and Bacteria in Blood of Schizophrenic Patients

> **Kut'ko, I. I.,** et al., "[The effect of endovascular laser therapy and antioxidants on the immune status and energy metabolism of patients with treatment-resistant forms of schizophrenia]." *Zhurnal Nevrologii I Psikhiatrii Imeni S.S. Korsakova / Ministerstvo Zdravookhraneniia I Meditsinskoĭ Promyshlennosti Rossiĭskoĭ Federatsii, Vserossiĭskoe Obshchestvo Nevrologov [i] Vserossiĭskoe Obshchestvo Psikhiatrov* 96, no. 2 (1996): 34–38., PMID: 8754337

> ➢ The influence of endovascular laser therapy and of antioxidants on clinical immunological indices and energy metabolism was analysed in 148 schizophrenic patients including 86 patients with shift-like progredient (first group) and 62 patients

with continuous-progredient (second group) forms of the disease. Positive trends in psychosis course were observed in 57% of cases in the first group and in 41.9% of patients of the second group. Pronounced improvement of the immunological indices was observed in patients with positive clinical dynamics: decreased peripheral blood immunocytes sensitization to the brain, hepatic, thymus tissue antigens as well as ATP elevation which was evidence of the improvement of energy metabolism.

Oxygen Treatment of Behavioral Problems

Hypobaric Oxygen Inhalation Reduces All Symptoms Relative to Mood and Attitude Significantly

Fraiberg, P. L., et al., "Oxygen Inhalation in the Control of Psychogeriatric Symptoms in Patients with Long-Term Illness." *Journal of the American Geriatrics Society* 21, no. 7 (July 1973): 321–24., Publisher: BLACKWELL PUBLISHING, INC., PMID: 4713288

> In general, the results of our study on the use of hypobaric oxygen inhalation upheld our impression of its usefulness in the treatment of behaviorally disturbed elderly patients. All of the psychogeriatric symptoms relative to mood and attitude were improved to a statistically significant degree. Usually the symptoms which were both severe and predominant showed the most improvement. These included nervous tension, withdrawal-apathy, restlessness, and confused states. There was a steady improvement throughout the treatment period. When treatment was discontinued, regression fol- lowed rapidly. In some instances the improvement in cognition was marked enough to arouse comment from the staff. No complications arising from the treatment were observed. Hypobaric oxygen therapy, although no panacea, is a useful procedure in the management of difficult geriatric behavioral problems.

Oxygen-enriched Air Inhalation has a Significant Improvement on Schizophrenia Patients Symptoms

Bloch, Yehudit, et al., "Normobaric Hyperoxia Treatment of Schizophrenia." *Journal of Clinical Psychopharmacology* 32, no. 4 (August 2012): 525–30. doi:10.1097/JCP.0b013e31825d70b8., Publisher: LIPPINCOTT WILLIAMS & WILKINS; PMID: 22722511

> There was significant improvement in total Positive and Negative Symptoms Scale score of patients who received oxygen compared with the control group. There were positive effects of oxygen on memory and attention in neuropsychological performance tests. The effect size is small despite the statistical significance, but the patient group was extremely chronic and severely impaired. These results are a proof of concept, and normobaric hyperoxia should be studied in patients with milder forms of the illness and earlier in the course of illness.

CODEX ALTERNUS

Hyperbaric Oxygen is Effective in Schizophrenic Patients Resistant to Pharmacotherapy Treatment

Kut'ko, I. I., et al., "[The use of hyperbaric oxygenation in treating mental patients resistant to psychopharmacotherapy]." *Zhurnal Nevrologii I Psikhiatrii Imeni S.S. Korsakova / Ministerstvo Zdravookhraneniia I Meditsinskoĭ Promyshlennosti Rossiĭskoĭ Federatsii, Vserossiĭskoe Obshchestvo Nevrologov [i] Vserossiĭskoe Obshchestvo Psikhiatrov* 96, no. 5 (1996): 47–51., Publisher: Media Sfera; PMID: 9012254

➤ "A positive clinical effect was marked in 72.5% of cases (in 67.4% of schizophrenic patients and in 77.4% of patients with vascular disease)."

Isakov, Iu V., et al., "[Clinical effectiveness of hyperbaric oxygenation in the combined treatment of patients with schizophrenia]." *Zhurnal Nevropatologii I Psikhiatrii Imeni S.S. Korsakova (Moscow, Russia: 1952)* 87, no. 12 (1987): 1832–35., Publisher: MEDIA SFERA; PMID: 3447399

➤ "The maximum therapeutic effect was observed after 10-12 sessions"

Stellate Ganglion Block Technique

Stellate Ganglion Block Technique Reduced the Severity and Frequency of Hallucinations in Schizophrenic Patient

Takano, Manami, et al., "Unexpected Beneficial Effect of Stellate Ganglion Block in a Schizophrenic Patient." *Canadian Journal of Anaesthesia = Journal Canadien D'anesthésie* 49, no. 7 (September 2002): 758–59. Publisher: CANADIAN ANAESTHETISTS' SOCIETY, doi:10.1007/BF03017464., PMID: 12193502

➤ Stellate ganglion block (SGB) is a technique widely used for treating chronic pain in the upper extremities, head, face and neck. Here we report a schizophrenic patient who presented with neck-shoulder pain in whom repeated SGB reduced the severity and frequency of hallucination as well as pain. The patient was a right-handed 37-yr-old man. At the age of 36 yr, he fell from a horse and developed intractable pain around the neck and left shoulder. After unsuccessful conventional therapies, a course of weekly left SGB was commenced. Before beginning SGB, the patient often felt that a third person was watching his work and criticizing him. After the first SGB, the third person in his mind became puzzled and less confident. One month later, he felt less noise, and auditory hallucinations changed from mandatory to recommendatory. With discontinuation of SGB, hallucinations worsened. During this period, no anti-psychotic medications were administered. The psychiatrist confirmed the diagnosis of schizophrenia, DSM-IV code 295.3. The Brief Psychiatric Rating Scale (BRPS), which assesses 18 objective and subjective symptoms through interview by a psychiatrist, was evaluated ten days after the last SGB. The BPRS score (min 18 - max 196) was 19, indicating the patient's mental state at this time was close to normal. Telaranta1 showed that pathognomonic symptoms of social phobia are alleviated by endoscopic thoracic sympathectomy. Comparable effects would be expected from SGB which blocks sympathetic efferents originating from the thoracic spinal cord. SGB is known to increase cerebral blood flow on the injected side. Modified blood flow to the cerebrum may have affected schizophrenia-related symptoms. The relaxing effect of SGB may have been additive. We were impressed with this unexpected, beneficial effect of SGB on psychiatric symptoms and suggest that more research in this direction may be warranted.

Stellate Ganglion Block is a Rapidly Effective Treatment for Psychosis

Ikeda, K., et al., "[Three case reports of the use of stellate ganglion block for the climacteric psychosis]." *Masui. The Japanese Journal of Anesthesiology* 42, no. 11 (November 1993): 1696–98. PMID: 8254884

> ➢ There are many reports of the use of stellate ganglion block (SGB) for the climacteric psychosis, which is considered to be sympathicotonic response to stress. We experienced three cases of the SGB therapy for the climacteric psychosis. We performed SGB three times per week by 1% lidocaine 5 ml, and observed improvements of the symptoms after doing SGB for five times. The patients reported psychological relaxation after receiving SGB therapy. We examined the changes of the serum concentrations of ACTH, LH, FSH, and catecholamines (epinephrine, norepinephrine) before and after SGB in 8 patients who were suffering from climacteric psychosis, because we wanted to know the endocrinological response to SGB. We observed a significant decrease in norepinephrine concentration after SGB, which is reasonable considering the sympathetic blockage. There were no significant changes of ACTH, LH, FSH, and epinephrine. We conclude that SGB therapy must be effective for the climacteric psychosis because of sympathetic blockade. But we could not clarify the influence of endocrinological response to SGB.

Insomnia Treatments

Salt of Gamma Hydroxbutyric Acid (GHB)

Sodium Salt of Gamma Hydroxbutyric Acid (GHB) Has Demonstrated Improvement in Objective Sleep Measures

Kantrowitz, Joshua T., et al., "The Importance of a Good Night's Sleep: An Open-Label Trial of the Sodium Salt of Gamma-Hydroxybutyric Acid in Insomnia Associated with Schizophrenia." *Schizophrenia Research* 120, no. 1–3 (July 2010): 225–26. Publisher: ELSEVIER BV; doi:10.1016/j.schres.2010.03.035., PMID: 20435443

> ➢ Although limited by an open-label design and small sample size, we demonstrate convergent improvement in subjective sleep, daytime sleepiness and objective sleep

measures. More broadly, we found an interrelationship between negative symptoms and measures of sleep. We are only aware of two previous trials specifically evaluating sleep in schizophrenia (Luthringer et al., 2007; Muller et al., 2004), neither of which reported an interrelationship with negative symptoms. Present findings suggest that SBX may improve objective sleep architecture and moreover, improvement in sleep may lead to downstream improvement in symptoms and function. Future double blind studies incorporating both symptoms and sleep-related cognitive measures appear warranted.

Acupuncture

Acupuncture is Effective on Insomnia and Psychopathology in Schizophrenia

> **Reshef, Alon,** et al., "The Effects of Acupuncture Treatment on Sleep Quality and on Emotional Measures among Individuals Living with Schizophrenia: A Pilot Study." *Sleep Disorders* 2013 (2013): 327820. Publisher: Hindawi Pub. Corp doi:10.1155/2013/327820., PMID: 24083027

➤ "Overall, the findings of this pilot study suggest that acupuncture has beneficial effects as a treatment for insomnia and psychopathology symptoms among patients with schizophrenia."

Melatonin

Melatonin is a Useful Short-term Hypnotic for Schizophrenic Patients

> **Suresh Kumar, P. N.,** et al., "Melatonin in Schizophrenic Outpatients with Insomnia: A Double-Blind, Placebo-Controlled Study." *The Journal of Clinical Psychiatry* 68, no. 2 (February 2007): 237–41., Publisher: PHYSICIANS POSTGRADUATE PRESS, INC. PMID: 17335321

➤ "Melatonin may be a useful short-term hypnotic for schizophrenic patients with insomnia. Melatonin could be considered for patients in whom conventional hypnotic drug therapy or higher sedative antipsychotic drug doses may be problematic."

➤ The modal stable dose of melatonin was 3mg. Relative to placebo, melatonin significantly improved the quality and depth of sleep of nighttime sleep, reduced the number of nighttime awaking's, and increased the duration of sleep without producing a morning hangover. Subjectively, melatonin also reduced sleep-onset latency, heightened freshness on awaking, improved mood, and improved daytime functioning.

Melatonin Improves Sleep Efficiency in Patients with Schizophrenia

> **Shamir, E.,** et al., "Melatonin Improves Sleep Quality of Patients with Chronic Schizophrenia." *The Journal of Clinical Psychiatry* 61, no. 5 (May 2000): 373–77., Publisher: PHYSICIANS POSTGRADUATE PRESS, INC. PMID: 10847313

> "Melatonin improves sleep efficiency in patients with schizophrenia whose sleep quality is low."

Music Relaxation

Music Relaxation is Beneficial for Insomnia and Anxiety in People with Schizophrenia

Bloch, Boaz, et al., "The Effects of Music Relaxation on Sleep Quality and Emotional Measures in People Living with Schizophrenia." *Journal of Music Therapy* 47, no. 1 (2010): 27–52., Publisher: NATIONAL ASSOCIATION FOR MUSIC THERAPY. PMID: 20635522

> Results showed an improvement in sleep latency and sleep efficiency after the music relaxation was played. Likewise, music relaxation was shown to improve participants' total psychopathology score (PANSS) as well as their level of depression. Moreover, a significant correlation was found between reduction in level of situational anxiety and improvement in sleep efficiency. The findings suggest the beneficial effect of music relaxation as a treatment both for insomnia and for emotional measures in people living with schizophrenia.

Mismatch Negativity Treatments

N-acetylcysteine

N-acetylcysteine Improves Mismatch Negativity

Lavoie, Suzie, et al., "Glutathione Precursor, N-Acetyl-Cysteine, Improves Mismatch Negativity in Schizophrenia Patients." *Neuropsychopharmacology: Official Publication of the American College of Neuropsychopharmacology* 33, no. 9 (August 2008): 2187–99. Publisher: NATURE PUBLISHING GROUP; doi:10.1038/sj.npp.1301624., PMID: 18004285

> "MMN improvement was observed in the absence of robust changes in assessments of clinical severity, thought the latter was observed in larger and more prolonged clinical study"

Glycine

High-dose Glycine Attenuates Mismatch Negativity

Leung, Sumie, et al., "Acute High-Dose Glycine Attenuates Mismatch Negativity (MMN) in Healthy Human Controls." *Psychopharmacology* 196, no. 3 (February 2008): 451–60. Publisher: SPRINGER-VERLAG; doi:10.1007/s00213-007-0976-8., PMID: 17952411

> "These findings suggest that an acute high dosage of glycine attenuates MMN in healthy controls, raising the possibility that optimal effects of glycine and other glycine agonists may depend on the integrity of the NMDA receptor system."

PrePulse Inhibition Treatments

Herbal Self-Heal (Heal All)

Herbal Self-Heal (Heal All) could be Useful for Treating Schizophrenia because it Ameliorates PPI and Attention Defects

Park, Se Jin, et al., "Prunella Vulgaris Attenuates Prepulse Inhibition Deficit and Attention Disruption Induced by MK-801 in Mice." *Phytotherapy Research: PTR* 27, no. 12 (December 2013): 1763–69. Publisher: JOHN/WILEY & SONS LTD. doi:10.1002/ptr.4929., PMID: 23348874

> "These results suggest that EEPV could be useful for treating schizophrenia because EEPV ameliorates prepulse inhibition disruption and attention deficits induced by MK-801."

Leptin

Leptin Significantly Increases Prepulse Inhibition and Has Antipsychotic Properties

Dashti, Somayeh, et al., "The Effect of Leptin on Prepulse Inhibition in a Developmental Model of Schizophrenia." *Neuroscience Letters* 555 (October 25, 2013): 57–61. Publisher: ELSEVIER IRELAND LTD; doi:10.1016/j.neulet.2013.09.027., PMID: 24055608

> In conclusion, our results reveal that leptin significantly increases PPI in socially-isolated rats. The findings of this study suggest possible antipsychotic properties for leptin. We suggest further studies on the possible disruption of leptin signaling in schizophrenia, and also the possible interaction of leptin with therapeutic effects of second generation antipsychotics.

Kami-ondam-tang

Kami-ondam-tang Attenuates MK-801-induced Pre Pulse Inhibition Disruption

Oh, Hee Kyong, et al., "Kami-Ondam-Tang, a Traditional Herbal Prescription, Attenuates the Prepulse Inhibition Deficits and Cognitive Impairments Induced by MK-801 in Mice." *Journal of Ethnopharmacology* 146, no. 2 (March 27, 2013): 600–607. Publisher: ELSEVIER IRELAND LTD; doi:10.1016/j.jep.2013.01.032., PMID: 23376282

> ➤ "These findings suggest that KODT attenuates MK-801-induced PPI disruption, social interaction deficits, and cognitive impairments, possibly, by regulating of cortical Akt and ERK signaling."

Sulforaphane

Sulforaphane Has Antipsychotic Activity in Animal Model of Schizophrenia

Shirai, Yumi, et al., "Effects of the Antioxidant Sulforaphane on Hyperlocomotion and Prepulse Inhibition Deficits in Mice after Phencyclidine Administration." *Clinical Psychopharmacology and Neuroscience: The Official Scientific Journal of the Korean College of Neuropsychopharmacology* 10, no. 2 (August 2012): 94–98. Publisher: KOREAN COLLEGE OF NEUROPSYCHOPHARMACOLOGY; doi:10.9758/cpn.2012.10.2.94., PMID: 23376282

> ➤ "These results suggest that SFN has antipsychotic activity in an animal model of schizophrenia. Therefore, it is likely that SFN may be a potential therapeutic drug for schizophrenia."

CDP-Choline

CDP-Choline Attenuates Scopolamine Induced Disruption of Prepulse Inhibition

Uslu, Gulsah, et al., "CDP-Choline Attenuates Scopolamine Induced Disruption of Prepulse Inhibition in Rats: Involvement of Central Nicotinic Mechanism." *Neuroscience Letters* 569 (May 21, 2014): 153–57. Publisher: ELSEVIER IRELAND LTD doi:10.1016/j.neulet.2014.03.070., PMID: 24708927

> ➤ "These results demonstrate that exogenous administration of CDP-choline attenuates scopolamine induced PPI disruption and show that the activation of central α7-nAChR may play a critical role in this effect."

Substance Abuse Treatments

Oxytocin

Oxytocin May Be a Treatment for Alcoholism in Schizophrenia

Pedersen, Cort A., et al., "Schizophrenia and Alcohol Dependence: Diverse Clinical Effects of Oxytocin and Their Evolutionary Origins." *Brain Research* 1580 (September 11, 2014): 102–23. Publisher: ELSEVIER BV; doi:10.1016/j.brainres.2014.01.050., PMID: 24508579

> ➤ In the ways discussed above, recent discoveries of clinical efficacy of OT in schizophrenia and alcohol withdrawal may provide new insights into OT mechanisms

which may have been selected for during the evolution of placental mammals to facilitate maternal-infant and other social attachments.

D-serine, Sarcosine, and Glycine

D-serine, Sarcosine, and Glycine May Work to Treat Substance Abuse in Schizophrenic Patients

Coyle, Joseph T., et al., "Substance Use Disorders and Schizophrenia: A Question of Shared Glutamatergic Mechanisms." *Neurotoxicity Research* 10, no. 3–4 (December 2006): 221–33., Publisher: F P/GRAHAM PUBLISHING COMPANY; PMID: 17197372

> ➤ Schizophrenia is noted for the remarkably high prevalence of substance use disorders (SUDs) including nicotine (>85%), alcohol and stimulants. Mounting evidence supports the hypothesis that the endophenotype of schizophrenia involves hypofunction of a subpopulation of cortico-limbic NMDA receptors. Low doses of NMDA receptor antagonists such as ketamine replicate in normal volunteers positive, negative and cognitive symptoms of schizophrenia as well as associated physiologic abnormalities such as eye tracking and abnormal event related potentials. Genetic studies have identified putative risk genes that directly or indirectly affect NMDA receptors including D-amino acid oxidase, its modulator G72, proline oxidase, mGluR3 and neuregulin. Clinical trials have shown that agents that directly or indirectly enhance the function of the NMDA receptor at its glycine modulatory site (GMS) reduce negative symptoms and in the case of D-serine and sarcosine improve cognition and reduce positive symptoms in schizophrenic subjects receiving concurrent anti-psychotic medications. Notably, the GMS partial agonist D-cycloserine exacerbates negative symptoms in clozapine responders whereas full agonists, glycine and D-serine have no effects, suggesting clozapine may act indirectly as a full agonist at the GMS of the NMDA receptor. Clozapine treatment is uniquely associated with decreased substance use in patients with schizophrenia, even without psychologic intervention. Given the role of NMDA receptors in the reward circuitry and in substance dependence, it is reasonable to speculate that NMDA receptor dysfunction is a shared pathologic process in schizophrenia and co-morbid SUDs.

Preventive Treatments

Antioxidants

Use of Antioxidants Before Psychosis Onset May Dramatically Improve Outcome of Illness

Mahadik, S. P., et al., "Oxidative Stress and Role of Antioxidant and Omega-3 Essential Fatty Acid Supplementation in Schizophrenia." *Progress in Neuro-Psychopharmacology & Biological Psychiatry* 25, no. 3 (April 2001): 463–93., Publisher: ELSEVIER INC. , PMID: 11370992

CODEX ALTERNUS

> "Since the oxidative stress exists at or before the onset of psychosis the use of antioxidants from the very onset of psychosis may reduce the oxidative injury and dramatically improve the outcome of illness."

Breast Feeding

Breast Feeding May Postpone the Onset of Schizophrenic Illness

Amore, M., et al., "Can Breast-Feeding Protect against Schizophrenia? Case-Control Study." *Biology of the Neonate* 83, no. 2 (2003): 97–101. Publisher: S./KARGER AG; doi:67960., PMID: 12576752

> "Breast-feeding is no less common in those who develop schizophrenia in later life. However, breast milk might postpone the onset of the illness in schizophrenic patients."

D-serine

D-serine May Prevent the Onset of Psychosis in Adults

Hagiwara, Hiroko, et al., "Neonatal Disruption of Serine Racemase Causes Schizophrenia-like Behavioral Abnormalities in Adulthood: Clinical Rescue by D-serine." *PloS One* 8, no. 4 (2013): e62438. Publisher: PUBLIC LIBRARY OF SCIENCE doi:10.1371/journal.pone.0062438., PMID: 23630632

> "This study shows that disruption of D-serine synthesis during developmental stages leads to behavioral abnormalities relevant to prodromal symptoms and schizophrenia, in later life. Furthermore, early pharmacological intervention with D-serine may prevent the onset of psychosis in adult."

Glycine

Glycine Treatment of Prodromal Symptoms No Patients Converted to Psychosis

Woods, Scott W., et al., "Glycine Treatment of the Risk Syndrome for Psychosis: Report of Two Pilot Studies." *European Neuropsychopharmacology: The Journal of the European College of Neuropsychopharmacology* 23, no. 8 (August 2013): 931–40. Publisher: ELSEVIER BV doi:10.1016/j.euroneuro.2012.09.008., PMID: 23089076

> Of seven completers, three met early remission criteria during the 8 weeks on glycine. No patients converted to psychosis. In MMRM analyses, patients improved significantly from baseline on SOPS total (-18.2+-9.9, $p<0.001$) and on positive symptom, disorganization, and general symptom subscales. Negative symptoms improved only at the trend level.

CODEX ALTERNUS

Long-Chain Polyunsaturated Fatty Acid

Perinatal Long-Chain Polyunsaturated Fatty Acid Supplementation May Prevent Schizophrenia in Adulthood

> **Das, Undurti N.,** et al., "Can Perinatal Supplementation of Long-Chain Polyunsaturated Fatty Acids Prevents Schizophrenia in Adult Life?" *Medical Science Monitor: International Medical Journal of Experimental and Clinical Research* 10, no. 12 (December 2004): HY33–37., Publisher: International Scientific Literature, Inc; PMID: 15567990

> ➤ It is suggested that perinatal supplementation of long-chain polyunsaturated fatty acids (LCPUFAs) especially; eicosapentaenoic and docosahexaenoic acids prevent schizophrenia in the adult. I propose that schizophrenia could be a low-grade systemic inflammatory disease with its origins in the perinatal period, probably triggered by maternal infection in a genetically susceptible individual that leads to excess production of pro-inflammatory cytokines both in the mother and the fetus. These cytokines, in turn, induce damage to the fetal neurons leading to the adult onset of schizophrenia. I suggest that maternal infection perse interferes with the metabolism of essential fatty acids (EFAs) resulting in deficiency of LCPUFAs that are known to have neuroprotective action. Alternatively, decreased formation of LCPUFAs as a result of decreased activity of D6 and D5 desaturases (due to prematurity) can result in neuronal damage due to the absence/decrease in the neuroprotective LCPUFAs. This is supported by the observation that LCPUFAs suppress the production of pro-inflammatory cytokines, have anti-inflammatory and neuroprotective actions. Furthermore, LCPUFAs are essential for brain growth and development. If this hypothesis is true, it implies that perinatal supplementation of appropriate amounts of LCPUFAs in the right combination is helpful in the prevention of schizophrenia in adult life.

N-acetylcysteine

N-acetylcysteine May Prevent Oxidative Damage from Early Life Environmental Insults

> **Cabungcal, Jan-Harry,** et al., "Early-Life Insults Impair Parvalbumin Interneurons via Oxidative Stress: Reversal by N-Acetylcysteine." *Biological Psychiatry* 73, no. 6 (March 15, 2013): 574–82. Publisher: ELSEVIER INC. doi:10.1016/j.biopsych.2012.09.020., PMID: 23140664

> ➤ In Gclm KO mice, early-life insults inducing oxidative stress are detrimental to immature parvalbumin interneurons and have long-term consequences. In analogy, individuals carrying genetic risks to redox dysregulation would be potentially vulnerable to early-life environmental insults, during the maturation of parvalbumin interneurons. Our data support the need to develop novel therapeutic approaches based

on antioxidant and redox regulator compounds such as N-acetylcysteine, which could be used preventively in young at-risk subjects.

N-acetylcysteine is a useful Medication to Prevent Conversion to Schizophrenia in at Risk Individuals

Asevedo, Elson, et al., "N-Acetylcysteine as a Potentially Useful Medication to Prevent Conversion to Schizophrenia in at-Risk Individuals." *Reviews in the Neurosciences* 23, no. 4 (2012): 353–62. Publisher: FREUND PUBLISHING HOUSE, LTD. doi:10.1515/revneuro-2012-0039., PMID: 22944654

> ➤ "In this article, we purpose that NAC could be a useful medication to prevent evolution of schizophrenia in individuals at risk for psychosis."

Omega-3 Fatty Acids

Omega-3 Fatty Acids May Help Prevent Most Psychotic Episodes

Saugstad, Letten F., et al., "Are Neurodegenerative Disorder and Psychotic Manifestations Avoidable Brain Dysfunctions with Adequate Dietary Omega-3?" *Nutrition and Health* 18, no. 2 (2006): 89–101., Publisher: A B ACADEMIC PUBLISHERS; PMID: 16859172

> ➤ The olfactory agnosia observed in schizophrenia supports an N-3 deficit as does a reduction of key ologodendrocyte- and myelin-related genes in this disorder and affective disorder, where a rise in dementia accords with a deficit of N-3 also in this disorder. N-3 normalizes cerebral excitability at all levels. That the two disorders are localized at the extremes of excitability is supported by their opposing treatments: convulsant neuroleptics and anti-epileptic anti-depressants. An adequate N-3 diet will probably prevent most psychotic episodes and prove that neurodegenerative disorder with dementia is also to a large extent not only preventable but avoidable.

Omega-3 Fatty Acids May Be Used in the Prevention of Psychotic Episodes

Mossaheb, Nilufar, et al., "Polyunsaturated Fatty Acids in Emerging Psychosis." *Current Pharmaceutical Design* 18, no. 4 (2012): 576–91., Publisher: BENTHAM SCIENCE PUBLISHERS LTD. PMID: 22239591

> ➤ Furthermore, we examine the available evidence in indicated prevention in emerging psychosis, monotherapy, add-on therapy and tolerability. The neuroprotective potential of n-3 LC-PUFAs for indicated prevention, i.e. delaying transition to psychosis in high-risk populations needs to be further explored.

CODEX ALTERNUS

Omega-3's May Reduce the Risk of Progression to Psychotic Disorder and May Prevent Subthreshold Psychotic States

> **Amminger, G. Paul**, et al., "Long-Chain Omega-3 Fatty Acids for Indicated Prevention of Psychotic Disorders: A Randomized, Placebo-Controlled Trial." *Archives of General Psychiatry* 67, no. 2 (February 2010): 146–54. Publisher: AMERICAN MEDICAL ASSOCIATION; doi:10.1001/archgenpsychiatry.2009.192., PMID: 20124114

> ➤ "Long-chain omega-3 PUFAs reduce the risk of progression to psychotic disorder and may offer a safe and efficacious strategy for indicated prevention in young people with subthreshold psychotic states."

Prenatal Choline

Prenatal Supplementation with Diets Rich in Choline Rich Food May Prevent Abnormal Fetal Brain Development

> **Freedman, Robert**, et al. "Prenatal Choline and the Development of Schizophrenia." *Shangh ai Archives of Psychiatry*, 2015, Vol. 27, No.2

> ➤ Prenatal dietary supplementation with phosphatidyl-choline and promotion of diets rich in choline-containing foods (meats, soybeans, and eggs) are possible interventions to promote fetal brain development and thereby decrease the risk of subsequent mental illnesses. The low risk and short (six month) duration of the intervention makes it especially conducive to population-wide adoption. Similar findings with folate for the prevention of cleft palate led to recommendations for prenatal pharmacological supplementation and dietary improvement. However, definitive proof of the efficacy of prenatal choline supplementation will not be available for decades (because of the 20-year lag until the onset of schizophrenia), so public health officials need to decide whether or not promoting choline supplementation is justified based on the limited information available.

Prenatal Vitamin D, Folic Acid and Iron

Adequate Prenatal Vitamin D, Folic Acid and Iron May Prevent Schizophrenia in Adulthood

> **McGrath, John**, et al., "Prevention and Schizophrenia--the Role of Dietary Factors." *Schizophrenia Bulletin* 37, no. 2 (March 2011): 272–83. Publisher: OXFORD UNIVERSITY PRESS; doi:10.1093/schbul/sbq121., PMID: 20974747

> ➤ Adequate prenatal nutrition is essential for optimal brain development. There is a growing body of evidence from epidemiology linking exposure to nutritional deprivation and increased risk of schizophrenia. Based on studies from the Netherlands

and China, those exposed to macronutrient deficiencies during famine have an increased risk of schizophrenia. With respect to micronutrients, we focus on 3 candidates where there is biological plausibility for a role in this disorder and at least 1 study of an association with schizophrenia. These nutrients include vitamin D, folic acid, and iron. While the current evidence is incomplete, we discuss the potential implications of these findings for the prevention of schizophrenia. We argue that schizophrenia can draw inspiration from public health interventions related to prenatal nutrition and other outcomes and speculate on relevant factors that bear on the nature, risks, impact, and logistics of various nutritional strategies that may be employed to prevent this disorder.

Vitamin D

Vitamin D Supplementation May Reduce the Incidence of Schizophrenia

> **McGrath, John,** et al., "Is It Time to Trial Vitamin D Supplements for the Prevention of Schizophrenia?" *Acta Psychiatrica Scandinavica* 121, no. 5 (May 2010): 321–24. Publisher: BLACKWELL MUNKSGAARD; doi:10.1111/j.1600-0447.2010.01551.x., PMID: 20525021

> ➢ Based on the accumulating evidence linking hypovitaminosis D and schizophrenia, and the potential that a simple, safe and cheap nutritional supplement could reduce the incidence of this disorder, I argue that we should move to randomized controlled trials promptly. In light of the substantial burden of disability associated with schizophrenia, we should undertake these studies with a sense of urgency.

Preventing Vitamin D Deficiency during Early Life May Prevent Schizophrenia

> **McGrath, John.,** et al., "Vitamin D Supplementation during the First Year of Life and Risk of Schizophrenia: A Finnish Birth Cohort Study." *Schizophrenia Research* 67, no. 2–3 (April 1, 2004): 237–45. Publisher: ELSEVIER BV; doi:10.1016/j.schres.2003.08.005., PMID: 14984883

> ➢ "Vitamin D supplementation during the first year of life is associated with a reduced risk of schizophrenia in males. Preventing hypovitaminosis D during early life may reduce the incidence of schizophrenia."

CODEX ALTERNUS

SECTION TWO

Bipolar Disorder Treatments

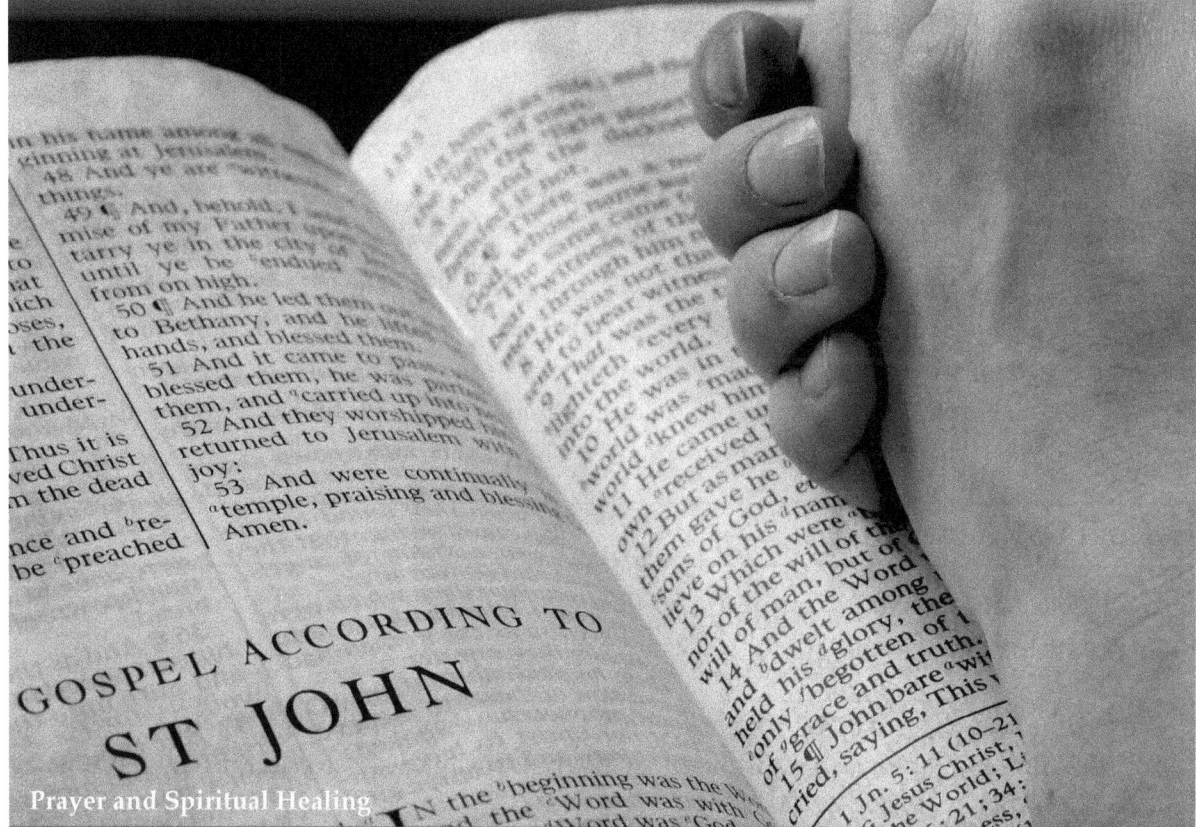

Prayer and Spiritual Healing

CODEX ALTERNUS

Dietary Changes

Dietary Tryptophan

Dietary Tryptophan Depletion as Treatment for Acute Mania

Applebaum, Julia, et al., "Rapid Tryptophan Depletion as a Treatment for Acute Mania: A Double-Blind, Pilot-Controlled Study." *Bipolar Disorders* 9, no. 8 (December 2007): 884–87. Publisher: BLACKWELL MUNKSGAARD; doi:10.1111/j.1399-5618.2007.00466.x., PMID: 18076538

> ➢ "Rapid tryptophan depletion may have an antimanic effect."

Fasting

Fasting during Ramadan has a Significant Decrease on Depression and Mania Rating Scales in Bipolar Patients on Lithium

Farooq, Saeed, et al., "Effect of Fasting during Ramadan on Serum Lithium Level and Mental State in Bipolar Affective Disorder." *International Clinical Psychopharmacology* 25, no. 6 (November 2010): 323–27. Publisher: LIPPINCOTT WILLIAMS & WILKINS doi:10.1097/YIC.0b013e32833d18b2., PMID: 20827213

> ➢ The scores on HDRS and YMRS showed significant decrease during Ramadan (F=34.12, P=0.00, for HDRS and F=15.6, P=0.000 for YMRS). The side effects and toxicity also did not differ significantly at three points. In conclusion, the patients who have stable mental state and lithium levels before Ramadan can be maintained on lithium during Ramadan. Fasting in an average temperature of 28°C for up to 12 h per day did not result in elevated serum lithium levels or more side effects and did not have adverse effects on mental state of patients suffering from bipolar affective disorder.

Inositol Deficiency Diet

Inositol Deficiency Diet had Major Effect on Reducing the Effect of Affective Disorder in Bipolar Patients

Shaldubina, Alona, et al., "Inositol Deficiency Diet and Lithium Effects." *Bipolar Disorders* 8, no. 2 (April 2006): 152–59. Publisher: BLACKWELL MUNKSGAARD; doi:10.1111/j.1399-5618.2006.00290.x., PMID: 16542185

> ➢ Dietary inositol restriction significantly augmented the inositol-reducing effect of Li in rat frontal cortex. Li reduced inositol levels by 4.7%, inositol-deficient diet by 5.1%, and Li plus inositol-deficient diet by 10.8%. However, feeding with the inositol-deficient diet

did not enhance the behavioral effect of Li in the Li-pilocarpine seizure model. Fifteen patients participated in an open clinical study of the inositol-deficient diet: six rapid cycling bipolar patients responding inadequately to Li or valproate in different phases of illness; two Li-treated bipolar outpatients with residual symptomatology, and seven inpatient Li-treated bipolar patients in non-responding acute mania. The diet had a major effect in reducing the severity of affective disorder in 10 of the patients within the first 7-14 days of treatment. These results suggest that dietary inositol restriction may be useful in some bipolar patients, but controlled replication is necessary.

Ketogenic Diet

Ketogenic Diet May Have Mood Stabilizing Properties

Phelps, James R. "The Ketogenic Diet for Type II Bipolar Disorder." *Neurocase* 19, no. 5 (2013): 423–26. Publisher: PSYCHOLOGY PRESS; doi:10.1080/13554794.2012.690421., PMID: 23030231

> Two woman with type II bipolar disorder were able to maintain ketosis for prolonged periods of time (2 and 3 years, respectively). Both experienced mood stabilization that exceeded that achieved with medication; experienced a significant subjective improvement that was directly related to ketosis and tolerated diet well. There was no significant adverse effects in either case. These cases demonstrate that the ketogenic diet is potentially sustainable option for mood stabilization in type II bipolar illness.

Ketogenic Diet has Antidepressant Properties

Murphy, Patricia, et al., "The Antidepressant Properties of the Ketogenic Diet." *Biological Psychiatry* 56, no. 12 (December 15, 2004): 981–83. Publisher: ELSEVIER INC. doi:10.1016/j.biopsych.2004.09.019., PMID: 15601609

> "The rats on the ketogenic diet spent less time immobile, suggesting that the rats on a ketogenic diet, like rats treated with antidepressants are less likely to exhibit "behayioral despair". It is concluded that the ketogenic diet has antidepressant properties."

The Ketogenic Diet May Have Mood Stabilizing Properties in Mood Disorders

El-Mallakh, R. S., et al., "The Ketogenic Diet May Have Mood-Stabilizing Properties." *Medical Hypotheses* 57, no. 6 (December 2001): 724–26. Publisher: CHURCHILL LIVINGSTONE doi:10.1054/mehy.2001.1446., PMID: 11918434

> The ketogenic diet, originally introduced in the 1920s, has been undergoing a recent resurgence as an adjunctive treatment for refractory epilepsy, particularly in children. In this difficult-to-treat population, the diet exhibits remarkable efficacy with two-thirds showing significant reduction in seizure frequency and one-third becoming nearly

seizure-free. There are several reasons to suspect that the ketogenic diet may also have utility as a mood stabilizer in bipolar illness. These include the observation that several anticonvulsant interventions may improve outcome in mood disorders. Furthermore, beneficial changes in brain-energy profile are noted in subjects on the ketogenic diet. This is important since global cerebral hypometabolism is a characteristic of the brains of depressed or manic individuals. Finally, the extracellular changes that occur in ketosis would be expected to decrease intracellular sodium concentrations, a common property of all effective mood stabilizers. Trials of the ketogenic diet in relapse prevention of bipolar mood episodes are warranted.

Vitamin Therapy

Micronutrients

Successful Treatment of Bipolar Disorder with Micronutrient Formula

Rucklidge, Julia J. "Successful Treatment of Bipolar Disorder II and ADHD with a Micronutrient Formula: A Case Study." *CNS Spectrums* 15, no. 5 (May 2010): 289–95., Publisher: MBL Communications; PMID: 20448519

> "After 8 weeks on the formula she showed significant improvements in mood, anxiety, and hyperactivity/impulsivity. Shen then choose to come off the formula; after 8 weeks her depression scores returned to baseline, and anxiety and ADHD symptoms worsened."

Empower Plus Microsupplement Resulted in Outcome Superior to Conventional Treatment

Frazier, Elisabeth A., et al., "Multinutrient Supplement as Treatment: Literature Review and Case Report of a 12-Year-Old Boy with Bipolar Disorder." *Journal of Child and Adolescent Psychopharmacology* 19, no. 4 (August 2009): 453–60. Publisher: MARY ANN/LIEBERT, INC. PUBLISHERS ;doi:10.1089/cap.2008.0157., PMID: 19702498

> " EMP+ [Empower Plus] resulted in outcome superior to conventional treatment."

Frazier, Elisabeth A., et al., "Nutritional and Safety Outcomes from an Open-Label Micronutrient Intervention for Pediatric Bipolar Spectrum Disorders." *Journal of Child and Adolescent Psychopharmacology* 23, no. 8 (October 2013): 558–67. Publisher: MARY ANN/LIEBERT, INC. PUBLISHERS; doi:10.1089/cap.2012.0098., PMID: 24138009

> "In this open prospective study. Short-term use of EMP+ in children with BPSD appeared safe and well-tolerated, with a side effect profile preferable to fist line psychotropic drugs for pediatric bipolar spectrum disorders."

Over Half the Adults with Bipolar Disorder Experienced Improvement Consuming a Micronutrient Supplement Formula at 6 Months

Gatley D., et al., "Database Analysis of Adults with Bipolar Disorder Consuming a Micronutrient Formula." *Clinical Medicine Psychiatry* 2009:4 3-16, Publisher: Libertas Academica

> "Mean symptom severity was 41% lower than baseline after 3 months (effect size =0.78), and 45% lower after 6 months (effect size= 0.76) (both paired t-tests significant. P< 0.001) In terms of responder status, 53% experienced >50% improvement at 6 months ."

Nutritional Supplements

Some Cases of Bipolar Disorder May Be Ameliorated by Nutritional Supplementation

Kaplan B. "Effective Mood Stabilization with Chelated Mineral Supplement: An Open-Label Trial in Bipolar Disorder." *J Clin Psychiatry* 2001;62:936-944, Publisher: PHYSICIANS POSTGRADUATE PRESS, INC.

> "Some cases of bipolar illness may be ameliorated by nutritional supplementation."

Vitamin B9 (Folate, Folic Acid)

Adjunctive Folic Acid is Effective for Treatment of Mania in Bipolar Disorder

Behzadi, A. H., et al., "Folic Acid Efficacy as an Alternative Drug Added to Sodium Valproate in the Treatment of Acute Phase of Mania in Bipolar Disorder: A Double-Blind Randomized Controlled Trial." *Acta Psychiatrica Scandinavica* 120, no. 6 (December 2009): 441–45. Publisher: BLACKWELL MUNKSGAARD; doi:10.1111/j.1600-0447.2009.01368.x., PMID: 19392814

> "Based on our findings, folic acid seems to be an effective adjunctive to sodium valproate in the treatment of the acute phase of mania in patients with bipolar disorder."

Folic Acid Enhances Lithium Prophylaxis

Coppen, A. "Folic Acid Enhances Lithium Prophylaxis." *Journal of Affective Disorders* 10, no. 1 (February 1986): 9–13., Publisher: ELSEVIER BV; PMID: 2939126

> "A double-blind trial was carried out to investigate the effect the effect on affective morbidity of a daily supplement of 200 micrograms folic acid or a matched placebo in a group of 75 patients on lithium therapy. During the trial the patients with the highest plasma folate concentrations showed a significant reduction in their affective morbidity. Patients who had their plasma folate increased to 13 ng/ml or above had a 40% reduction in their affective morbidity. It is suggested that a daily supplement of 300-400 micrograms folic acid would be useful in long term lithium prophylaxis."

Choline

Choline is Effective in the Treatment of Rapid-Cycling Bipolar Disorder

Stoll, A. L., et al., "Choline in the Treatment of Rapid-Cycling Bipolar Disorder: Clinical and Neurochemical Findings in Lithium-Treated Patients." *Biological Psychiatry* 40, no. 5 (September 1, 1996): 382–88. Publisher: ELSEVIER INC. doi:10.1016/0006-3223(95)00423-8., PMID: 8874839

> The study examined choline augmentation of lithium for rapid cycling bipolar disorder. Choline bitartrate was given openly to 6 consecutive lithium-treated outpatients with rapid-cycling bipolar disorder. Five patients also underwent brain proton magnetic resonance spectroscopy. Five of 6 rapid-cycling patients had a substantial reduction in manic symptoms, and 4 patients had marked reduction in all mood symptoms during choline therapy."…"Choline, in the presence of lithium, was a safe and effective treatment for 4 of the 6 rapid-cycling patients in our series.

Vitamin C

Vitamin C Produced Statically Significant Improvement in Depressive, Manic and Paranoid symptom Complexes in Chronic Psychiatric Patients

Milner G., et al., "Ascorbic Acid in Chronic Psychiatric Patients—A Controlled Trial." *Brit J Psychiat* (1963), 109, 294-299, Publisher: ROYAL MEDICO-PSYCHOLOGICAL ASSOCIATION

> "Statistically significant improvement in depressive, manic and paranoid symptom complexes, together with an improvement in overall personality functioning, was obtained following saturation with ascorbic acid."

Fatty Acids

Omega-3

Omega-3's May Be Effective for the Treatment of Bipolar Disorder Depression

CODEX ALTERNUS

Sarris, Jerome, et al., "Omega-3 for Bipolar Disorder: Meta-Analyses of Use in Mania and Bipolar Depression." *The Journal of Clinical Psychiatry* 73, no. 1 (January 2012): 81–86. Publisher: PHYSICIANS POSTGRADUATE PRESS, INC. doi:10.4088/JCP.10r06710., PMID: 21903025

> ➤ "The meta-analytic findings provide strong evidence that bipolar depressive symptoms may be improved by adjunctive use of omega-3. The evidence, however, does not support its adjunctive use in attenuating mania."

Omega-3 Fatty Acids Decrease Irritability in Bipolar Disorder

Sagduyu, Kemal, et al., "Omega-3 Fatty Acids Decreased Irritability of Patients with Bipolar Disorder in an Add-On, Open Label Study." *Nutrition Journal* 4 (2005): 6. Publisher: BIOMED CENTRAL LTD; doi:10.1186/1475-2891-4-6., PMID: 15703073

> ➤ Omega-3 Fatty Acid intake helped with irritability component of patients suffering from bipolar disorder with significant presenting sign of irritability. Low dose (to 2 grams per day), add-on O-3FA may also help with the irritability component of different clinical conditions, such as schizophrenia, borderline personality disorder and other psychiatric conditions with a common presenting sign of irritability.

Omega-3 Fatty Acid Supplementation May Be Helpful Adjunct in Selected Patients with Bipolar Disorder

Turnbull, Teresa, et al., "Efficacy of Omega-3 Fatty Acid Supplementation on Improvement of Bipolar Symptoms: A Systematic Review." *Archives of Psychiatric Nursing* 22, no. 5 (October 2008): 305–11. Publisher: W.B./SAUNDERS CO. doi:10.1016/j.apnu.2008.02.011., PMID: 18809123

> ➤ Those using an omega-3 combination of eicosapentaenoic acid and docosahexanoic acid demonstrated a statistically significant improvement in bipolar symptoms, whereas those using a single constituent did not. Dosage variations did not demonstrate statistically significant differences. Due to its benign side effect profile and some evidence supporting its usefulness in bipolar illness, omega-3 may be a helpful adjunct in treatment of selected patients. Future studies are needed to conclusively confirm the efficacy of omega-3s in bipolar disorder, uncovering a new well-tolerated treatment option.

Adjunctive Omega-3 Fatty Acids are Effective for Depressive Symptoms in Bipolar Disorder

Montgomery, P., et al., "Omega-3 Fatty Acids for Bipolar Disorder." *The Cochrane Database of Systematic Reviews,* no. 2 (2008): CD005169. doi:10.1002/14651858.CD005169.pub2., Publisher: WILEY INTERSCIENCE; PMID: 18425912

> Results from one study showed positive effects of omega-3 as an adjunctive treatment for depressive but not manic symptoms in bipolar disorder. These findings must be regarded with caution owing to the limited data available. There is an acute need for well-designed and executed randomised controlled trials in this field.

Flax Oil

Flax Oil May Decrease the Severity of Illness in Children with Bipolar Disorder

Gracious, Barbara L., et al., "Randomized, Placebo-Controlled Trial of Flax Oil in Pediatric Bipolar Disorder." *Bipolar Disorders* 12, no. 2 (March 2010): 142–54. Publisher: BLACKWELL MUNKSGAARD; doi:10.1111/j.1399-5618.2010.00799.x., PMID: 20402707

> Although flax oil may decrease severity of illness in children and adolescents with bipolar disorder who have meaningful increases in serum EPA percent levels and/or decreased AA and DPA-n6 levels, individual variations in conversion of a-LNA to EPA and DHA as well as dosing burden favor the use of fish oil both for clinical trials and clinical practice.

Amino Acids

5-HTP

Antidepressant Potentiation by 5-HTP Showed Greater Clinical Improvement

Mendlewicz, J., et al., "Antidepressant Potentiation of 5-Hydroxytryptophan by L-Deprenil in Affective Illness." *Journal of Affective Disorders* 2, no. 2 (June 1980): 137–46., Publisher: ELSEVIER BV; PMID: 6448885

> In an open label study, L-Deprenil, an irreversible selective MAO-B inhibitor without 'cheese effect' was given to 14 patents with unipolar and bipolar depression receiving L-5-Hydroxytryptophan (L-5-HTP) and benzerazide. Ten out of 14 patients showed a good response to the combination of drugs and correlation was found between the degree of platelet MAO inhibition and clinical response. In a double-blind controlled study, 18 affectively ill patients were randomly allocated to L-Deprenil plus L-5-HTP and benzerazide, 21 patients were treated with L-5-HTP and benzerazide and 19 patients placebo only. Patients treated with combination of L-Deprenil and L-5-HTP showed a significantly greater clinical improvement than placebo patients but this was not the case with 5-HTP alone.

Branched Amino Acids

Branched Amino Acid Drink Ameliorate Manic Symptoms

CODEX ALTERNUS

Scarna, A., et al., "Effects of a Branched-Chain Amino Acid Drink in Mania." *The British Journal of Psychiatry: The Journal of Mental Science* 182 (March 2003): 210–13., Publisher: ROYAL MEDICO-PSYCHOLOGICAL ASSOCIATION; PMID: 12611783

> "A nutritional intervention that decreases tyrosine availability to the brain acutely ameliorating's manic symptoms."

L-tryptophan

Tryptophan Combined with Lithium Results in Significantly Greater Improvement in Bipolar and Schizoaffective Disorders

Brewerton, T. D., et al.,"Lithium Carbonate and L-Tryptophan in the Treatment of Bipolar and Schizoaffective Disorders." *The American Journal of Psychiatry* 140, no. 6 (June 1983): 757–60., Publisher: AM PSYCHIATRIC ASSN; PMID: 6405638

> The authors review theoretical and clinical data supporting the hypothesis that L-tryptophan may potentiate the effects of lithium carbonate and report on a double-blind clinical comparison of lithium plus L-tryptophan and lithium plus placebo in 9 bipolar and 7 schizoaffective patients. Overall the combination of lithium and L-tryptophan resulted in significantly greater improvement. However, the results may have been confounded by the greater, although nonsignificant, doses of neuroleptics administered to the group receiving L-tryptophan. The authors discuss the interactions of lithium and L-trypotophan with the serotonin system.

L-tryptophan Has Some Therapeutic Effect for Treatment of Acute Mania

Chouinard, G., et al., "A Controlled Clinical Trial of L-Tryptophan in Acute Mania." *Biological Psychiatry* 20, no. 5 (May 1985): 546–57., Publisher: ELSEVIER INC; PMID: 3886024

> In a 2 week study, 24 newly admitted manic patients were treated for 1 week with L-tryptophan (12g/day); during the second week, half the patients, chosen at random, continued to receive tryptophan, while placebo was substituted in the other half under double-blind conditions. In the open phase of the study, there was a clinically and statistically (p less than 0.001) significant reduction in manic symptom scores, with little need for haloperidol prn. Patients who continued to be treated with tryptophan showed no significant change in mean scores during the second week, but those who were switched to placebo tended (p less than 0.10) to show an increase in mean scores for manic symptoms."..."These results suggest that increasing the synthesis of 5-hydroxytyptamine has some therapeutic effect in mania.

L-Tryptophan is a Safe Alternative for Maintenance Treatment of Bipolar II Disorder

Beitman, B. D., et al., "L-Tryptophan in the Maintenance Treatment of Bipolar II Manic-Depressive Illness." *The American Journal of Psychiatry* 139, no. 11 (November 1982): 1498–99., Publisher: AM PSYCHIATRIC ASSN; PMID: 7137405

> ➤ Although tryptophan is quite expensive and may require concomitant ascorbic acid and/or nicotinamide, it appears safe and may be considered an alternative maintenance treatment in bipolar patients who are unresponsive to or unable to take lithium. The effective dose range appears to be quite wide (2-12 g/day), which may indicate the absence of a therapeutic window.

Tryptophan for Treatment of Rapid-Cycling Bipolar Disorder Comorbid with Fibromyalgia in Middle-aged Woman

Sharma, V., et al., "Tryptophan for Treatment of Rapid-Cycling Bipolar Disorder Comorbid with Fibromyalgia." *Canadian Journal of Psychiatry. Revue Canadienne De Psychiatrie* 46, no. 5 (June 2001): 452–53., Publisher: CANADIAN PSYCHIATRIC ASSOCIATION., PMID: 11441787

> ➤ Ms. A is a 40-year-old lady who has presented with a history of recurrent episodes of depression since her mid-teens. She questioned the effectiveness of various treatment interventions and became increasingly frustrated with her ongoing mood instability, chronic pain condition, and poor psychosocial functioning. At this time, it was decided to prescribe a trial of tryptophan. The dosage was gradually increased over a couple of weeks to 4 g daily. She remained on lorazepam 1mg and oxazepam 25mg daily, which she had taken for years. Within 2 weeks of reaching the 4 g dosage, she developed a mixed state characterized by symptoms of feeling "revved up, "irritable, agitated, with racing thoughts, preoccupation with thoughts of suicide, and dysphroia. The tryptophan dosage was gradually lowered to 2 g, and her mood has been quite stable for a least 18 months. She continues to experience symptoms of fibromyalgia, but these are not as intense or disabling as before. She has been gainfully employed for more than 1 year and remains on the drug regimen of tryptophan 2g, lorazepam 1mg, and oxazepam 25mg daily.

Tryptophan for Refractory Bipolar Disorder and Sleep Phase Delay

Cooke, Robert G., et al., "Tryptophan for Refractory Bipolar Spectrum Disorder and Sleep-Phase Delay." *Journal of Psychiatry & Neuroscience: JPN* 35, no. 2 (March 2010): 144., Publisher: CANADIAN MEDICAL ASSOCIATION; PMID: 20184811

> ➤ A trial of L-tryptophan, starting at a dose of 1 g in the evening was begun in June 2007, and within 3 weeks she began to report an improvement in her ability to get to sleep and

wake in time on the morning. Over a few more weeks, the dosage was increased to 3.5g daily combined with over –the-counter pyridoxine to limit the toxic metabolites of tryptophan. After about 10 weeks of treatment, she began to consistently arrive at work at 9 am, and her depressive symptoms cleared. Two years after L-tryptophan was initiated, she continued to show a normal sleep-wake pattern and remained free of depressive and hypomanic symptoms. She was taking no prescribed medications except L-tryptophan and pyridoxine.

L-tryptophan and Niacin

Potentiation of Lithium by L-Tryptophan/Niacin Combination Results in Complete Remission in Patient with Bipolar Disorder

> **Chouinard, G.,** et al., "Potentiation of Lithium by Tryptophan in a Patient with Bipolar Illness." *The American Journal of Psychiatry* 136, no. 5 (May 1979): 719–20., Publisher: AM PSYCHIATRIC ASSN; PMID: 155408

> ➤ "It was decided to add L-tryptophan, 3 g p.o. b.i.d., and nicotinamide, 750mg p.o. b.i.d., to her treatment regimen…"
> ➤ In this case described here, the patient had been treated with tryciclics, lithium alone, and subsequently with lithium in combination with a neuroleptic. These treatment regimens had not adequately controlled her manic or depressive symptoms or altered her cycles length. However, the addition of tryptophan-nicotinamide to lithium resulted in an almost complete remission of symptoms. The first effect was seen 7 weeks after addition of tryptophan-nicotinamide, with a reduction in the severity of the depressed phase. After 10 weeks the patient entered her first extended period of normality since the illness began 4 years ago.

Tyrosine

Dietary Tyrosine Depletion Attenuates Symptoms of Mania

> **McTavish, S. F.,** et al., "Antidopaminergic Effects of Dietary Tyrosine Depletion in Healthy Subjects and Patients with Manic Illness." *The British Journal of Psychiatry: The Journal of Mental Science* 179 (October 2001): 356–60., Publisher: ROYAL MEDICO-PSYCHOLOGICAL ASSOCIATION; PMID: 11581118

> ➤ We also obtained preliminary evidence that the TYR-free mixture is capable of attenuating the symptoms of acute mania. As is common in the in-patient treatment of manic illness, our subjects were receiving treatment with antipsychotic drugs at doses likely to produce a high degree of dopamine D2 receptor occupancy. Despite this, they continued to experience clinically significant manic symptomology that was diminished by tyrosine depletion.

CODEX ALTERNUS

Hormones

Estrogen and Progesterone

Estrogen-Progesterone Combination May Be Effective As Mood Stabilizers for Bipolar Disorder

> **Chouinard, G.,** et al., "Estrogen-Progesterone Combination: Another Mood Stabilizer?" *The American Journal of Psychiatry* 144, no. 6 (June 1987): 826., Publisher: AM PSYCHIATRIC ASSN; PMID: 3592013

> ➢ The mechanism of mood stabilization is unknown but may involve noradrenergic, dopaminergic, and/or serotonergic systems. Estrogen, administered chronically, increases dopaminergic receptor density (1) and decreases dopaminergic concentration in the limbic structures (2), while progesterone inhibits reuptake of serotonin and decreases its metabolism, resulting in enhanced serotonergic activity in the CNS. Chronic estrogen treatment also increases progesterone receptors in target organs, possibly augmenting the activity of progesterone in the CNS. Thus, the modulation of mood appears to be mediated through progesterone. These cases suggest that hormones may be effective as mood stabilizers in bipolar patients resistant to standard treatments.

Estrogen-Progesterone Combination is Effective in Treatment of Post-partum Mania

> **Huang, Ming-Chyi,** et al., "Estrogen-Progesterone Combination for Treatment-Refractory Post-Partum Mania." *Psychiatry and Clinical Neurosciences* 62, no. 1 (February 2008): 126. Publisher: BLACKWELL PUBLISHING ASIA; doi:10.1111/j.1440-1819.2007.01782.x., PMID: 18289153

> ➢ Estrogen modulates various systems of neurotransmission, especially dopaminergic transmission. A low rate of relapse is reported under prophylaxis of estrogen in patients with histories of post-partum affective disorder. The beneficial effect of estradiol treatment in post-partum psychosis could be related to low serum estradiol level. Combined estrogen and progesterone appeared effective as adjuvant treatment for mood stabilization. A recent pilot study also suggested that medroxyprogesterone may have benefits in the management of manic symptoms. In the present patient the prolonged post-partum manic episode might have been due to rapid decrease of both estrogen and progesterone levels, and which then subsided following HRT. To our knowledge this is the first report regarding the role of HRT in the treatment of post-partum mood swings.

Insulin

Intranasal Insulin Significantly Improved a Single Measure of Executive Function in Bipolar Disorder

CODEX ALTERNUS

McIntyre, Roger S., et al., "A Randomized, Double-Blind, Controlled Trial Evaluating the Effect of Intranasal Insulin on Neurocognitive Function in Euthymic Patients with Bipolar Disorder." *Bipolar Disorders* 14, no. 7 (November 2012): 697–706. Publisher: BLACKWELL MUNKSGAARD; doi:10.1111/bdi.12006., PMID: 23107220

> ➢ Adjunctive intranasal insulin administration significantly improved a single measure of executive function in bipolar disorder. We were unable to detect between-group differences on other neurocognitive measures, with improvement noted in both groups. Subject phenotyping on the basis of pre-existing neurocognitive deficits and/or genotype [e.g., apolipoprotein E (ApoE)] may possibly identify a more responsive subgroup.

Melatonin

Melatonin Treatment Leads to Rapid Relief of Insomnia and Aborts Manic Episode in Boy with Bipolar Disorder

Robertson, J. M., et al., "Case Study: The Use of Melatonin in a Boy with Refractory Bipolar Disorder." *Journal of the American Academy of Child and Adolescent Psychiatry* 36, no. 6 (June 1997): 822–25. Publisher: LIPPINCOTT WILLIAMS & WILKINS doi:10.1097/00004583-199706000-00020., PMID: 9183138

> ➢ "A trial of melatonin led to rapid relief of insomnia and aborted a manic episode. He continued to take melatonin and adjunctive alprazolam for 15 months without reoccurrence of insomnia or mania."

Pregnenolone

Pregnenolone May Improve Depressive Symptoms in Patients with Bipolar Disorder

Brown, E. Sherwood, et al., "A Randomized, Double-Blind, Placebo-Controlled Trial of Pregnenolone for Bipolar Depression." *Neuropsychopharmacology: Official Publication of the American College of Neuropsychopharmacology* 39, no. 12 (November 2014): 2867–73. Publisher: NATURE PUBLISHING GROUP; doi:10.1038/npp.2014.138., PMID: 24917198

> ➢ Depression remission rates were greater in the pregnenolone group (61%) compared with the placebo group (37%), as assessed by the IDS-SR ($\chi(2)(1)=3.99$, p=0.046), but not the HRSD. Large baseline-to-exit changes in neurosteroid levels were observed in the pregnenolone group but not in the placebo group. In the pregnenolone group, baseline-to-exit change in the HRSA correlated negatively with changes in allopregnanolone (r(22)=-0.43, p=0.036) and pregNANolone (r(22)=-0.48, p=0.019) levels. Pregnenolone was well tolerated. The results suggest that pregnenolone may improve depressive symptoms in patients with BPD and can be safely administered.

CODEX ALTERNUS

Traditional Ayurvedic/Asian/Chinese/Kampo Medicine

Ashwagandha (Indian Ginseng)

Ashwagandha Appears to Improve Auditory Verbal Working Memory in Bipolar Disorder

> **Chengappa, K. N. Roy,** et al., "Randomized Placebo-Controlled Adjunctive Study of an Extract of Withania Somnifera for Cognitive Dysfunction in Bipolar Disorder." *The Journal of Clinical Psychiatry* 74, no. 11 (November 2013): 1076–83. Publisher: PHYSICIANS POSTGRADUATE PRESS, INC.; doi:10.4088/JCP.13m08413., PMID: 24330893

> ➢ Although results are preliminary, WSE appears to improve auditory-verbal working memory (digit span backward), a measure of reaction time, and a measure of social cognition in bipolar disorder. Given the paucity of data for improving cognitive capacity in bipolar disorder, WSE offers promise, appears to have a benign side-effects profile, and merits further study.

Free and Easy Wanderer Plus

Adjunctive Free and Easy Wanderer Plus Results in Significant Improvement of Depression for the Treatment of Bipolar Disorder

> **Zhang, Zhang-Jin,** et al., "Adjunctive Herbal Medicine with Carbamazepine for Bipolar Disorders: A Double-Blind, Randomized, Placebo-Controlled Study." *Journal of Psychiatric Research* 41, no. 3–4 (June 2007): 360–69. Publisher: PERGAMON doi:10.1016/j.jpsychires.2005.06.002., PMID: 16081106

> ➢ "Compared to CBZ momotherapy, adjunctive FEWP with CBZ resulted in significantly greater improvement on depressed subjects (84.8% vs. 63.8%, p=.032), but failed to produce significantly greater improvement on manic measures and the response rate in manic subjects."

> **Zhang, Zhang-Jin,** et al., "The Beneficial Effects of the Herbal Medicine Free and Easy Wanderer Plus (FEWP) for Mood Disorders: Double-Blind, Placebo-Controlled Studies." *Journal of Psychiatric Research* 41, no. 10 (November 2007): 828–36. Publisher: PERGAMON; doi:10.1016/j.jpsychires.2006.08.002., PMID: 17010995

> ➢ "Both unipolar and bipolar patients assigned to FEWP displayed significantly greater improvement on the three efficiency indices and significantly higher clinical response rate (74%) than those treated with placebo (42%) at endpoint."

CODEX ALTERNUS

Siberian Ginseng

Siberian Ginseng as Adjunctive Therapy for Lithium in Pediatric Bipolar Disorder is as effective as Prozac

> **Weng, Shenhong,** et al., "Comparison of the Addition of Siberian Ginseng (Acanthopanax Senticosus) Versus Fluoxetine to Lithium for the Treatment of Bipolar Disorder in Adolescents: A Randomized, Double-Blind Trial." *Current Therapeutic Research, Clinical and Experimental* 68, no. 4 (July 2007): 280–90. Publisher: EXCERPTA MEDICA, INC. doi:10.1016/j.curtheres.2007.08.004., PMID: 24683218

> ➤ "Our study found no significant differences in these adolescents with BD treated with lithium plus adjunctive A. senticosus or fluoxetine. All treatments were generally well tolerated."

Xiao Yao San Jia Wei

Xiao Yao San Jia Wei for Marked Improvement of Bipolar Disorder

> **Zhang, L. D.,** et al., "Traditional Chinese Medicine Typing of Affective Disorders and Treatment." *The American Journal of Chinese Medicine* 22, no. 3–4 (1994): 321–27. Publisher: INST FOR ADVANCED RES IN ASIAN; doi:10.1142/S0192415X94000383. , PMID: 7872244

> ➤ "The results are 26 patients with marked improvement, 17 patients with improvement, 7 patients with no improvement."

Other Natural Compounds

Acetyl-L-carnitine

Acetyl-L-carnitine May Have Antidepressant Effects in Depressed Elderly Populations

> **Soczynska, Joanna K.,** et al., "Acetyl-L-Carnitine and Alpha-Lipoic Acid: Possible Neurotherapeutic Agents for Mood Disorders?" *Expert Opinion on Investigational Drugs* 17, no. 6 (June 2008): 827–43. doi:10.1517/13543784.17.6.827., PMID: 18491985

> ➤ L-carnitine and alpha-lipoic acid may offer neurotherapeutic effects (e.g., neurocognitive enhancement) via disparate mechanisms including antioxidant, anti-inflammatory, and metabolic regulation. Preliminary controlled trials in depressed geriatric populations also suggest an antidepressant effect with acetyl-L-carnitine.

CODEX ALTERNUS

Alpha-lipoic Acid

Alpha-lipoic Acid Has an Anti-Manic Effect

Macêdo, Danielle S., et al., "Effects of Alpha-Lipoic Acid in an Animal Model of Mania Induced by D-Amphetamine." *Bipolar Disorders* 14, no. 7 (November 2012): 707–18. doi:10.1111/j.1399-5618.2012.01046.x., PMID: 22897629

> ➤ Our findings showed that ALA, similarly to Li, is effective in reversing and preventing AMPH-induced behavioral and neurochemical alterations, providing a rationale for the design of clinical trials investigating ALA's possible antimanic effect.

Calabar Bean (Physostigmine)

Physostigmine Can Dramatically Reverse Mania for a Temproray Period

Khouzam, H. R. et al., "Physostigmine Temporarily and Dramatically Reversing Acute Mania." *General Hospital Psychiatry* 18, no. 3 (May 1996): 203–4., PMID: 8739014

> ➤ Physostigmine is contraindicated in patients with unstable vital signs, asthma, or history of cardiac abnormalities. It is also clinically important to know that physostigmine effects on reversing mania, although they may be dramatic, are usually temporary, lasting 20-90 minutes, and may paradoxically lead to rebounding agitation and mania. Physostigmine is useful in the treatment of mania as long as comprehensive medical and psychiatric assessment and emergency cardiac monitoring and life-support services are available.

Cannabis

Cannabis as a Mood Stabilizer in Bipolar Disorder

Grinspoon, L., et al., "The Use of Cannabis as a Mood Stabilizer in Bipolar Disorder: Anecdotal Evidence and the Need for Clinical Research." *Journal of Psychoactive Drugs* 30, no. 2 (June 1998): 171–77. Publisher: HAIGHT-ASHBURY PUBLICATIONS doi:10.1080/02791072.1998.10399687., PMID: 9692379

> ➤ The authors present case histories indicating that a number of patients find cannabis (marihuana) useful in the treatment of their bipolar disorder. Some used it to treat mania, depression, or both. They stated that it was more effective than conventional drugs, or helped relieve the side effects of those drugs. One woman found that cannabis curbed her manic rages; she and her husband have worked to make it legally available as a medicine. Others described the use of cannabis as a supplement to lithium (allowing reduced consumption) or for relief of lithium's side effects. Another case illustrates the

fact that medical cannabis users are in danger of arrest, especially when children are encouraged to inform on parents by some drug prevention programs. An analogy is drawn between the status of cannabis today and that of lithium in the early 1950s, when its effect on mania had been discovered but there were no controlled studies. In the case of cannabis, the law has made such studies almost impossible, and the only available evidence is anecdotal. The potential for cannabis as a treatment for bipolar disorder unfortunately can not be fully explored in the present social circumstances.

Cannabinoids

Cannabinoids have Pharmacological Properties that Could Be Therapeutic in Patients with Bipolar Disorder

> **Ashton, C. H.,** et al., "Cannabinoids in Bipolar Affective Disorder: A Review and Discussion of Their Therapeutic Potential." *Journal of Psychopharmacology (Oxford, England)* 19, no. 3 (May 2005): 293–300. Publisher: SAGE SCIENCE PRESS (UK) doi:10.1177/0269881105051541., PMID: 15888515

> ➤ "Despite the sparse anecdotal data in humans and the absence of controlled clinical trials, the evidence discussed above shows that both THC and CBD have pharmacological properties that could be therapeutic in patients with BAD."

Carboxylic Acids

Carboxylic Fatty Acids Have Potent Anticonvulsant Activity Which Might Possess Mood Stabilizing Effects

> **Azab, Abed N.,** et al., "Anticonvulsant Efficacy of Valproate-like Carboxylic Acids: A Potential Target for Anti-Bipolar Therapy." *Bipolar Disorders* 9, no. 3 (May 2007): 197–205. doi:10.1111/j.1399-5618.2007.00351.x., PMID: 17430293

> ➤ In summary, these data demonstrate that some dietary fatty acids and other valproate-like acids have potent anticonvulsant activity and might also possess mood stabilizing effects that may expand the treatment options for bipolar disorder.

Show Here is that Hexanoic Acid, Heptanoic Acid, Otanoic Acid, Nonanoic Acid, Decanoic Acid, and Ethhexanoate Decrease Intracellular Inositol Levels

> **Ding, Daobin**, et al., "Yeast Bioassay for Identification of Inositol Depleting Compounds." *The World Journal of Biological Psychiatry: The Official Journal of the World Federation of Societies of Biological Psychiatry* 10, no. 4 Pt 3 (2009): 893–99. doi:10.1080/15622970802485276., PMID: 18979283

> We have previously shown that valproate, like lithium, decreases intracellular inositol, which supports the inositol depletion hypothesis. We employed inositol depletion in yeast as a sceening tool to identify potential new anti-bipolar medications. We show here that hexanoic acid, heptanoic acid, otanoic acid, nonanoic acid, decanoic acid, ethhexanoate decrease intracellular inositol levels and increase the expression on *INO1*, the gene encoding myo-inositol-3-phosphate synathe (MIPS). Similar to valproate, these inositol-depleting carboxylic acids+ inhibited MIPS indirectly. A correlation was shown between cell growth inhibition and the increase in *INO1* expression by the carboxylic acids, factors that were reversed in the presence of inositol. Inositol depletion in yeast may be exploited as an easy and inexpensive screening test for potential new inositol depleting compounds.

Chelation

Control of Mania in Wilson 's disease by Chelation Only

Mitra, Saikat, et al., "Control of Mania with Chelation-Only in a Case of Wilson's Disease." *The Journal of Neuropsychiatry and Clinical Neurosciences* 26, no. 1 (2014): E6. Publisher: AMERICAN PSYCHIATRIC PUBLISHING, INC. doi:10.1176/appi.neuropsych.12110271., PMID: 24515687

> In this case, psychiatric manifestations appeared in the course of WD without any worsening of motor manifestations, which is quite rare. Emergence of manic symptoms on omission of penicillamine and remission after reinstitution confirms it to be a primary neuropsychiatric manifestation of WD. This case also signifies that only optimization of primary management with chelating agents may suffice for controlling psychiatric manifestations in WD. This agrees well with the concept of organic psychosis. This is important to reduce unnecessary health costs and the burden of side effects of psychotropics in these cases.

Chelation of Vanadium with Vitamin C and EDTA is Effective as Standard Drugs for Depressive Symptoms in Bipolar Patients, But Not for Mania

Kay, D. S., et al., "The Therapeutic Effect of Ascorbic Acid and EDTA in Manic-Depressive Psychosis: Double-Blind Comparisons with Standard Treatments." *Psychological Medicine* 14, no. 3 (August 1984): 533–39., PMID: 6436854

> It is worthy of not that patients receiving ascorbic acid and EDTA tended to complain of fewer side effects and there was a suggestion that such a drug combination produced an earlier onset of action. It is also possible that treatment with ascorbic acid and EDTA is beneficial clinically but through an effect which in unrelated to vanadium metabolism. However, the results of this study are consistent with the suggestion that, in depressive psychosis, changes in vanadate metabolism are eatiologically related to the changes in mood and that ascorbic acid and EDTA may be of clinical use in treating such states. Any possible side-effects associated with the long-term use of such drugs is not yet known.

> In mania, however, treatment approaches aimed at reducing the concentration of intracellular vanadate were found to be less effective than lithium. The design of the trial was such that it could not demonstrate whether ascorbic acid and EDTA had any effect in reducing the severity of manic symptomology, but only demonstrated that the combination of ascorbic acid and EDTA was less effective than lithium. The results therefore provide no evidence to support the suggestion that vanadium metabolism is of aetiological significance in mania, a finding which contrasts with previous studies. However, there is less agreement on the biochemical changes occurring in mania than those occurring in depression and the detailed metabolism of vanadium in manic depressive disorders is probably complex—for example, in mania the vanadium content of hair is high but those of plasma and of whole blood are normal, whereas in depression the vanadium contents of whole blood and plasma are high.

Chelerythrine

PKC Inhibitor Chelerythrine May Have Antimanic Effects

Einat, Haim, et al., "Partial Effects of the Protein Kinase C Inhibitor Chelerythrine in a Battery of Tests for Manic-like Behavior in Black Swiss Mice." *Pharmacological Reports: PR* 66, no. 4 (August 2014): 722–25. Publisher: INSTITUTE OF PHARMACOLOGY, POLISH ACADEMY OF SCIENCES; doi:10.1016/j.pharep.2014.03.013., PMID: 24948079

> The partial effects in the battery are not unique as previous studies showed that lithium, valproate and risperidone, all used in the treatment of bipolar disorder, have distinct profiles in the battery. It is therefore concluded that chelerythrine may have antimanic effects and additional dose and time response studies are warranted to further evaluate its range of activity.

Chromium

Chromium is Well Tolerated for Treatment Resistant Rapid-Cycling Bipolar Disorder

Amann, Benedikt L., et al., "A 2-Year, Open-Label Pilot Study of Adjunctive Chromium in Patients with Treatment-Resistant Rapid-Cycling Bipolar Disorder." *Journal of Clinical Psychopharmacology* 27, no. 1 (February 2007): 104–6. Publisher: LIPPINCOTT WILLIAMS & WILKINS; doi:10.1097/JCP.0b013e31802e744b., PMID: 17224731

> Six of 7 patients showed a reduction in the numbers of affective episodes within 1 year. The mean number of affective episodes in 7 patients before entry decreased from 6 (SD, 4.0; range , 4]5) to 2.6 (SD, 2.0; range, 0]6) after 1 year having received add-on CC. This reduction in 6 of 7 patients was also evident in the analysis of the CGI-BP. The mean overall CGI changed from 3.9 (SD, 1.4; range. 1]6) to 3.2 (SD, 1.8; range 1]6)…In general , chromium in doses up to 800 Ag/d was very well tolerated by all patients. However,

some patients reported side effects, which were in general mild and did not lead to any dropout during the study.

Citicoline

Citicoline Add-on Therapy was Associated with Improvement in Declarative Memory and Cocaine Use in Bipolar Disorder

> **Brown, E. Sherwood,** et al., "A Randomized, Placebo-Controlled Trial of Citicoline Add-on Therapy in Outpatients with Bipolar Disorder and Cocaine Dependence." *Journal of Clinical Psychopharmacology* 27, no. 5 (October 2007): 498–502. Publisher: LIPPINCOTT WILLIAMS & WILKINS doi:10.1097/JCP.0b013e31814db4c4., PMID: 17873684

> ➤ "The use of citicoline was associated with improvement relative to placebo in some aspects of declarative memory and cocaine use, but not for mood. The findings are promising and suggest that larger trials of citicoline are warranted. "

Citicoline Add-on Therapy May Have Antidepressant Properties in Bipolar Methamphetamine Users

> **Brown, E. Sherwood,** et al., "A Randomized, Double-Blind, Placebo-Controlled Trial of Citicoline for Bipolar and Unipolar Depression and Methamphetamine Dependence." *Journal of Affective Disorders* 143, no. 1–3 (December 20, 2012): 257–60. Publisher: ELSEVIER BV; doi:10.1016/j.jad.2012.05.006., PMID: 22974472

> ➤ To our knowledge this is the first placebo-controlled trial in a dual diagnosis sample with methamphetamine use disorders. Findings suggest that citicoline may have antidepressant properties in this population. Greater treatment retention with citicoline is also noteworthy in a patient population with substance dependence. Larger trials targeting depressive symptoms and treatment retention seem warranted.

Coenzyme Q10

Coenzyme Q10 was Found to Reduce Depressive Symptom Severity for Older Adults with Bipolar Disorder

> **Forester, Brent P.,** et al., "Coenzyme Q10 Effects on Creatine Kinase Activity and Mood in Geriatric Bipolar Depression." *Journal of Geriatric Psychiatry and Neurology* 25, no. 1 (March 2012): 43–50. doi:10.1177/0891988712436688.

> ➤ This study employing the novel MRS technique of MT did not demonstrate significance between group differences in the k(for) of CK but did observe a trend that would require confirmation in a larger study. An exploratory analysis suggested a reduction in depression symptom severity during treatment with high-dose CoEnzyme Q10 for older

adults with BPD. Further studies exploring alterations of high-energy phosphate metabolites in geriatric BPD and efficacy studies of CoQ10 in a randomized controlled trial are both warranted.

Curcumin

Curcumin Has Anti-inflammatory and Antioxidant Properties in the Treatment of Bipolar Disorder

> **Brietzke, Elisa,** et al., "Is There a Role for Curcumin in the Treatment of Bipolar Disorder?" *Medical Hypotheses* 80, no. 5 (May 2013): 606–12. Publisher: CHURCHILL LIVINGSTONE doi:10.1016/j.mehy.2013.02.001., PMID: 23484676

> ➢ Curcumin putative targets, known based on studies of diverse central nervous system disorders other than bipolar disorders (BD) include several proteins currently implicated in the pathophysiology of BD. These targets include, but are not limited to, transcription factors activated by environmental stressors and pro-inflammatory cytokines, protein kinases (PKA, PKC), enzymes, growth factors, inflammatory mediators, and anti-apoptotic proteins (Bcl-XL). Herein, we review previous studies on the anti-inflammatory and antioxidant properties of curcumin and discuss its therapeutic potential in BD.

Cucumin May Be a Preventative Intervention in Bipolar Disorder Reducing Episode Relapse

> **Gazal, Marta,** et al., "Neuroprotective and Antioxidant Effects of Curcumin in a Ketamine-Induced Model of Mania in Rats." *European Journal of Pharmacology* 724 (February 5, 2014): 132–39. doi:10.1016/j.ejphar.2013.12.028., PMID: 24384407

> ➢ Our research investigates the protective effects of curcumin, the main curcuminoid of the Indian spice turmeric, in a model of mania induced by ketamine administration in rats. Our results indicated that ketamine treatment (25 mg/kg, for 8 days) induced hyperlocomotion in the open-field test and oxidative damage in prefrontal cortex (PFC) and hippocampus (HP), evaluated by increased lipid peroxidation and decreased total thiol content. Moreover, ketamine treatment reduced the activity of the antioxidant enzymes superoxide dismutase and catalase in the HP. Pretreatment of rats with curcumin (20 and 50 mg/kg, for 14 days) or with lithium chloride (45 mg/kg, positive control) prevented behavioral and pro-oxidant effects induced by ketamine. These findings suggest that curcumin might be a good compound for preventive intervention in BD, reducing the episode relapse and the oxidative damage associated with the manic phase of this disorder.

CODEX ALTERNUS

Cytidine

Cytidine is Effective in Treating Bipolar Depression

Yoon, Sujung J., et al. "Decreased Glutamate/glutamine Levels May Mediate Cytidine's Efficacy in Treating Bipolar Depression: A Longitudinal Proton Magnetic Resonance Spectroscopy Study." *Neuropsychopharmacology: Official Publication of the American College of Neuropsychopharmacology* 34, no. 7 (June 2009): 1810–18. doi:10.1038/npp.2009.2.

> ➤ In conclusion, we report that cytidine supplementation of valproate is associated with an earlier response in treating bipolar depression and with greater and earlier reductions in cerebral glutamate/glutamine levels. In light of the need for developing improved therapeutics targeting the symptoms of bipolar depression, cytidine augmentation, which may alter the glutamatergic system potentially through a novel mechanism, appears to be a promising option for further study for treating severe depressive episodes in bipolar patients.

Dopamine Beta-Hydroxylase Inhibition

Fusaric Acid Dopamine Beta-Hydroxylase Inhibition Decreased a Patient's Manic Symptoms

Pandey, R. S., et al., "Dopamine Beta-Hydroxylase Inhibition in a Patient with Wilson's Disease and Manic Symptoms." *The American Journal of Psychiatry* 138, no. 12 (December 1981): 1628–29., Publisher: AM PSYCHIATRIC ASSN; PMID: 7304799

> ➤ The authors studied the effect of dopamine beta-hydroxylase inhibition on the manic symptoms of a 34-year-old man. They found that fusaric acid decreased the patient's manic symptoms and that his symptoms approximately reverted to their previous state when a placebo was reinstituted.

Herbal Medicines

Herbal Medicines Have Potential to Alleviate Symptoms of Anxiety and Insomnia in Bipolar Disorder

Baek, Ji Hyun, et al., "Clinical Applications of Herbal Medicines for Anxiety and Insomnia; Targeting Patients with Bipolar Disorder." *The Australian and New Zealand Journal of Psychiatry* 48, no. 8 (June 19, 2014): 705–15. Publisher: BLACKWELL PUBLISHING ASIA doi:10.1177/0004867414539198., PMID: 24947278

> ➤ "Adjunctive herbal medicines may have the potential to alleviate these symptoms and improve the outcomes of standard treatment, despite limited evidence. Physicians need to have a more in-depth understanding of the evidence of benefits, risks, and drug interactions of alternative treatments."

CODEX ALTERNUS

Homeopathy

Homeopathy is an Effective Adjunctive Treatment for Bipolar Disorder

Merizalade, Bernardo, "Bipolar Disorder: A Presentation of Three Cases. (*Presented at the American Institute of Homeopathy Case Conference*, New Orleans, September 19-21, 2003)

> ➢ I have found homeopathic remidies to be helpful adjuncts in the treatment of bipolar disorder they help to relieve acute symptoms, prevent further deterioration of the patient and may be adjunct to conventional medications. It may help reduce the number of medications necessary in the treatment of some patients with bipolar disorder.

Hydrogen Gas

Hydrogen Gas is a Potential Novel Therapy for Treatment of Schizophrenia and Bipolar Disorder

Ghanizadeh, Ahmad, et al. "Molecular Hydrogen: An Overview of Its Neurobiological Effects and Therapeutic Potential for Bipolar Disorder and Schizophrenia." Medical Gas Research 3, no. 1 (2013): 11. doi:10.1186/2045-9912-3-11., PMID: 23742229

> ➢ Hydrogen gas is a bioactive molecule that has a diversity of effects, including anti-apoptotic, anti-inflammatory and anti-oxidative properties; these overlap with the process of neuroprogression in major psychiatric disorders. Specifically, both bipolar disorder and schizophrenia are associated with increased oxidative and inflammatory stress. Moreover, lithium which is commonly administered for treating bipolar disorder has effects on oxidative stress and apoptotic pathways, as do valproate and some atypical antipsychotics for treating schizophrenia. Molecular hydrogen has been studied pre-clinically in animal models for the treatment of some medical conditions including hypoxia and neurodegenerative disorders, and there are intriguing clinical findings in neurological disorders including Parkinson's disease. Therefore, it is hypothesized that administration of hydrogen molecule may have potential as a novel therapy for bipolar disorder, schizophrenia, and other concurrent disorders characterized by oxidative, inflammatory and apoptotic dysregulation.

Inositol

Inositol is Effective for Treatment of Bipolar Depression

Chengappa, K. N., et al., "Inositol as an Add-on Treatment for Bipolar Depression." *Bipolar Disorders* 2, no. 1 (March 2000): 47–55., Publisher: BLACKWELL MUNKSGAARD; PMID: 11254020

> Among 22 subjects who completed the trial, six (50%) of the inositol-treated subjects responded with a 50% of greater decrease in baseline Hamilton Depression Rating Scale (HAM-D) score and a Clinical Global Improvement (CGI) scale score change of much or very much improved, as compared to three subjects assigned to placebo, a statistically non-significant difference.

Kava Pyrones

Kava Pyrones Exhibit a Profile Similar to Mood Stabilizers

Grunze, H., et al. "Kava Pyrones Exert Effects on Neuronal Transmission and Transmembraneous Cation Currents Similar to Established Mood Stabilizers--a Review." *Progress in Neuro-Psychopharmacology & Biological Psychiatry* 25, no. 8 (November 2001): 1555–70. PMID: 11642654

> In summary, kava pyrones exhibit a profile of cellular actions that shows a large overlap with several mood stabilizers, especially lamotrigine.

Lecithin

Attenuation of Mania with Lecithin

Cohen, B. M., et al., "Lecithin in Mania: A Preliminary Report." *The American Journal of Psychiatry* 137, no. 2 (February 1980): 242–43., Publisher: AM PSYCHIATRIC ASSN ; PMID: 6101528

> The design of this preliminary study does not permit definite conclusions as to the efficiency of lecithin in mania. However, the results are consistent with a beneficial effect. All subjects who received Phosophilipon 100 improved rapidly, and three of four showed some worsening following withdrawal of lecithin.

Lithium Orotate: See Appendix B

Lithium Orotate Has Therapeutic Effect in Alcoholics with Manic Depression

Sartori, H. E. "Lithium Orotate in the Treatment of Alcoholism and Related Conditions." Alcohol (Fayetteville, N.Y.) 3, no. 2 (April 1986): 97–100.; PMID: 3718672

> There was an improvement in the depressive mood of all patients. In addition, irritability, particularly in male patients prone to resort to violence, was improved markedly after a few weeks of the lithium orotate. The spouses reported that their husbands were less irritable and consequently were less violent in general. No recurrence of manic episodes was experienced during lithium orotate therapy by the three patients with major affective disorders and previous manic episodes.

> Chronic alcohol-induced depression of the majority of the patients showed favorable response to lithium orotate and the patients seemed cheerful and less tense. The three patients with manic depressive psychosis showed moderation of the depressive phase and the depression disappeared in one case. No manic episodes were evident in any of the three patients during the Li orotate treatment.

Magnesium oxide

Magnesium Augmentation in Mania May Increase Antimanic Efficacy of Verapamil

> **Giannini, A. J.,** et al., "Magnesium Oxide Augmentation of Verapamil Maintenance Therapy in Mania." *Psychiatry Research* 93, no. 1 (February 14, 2000): 83–87., Publisher: ELSEVIER IRELAND LTD; PMID: 10699232

> The authors compared the antimanic effects of verapamil-magnesium (V-M) combination with verapamil-placebo combination (V-P) in patients pretreated with verapamil. BPRS scores and serum magnesium levels were compared. The V-M combination was found to be significantly more effective the V-P in reducing manic symptoms (P=0,015). Serum magnesium levels were significantly higher in V-M group (P<0.04). These data suggest that magnesium may increase antimanic efficacy of verapamil by mechanisms which may operate at the intercellar level.

Magnesiocard

Magnesiocard as a Mood Stabilizer for Rapid Cycling Bipolar Disorder Has Found to Have Clinical Results Equivalent to Those of Lithium

> **Chouinard, G.,** et al., "A Pilot Study of Magnesium Aspartate Hydrochloride (Magnesiocard) as a Mood Stabilizer for Rapid Cycling Bipolar Affective Disorder Patients." *Progress in Neuro-Psychopharmacology & Biological Psychiatry* 14, no. 2 (1990): 171–80., Publisher: ELSEVIER INC. PMID: 2309035

> Nine severe rapid cycling manic-depressive patients were treated with magnesium preparation, Magnesiocard 40mEq/day in an open label study for a period up to 32 weeks.. Magnesiocard was found to have clinical results at least equivalent to those of lithium in about 50% of these patients. These results were obtained in an exploratory study and should be interpreted with caution.

Magnesium Sulphate (Epsom Salt)

Intravenous Magnesium Sulphate (Epsom Salt) May Be Used for Clinical Management of Severe Manic Agitation

CODEX ALTERNUS

Heiden, A., et al., "Treatment of Severe Mania with Intravenous Magnesium Sulphate as a Supplementary Therapy." *Psychiatry Research* 89, no. 3 (December 27, 1999): 239–46., Publisher: ELSEVIER IRELAND LTD; PMID: 10708270

> ➤ Ten patients with severe, therapy-resistant manic agitation received magnesium sulphate infusions with continuous magnesium (Mg) flow of approximately 200mg/h (4353+/-836mg/day; daily monitored Mg plasma level: 2.44+/-0.34 mmol/l) for periods ranging from 7 to 23 days." "Seven patients showed a marked improvement in the Clinical Global Impression Scale. In case of bradycardia detected by the ECG monitor (n=5), mg flow was reduced and bradycardia disappeared promptly. Mg i.v. may be a useful supplemental therapy for the clinical management of severe manic agitation.

Epsom Salt May Be a Potential Treatment for Acute Mania

Barbosa, Francisco J., et al., "Magnesium Sulfate and Sodium Valproate Block Methylphenidate-Induced Hyperlocomotion, an Animal Model of Mania." *Pharmacological Reports: PR* 63, no. 1 (2011): 64–70., PMID: 21441612

> ➤ In conclusion, the present results indicate that acute MgSO exerts an antimanic-like effect on methylphenidate-induced hyperlocomotion and support future investigations of MgSO as a potential treatment for acute mania.

N-acetylcysteine

N-acetyl cysteine Add-on Treatment for Bipolar Disorder Achieves Full Remission of Both Depressive and Manic Symptoms

Magalhães, P. V., et al., "N-Acetyl Cysteine Add-on Treatment for Bipolar II Disorder: A Subgroup Analysis of a Randomized Placebo-Controlled Trial." *Journal of Affective Disorders* 129, no. 1–3 (March 2011): 317–20. Publisher: ELSEVIER BV doi:10.1016/j.jad.2010.08.001., PMID: 20800897

> ➤ "Fourteen individuals were available for this report, seven in each group. Six people achieved full remission of both depressive and manic symptoms in the NAC group; this was true for only two people in the placebo group."

N-acetylcysteine as Adjunctive Treatment Demonstrates a Robust Decrease in Bipolar Depression

Berk, Michael, et al., "The Efficacy of N-Acetylcysteine as an Adjunctive Treatment in Bipolar Depression: An Open Label Trial." *Journal of Affective Disorders* 135, no. 1–3 (December 2011): 389–94. Publisher: ELSEVIER BV; doi:10.1016/j.jad.2011.06.005., PMID: 21719110

> In this trial, the estimated mean baseline Bipolar Depression Rating Scale (BDRS) score was 19.7 (SE=0.8), and the mean BDRS score at the end of the 8 week open label treatment phase was 11.1 (SE=0.8). This reduction was statistically significant (p<0.001). Improvements in functioning and quality of life were similarly evident. These open label data demonstrate a robust decrement in depression scores with NAC treatment.

Berk, Michael, et al., "N-Acetyl Cysteine for Depressive Symptoms in Bipolar Disorder--a Double-Blind Randomized Placebo-Controlled Trial." *Biological Psychiatry* 64, no. 6 (September 15, 2008): 468–75. Publisher: ELSEVIER INC. doi:10.1016/j.biopsych.2008.04.022., PMID: 18534556

> "NAC appears a safe and effective augmentation strategy for depressive symptoms in bipolar disorder."

Palmitoylethanolamide

Palmitoylethanolamide May Be an Effective Antidepressant for Bipolar Depression

Coppola, M., et al., "Is There a Role for Palmitoylethanolamide in the Treatment of Depression?" *Medical Hypotheses* 82, no. 5 (May 2014): 507–11. doi:10.1016/j.mehy.2013.12.016.

> "Considering the recent findings about the antidepressant effect of palmitoylethanolamide in animal model, we have hypothesized the potential antidepressant effect of this fatty acid amide in unipolar and bipolar depressed patients."

Prolyl Oligopeptidase Inhibitors

Tarrago, Teresa, et al., "The Natural Product Berberine Is a Human Prolyl Oligopeptidase Inhibitor." *ChemMedChem* 2, no. 3 (March 2007): 354–59. Publisher: WILEY-VCH doi:10.1002/cmdc.200600303., PMID: 17295371

> "As berberine is a natural compound that has been safely administered to humans, it opens up new perspectives for the treatment of neuropsychiatric diseases."

Tarragó, Teresa, et al., "Identification by 19F NMR of Traditional Chinese Medicinal Plants Possessing Prolyl Oligopeptidase Inhibitory Activity." *Chembiochem: A European Journal of Chemical Biology* 7, no. 5 (May 2006): 827–33. Publisher: WILEY - V C H VERLAG GMBH & CO. KGAA; doi:10.1002/cbic.200500424., PMID:16628753

> "This peptidase has been associated with schizophrenia, bipolar affective disorder, and related neuropsychiatric disorders and might therefore have important clinical implications."

Sodium Butyrate

Sodium Butyrate May Be a Potential Mood Stabilizer for Bipolar Disorder

Resende, Wilson R., et al., "Effects of Sodium Butyrate in Animal Models of Mania and Depression: Implications as a New Mood Stabilizer." *Behavioural Pharmacology*, August 29, 2013. Publisher: LIPPINCOTT WILLIAMS & WILKINS doi:10.1097/FBP.0b013e32836546fc., PMID: 23994816

> ➤ Bipolar disorder is a severe mood disorder with high morbidity and mortality. Despite adequate treatment, patients continue to have recurrent mood episodes, residual symptoms, and functional impairment. Some preclinical studies have shown that histone deacetylase inhibitors may act on depressive-like and manic-like behaviors. Therefore, the aim of the present study was to evaluate the effects of sodium butyrate (SB) on behavioral changes in animal models of depression and mania. The animals were submitted to protocols of chronic mild stress or maternal deprivation for induction of depressive-like behaviors and subjected to amphetamine, or ouabain administration for induction of manic-like behaviors. SB reversed the depressive-like and manic-like behaviors evaluated in the animal models. From these results we can suggest that SB may be a potential mood stabilizer.

Sodium Butyrate May Be New Medication for the Treatment of Mania

Moretti, Morgana, et al., "Behavioral and Neurochemical Effects of Sodium Butyrate in an Animal Model of Mania." *Behavioural Pharmacology* 22, no. 8 (December 2011): 766–72. Publisher: LIPPINCOTT WILLIAMS & WILKINS; doi:10.1097/FBP.0b013e32834d0f1b., PMID: 21989497

> ➤ The present study investigated the effect of the histone deacetylase inhibitor, sodium butyrate (SB), on locomotor behavior and on mitochondrial respiratory-chain complexes activity in the brain of rats subjected to an animal model of mania induced by d-amphetamine (d-AMPH). In the reversal treatment, Wistar rats were first treated with d-AMPH or saline (Sal) for 14 days. Thereafter, between days 8 and 14, rats were administered SB or Sal. In the prevention treatment, rats were treated with SB or Sal for 14 days and received d-AMPH or Sal between days 8 and 14. The d-AMPH treatment increased locomotor behavior in Sal-treated rats under reversion and prevention treatment, and SB reversed and prevented d-AMPH-related hyperactivity. Moreover, d-AMPH decreased the activity of mitochondrial respiratory-chain complexes in Sal-treated rats in the prefrontal cortex, hippocampus, striatum, and amygdala in both experiments, and SB was able to reverse and prevent this impairment. The present study suggests that the mechanism of action of SB involves induction of mitochondrial function in parallel with behavioral changes, reinforcing the need for more studies on

histone deacetylase inhibitors as a possible target for new medications for bipolar disorder treatment.

Sodium Butyrate Reversed Ouabain-Induced Manic Behavior and Increased Neurotrophins in Animal Model of Bipolar Disorder

Varela, Roger B., et al., "Sodium Butyrate and Mood Stabilizers Block Ouabain-Induced Hyperlocomotion and Increase BDNF, NGF and GDNF Levels in Brain of Wistar Rats." *Journal of Psychiatric Research,* November 21, 2014. Publisher: PERGAMON doi:10.1016/j.jpsychires.2014.11.003., PMID: 25467060

> ➤ Bipolar Disorder (BD) is one of the most severe psychiatric disorders. Despite adequate treatment, patients continue to have recurrent mood episodes, residual symptoms, and functional impairment. Some preclinical studies have shown that histone deacetylase inhibitors may act on manic-like behaviors. Neurotrophins have been considered important mediators in the pathophysiology of BD. The present study aims to investigate the effects of lithium (Li), valproate (VPA), and sodium butyrate (SB), an HDAC inhibitor, on BDNF, NGF and GDNF in the brain of rats subjected to an animal model of mania induced by ouabain. Wistar rats received a single ICV injection of ouabain or artificial cerebrospinal fluid. From the day following ICV injection, the rats were treated for 6 days with intraperitoneal injections of saline, Li, VPA or SB twice a day. In the 7th day after ouabain injection, locomotor activity was measured using the open-field test. The BDNF, NGF and GDNF levels were measured in the hippocampus and frontal cortex by sandwich-ELISA. Li, VPA or SB treatments reversed ouabain-related manic-like behavior. Ouabain decreased BDNF, NGF and GDNF levels in hippocampus and frontal cortex of rats. The treatment with Li, VPA or SB reversed these impairment induced by ouabain. In addition, Li, VPA and SB per se increased NGF and GDNF levels in hippocampus of rats. Our data support the notion that neurotrophic factors play a role in BD and in the mechanisms of the action of Li, VPA and SB.

Triacetyluridine

Triacetyluridine Decreased Clinical Depressive Symptoms and Lowers Brain Acidity

Jensen, J. Eric, et al., "Triacetyluridine (TAU) Decreases Depressive Symptoms and Increases Brain pH in Bipolar Patients." *Experimental and Clinical Psychopharmacology* 16, no. 3 (June 2008): 199–206. doi:10.1037/1064-1297.16.3.199. , PMID: 18540779

> ➤ Triacetyluridine (TAU) taken orally for a 6 week period decreased clinical depressive symptoms and lowered brain acidity (increased brain-tissue pH and thus alkalosis) in patients with bipolar disorder who showed treatment response. As acidity (pH) is related to mitochondrial function and TAU alters this measure in bipolar disorder, it is speculated that uridine therapy may exert its effect through a metabolic "readjustment"

CODEX ALTERNUS

by ameliorating the mitochondrial dysfunction thought to be present in bipolar disorder in such a way as to relieve symptoms and improve neuronal functioning. This study showed an early, short-term improvement in depressive symptoms. Further study of the mechanism of TAU may be necessary to understand the underlying reason for this effect.

Vitamin D

Youth with Bipolar Disorder using Vitamin D Had a Significant Decrease In Their YMRS Scores

Sikoglu, Elif M., et al., "Vitamin D3 Supplemental Treatment for Mania in Youth with Bipolar Spectrum Disorders." *Journal of Child and Adolescent Psychopharmacology* 25, no. 5 (June 2015): 415–24. doi:10.1089/cap.2014.0110., PMID: 26091195

> Baseline ACC GABA/creatine (Cr) was lower in BSD than in TD (F[1,31]=8.91, p=0.007). Following an 8 week Vitamin D3 supplementation, in BSD patients, there was a significant decrease in YMRS scores (t=-3.66, p=0.002, df=15) and Children's Depression Rating Scale (CDRS) scores (t=-2.93, p=0.01, df=15); and a significant increase in ACC GABA (t=3.18, p=0.007, df=14). Following an 8 week open label trial with Vitamin D3, BSD patients exhibited improvement in their mood symptoms in conjunction with their brain neurochemistry.

Vitis Labrusca

Grape Extract Exhibits Protective Properties against Oxidative Stress in Bipolar Disorder

Scola, Gustavo, et al., "Vitis Labrusca Extract Effects on Cellular Dynamics and Redox Modulations in a SH-SY5Y Neuronal Cell Model: A Similar Role to Lithium." *Neurochemistry International* 79 (December 2014): 12–19. Publisher: ELSEVIER LTD. doi:10.1016/j.neuint.2014.10.002., PMID: 25445986

> "The findings of this study suggest that VLE exhibits protective properties against oxidative stress-induced alterations similar to that of lithium. These findings suggest that VLE may be an attractive potential candidate as a novel therapeutic agent for BD."

Uridine

Uridine is a Safe and Effective Treatment for Bipolar Depression

Kondo, Douglas G., et al., "Open-Label Uridine for Treatment of Depressed Adolescents with Bipolar Disorder." *Journal of Child and Adolescent Psychopharmacology* 21, no. 2 (April 2011): 171–75. doi:10.1089/cap.2010.0054., PMID: 21486171

> The authors report results of what we believe to be the first study of uridine as a treatment for depressed adolescents with bipolar disorder. Open-label uridine 500 mg twice daily for 6 weeks was associated with a mean decrease in CDRS-R raw score of 35.6, representing a reduction of 54% compared with baseline scores at study entry. The benefit associated with uridine was not associated with switches to mania, treatment-emergent suicidal behavior, or serious adverse events. No clinically significant laboratory abnormalities were associated with uridine in our study. Although not measured systematically, improvement in psychosocial domains such as school performance, peer relations, and family function appeared to be associated with uridine treatment as well. Feedback from participants and parents suggests that uridine would score well on measures of patient acceptability and patient satisfaction.

Zinc

Zinc is Beneficial in Altering the Cognitive Function and Short-term Memory of Animals Treated with Lithium

Bhalla, Punita, et al., "Effectiveness of Zinc in Modulating Lithium Induced Biochemical and Behavioral Changes in Rat Brain." *Cellular and Molecular Neurobiology* 27, no. 5 (August 2007): 595–607. Publisher: SPRINGER NEW YORK LLC; doi:10.1007/s10571-007-9146-0., PMID: 17458692

> Further, lithium-treated rats showed an increase in depression time as compared to normal controls both after 1 and 4 months of treatment. Short-term memory significantly improved in lithium-treated rats in all treatment groups. However, no change in the cognitive behavior of the animals was reported after lithium treatment. Zinc co-administration with lithium significantly improved the short-term memory and cognitive functions of the animals. From the above results it can be concluded that zinc proved beneficial in altering the status of neurotransmitters as well as the behavior patterns of the animals treated with both short and long-term lithium therapy.

Sensory Therapies

Ambient Air Anionization

Treatment with Ambient Air Anionization Produces Significant Antimanic Effect

Giannini, A. James, et al., "Treatment of Acute Mania with Ambient Air Anionization: Variants of Climactic Heat Stress and Serotonin Syndrome." *Psychological Reports* 100, no. 1 (February 2007): 157–63. Publisher: AMMONS SCIENTIFIC LTD. doi:10.2466/pr0.100.1.157-163., PMID: 17451018

> High concentrations of ambient anions (O2-) were used to augment treatment for 20 acutely manic male patients. Anions were produced by anion generator in sealed room. A double-blind crossover design was used and responses were evaluated with Brief Psychiatric Rating Scale by 2 blinded raters. This produced significant antimanic effect: total rating scores declined with anion treatment. Presham and postsham total scores for these 5 were 31.3 and 31.6, respectively. Pretreatment and posttreatemnt total scores were 31.6 and 26.3, respectively.

Chronotherapy

Chronotherapy Accelerates the Antidepressant Response in Bipolar Disorder

Wu, Joseph C., et al.,"Rapid and Sustained Antidepressant Response with Sleep Deprivation and Chronotherapy in Bipolar Disorder." *Biological Psychiatry* 66, no. 3 (August 1, 2009): 298–301. Publisher: ELSEVIER INC. doi:10.1016/j.biopsych.2009.02.018., PMID: 19358978

> Significant decreases in depression in the CAT versus MED patients were seen within 48 hours of SD and were sustained over a 7-week period. This is the first study to demonstrate the benefit of adding three noninvasive circadian-related interventions to SD in medicated patients to accelerate and sustain antidepressant responses and provides a strategy for the safe, fast-acting, and sustainable treatment of BPD.

Chronobiological Treatment is enhanced by Lithium in Bipolar Depression

Benedetti, F., et al., "Sleep Phase Advance and Lithium to Sustain the Antidepressant Effect of Total Sleep Deprivation in Bipolar Depression: New Findings Supporting the Internal Coincidence Model?" *Journal of Psychiatric Research* 35, no. 6 (December 2001): 323–29., Publisher: PERGAMON; PMID: 11684139

> Recent European studies suggested that sleep phase advance (SPA) could sustain the effects of total sleep deprivation (TSD) both with or without a combined antidepressant drug treatment. Previous studies by our group showed that an ongoing lithium treatment could enhance and sustain the effect of repeated TSD. In the present study we studied the effect of a single TSD followed by 3 days SPA (beginning with sleep allowed from 17:00 until 24:00, with daily shiftbacks of 2 h) in consecutively admitted bipolar depressed inpatients who were taking a chronic lithium salts treatment (n=16) or who were devoid of psychotropic medications (n=14). Changes in mood during treatment were recorded with self administered visual analogue scales and with Hamilton rating scale for depression. Results showed that SPA could sustain the acute antidepressant effect of TSD, and that lithium enhanced the effect of the chronobiological treatment. According to the internal coincidence model, the better clinical effects observed in lithium-treated patients could be due to the phase delaying effect of lithium on

biological rhythms, leading to a better synchronization of biological rhythms with the sleep-wake cycle.

Light and Dark Therapy

Blue Light Blockade is Effective for Mania and Sleep in Patient with Bipolar Disorder

Henriksen, Tone EG, et al., "Blocking Blue Light during Mania - Markedly Increased Regularity of Sleep and Rapid Improvement of Symptoms: A Case Report." *Bipolar Disorders* 16, no. 8 (December 2014): 894–98. Publisher: BLACKWELL MUNKSGAARD doi:10.1111/bdi.12265., PMID: 25264124

> Manic symptoms were unaltered during the first seven days. The transition to the blue-blocking regime was followed by a rapid and sustained decline in manic symptoms accompanied by a reduction in total sleep, a reduction in motor activity during sleep intervals, and markedly increased regularity of sleep intervals. The patient's total length of hospital stay was 20 days shorter than the average time during his previous manic episodes.

Morning Sunlight Reduces Length of Hospital Stay in Bipolar Depression

Benedetti, F., et al., "Morning Sunlight Reduces Length of Hospitalization in Bipolar Depression." *Journal of Affective Disorders* 62, no. 3 (February 2001): 221–23., Publisher: ELSEVIER BV; PMID: 11223110

> Bipolar inpatients in E rooms (exposed to direct sunlight in the morning) had a mean 3.67-day shorter hospital stay than patients in W rooms. No effect was found in unipolar inpatients. Natural sunlight can be an underestimated and uncontrolled light therapy for bipolar depression.

Phototherapy is Effective in Bipolar Disorder at 3 Month Follow-up

Deltito, J. A., et al., "Effects of Phototherapy on Non-Seasonal Unipolar and Bipolar Depressive Spectrum Disorders." *Journal of Affective Disorders* 23, no. 4 (December 1991): 231–37., Publisher: ELSEVIER BV; PMID: 1791269

> In a group of 17 patients with non-SAD depressive disorders we compared the response of bipolar spectrum versus unipolar patients to treatment with light therapy. The main hypothesis was that bipolar spectrum depressed patients would preferentially respond to bright light therapy as compared to unipolar depressed patients. All patients were treated with either 400 or 2500 lux phototherapy for 2 h on seven consecutive days. All outcome measures, which included the SIGH-SAD, CGI, and the Anxiety and Depressive Factors of the SCL-90, showed significant improvement in the bipolar vs. the unipolar spectrum patients. Unexpected this occurred regardless of the intensity of the

light. These changes were judged to be quite clinically significant. All patients showing response were noted to have maintained their response at a 3-month follow-up.

Phototherapy Treatment Decreases Depression and Anxiety and Normalizes Sleep Behavior in Affective Psychosis

Peter, K., et al., "[Initial results with bright light (phototherapy) in affective psychoses]." *Psychiatrie, Neurologie, Und Medizinische Psychologie* 38, no. 7 (July 1986): 384–90., Publisher: S. HIRZEL VERLAG LEIPZIG; PMID: 3763766

> The biological foundations of light-treatment and their relation to neurophysiological and biochemical mechanisms were discussed. We developed an apparatus for treatment and report of first experiences in affective psychosis. In addition to a decrease of depressivity and anxiety we found an unequivocal tendency to normalization of sleep-behaviour. The farther clinical and paraclinical investigations has to show the position of this method of treatment in the total conception of a biological therapy.

Bright Light Therapy for Bipolar Disorder Treats Depressive Symptoms

Papatheodorou, G., et al., "The Effect of Adjunctive Light Therapy on Ameliorating Breakthrough Depressive Symptoms in Adolescent-Onset Bipolar Disorder." *Journal of Psychiatry & Neuroscience: JPN* 20, no. 3 (May 1995): 226–32., Publisher: CANADIAN MEDICAL ASSOCIATION; PMID: 7786884

> "These preliminary results indicate that some bipolar adolescents with breakthrough depressive symptoms could benefit from light therapy as an adjunct to their continued thymoleptic treatment."

Dark Therapy for Mania Results in a Significant Decrease in YMRS Scores

Barbini, Barbara, et al., "Dark Therapy for Mania: A Pilot Study." *Bipolar Disorders* 7, no. 1 (February 2005): 98–101. Publisher: BLACKWELL MUNKSGAARD; doi:10.1111/j.1399-5618.2004.00166.x., PMID: 15654938

> "Adding DT to TAU [therapy as usual] resulted in a significantly faster decrease of YMRS scores when patients were treated within 2 weeks from onset of the current manic episode."

Dark Therapy May Work for Rapid Cycling Bipolar Disorder

Phelps, James, "Dark Therapy for Bipolar Disorder Using Amber Lenses for Blue Light Blockade." *Medical Hypotheses* 70, no. 2 (2008): 224–29. Publisher: CHURCHILL LIVINGSTONE; doi:10.1016/j.mehy.2007.05.026., PMID: 17637502

> If amber lenses can effectively simulate darkness, a broad range of conditions might respond to this inexpensive therapeutic tool: common forms of insomnia; sleep

deprivation in nursing mothers; circadian rhythm disruption in shift workers; and perhaps even rapid cycling bipolar disorder, a difficult-to-treat variation of common illness.

Negative Air Ions

There May Be a Calming Effect of Negative Air Ions on Manic Patients

> **Misiaszek, J.,** et al., "The Calming Effects of Negative Air Ions on Manic Patients: A Pilot Study." *Biological Psychiatry* 22, no. 1 (January 1987): 107–10., Publisher: ELSEVIER INC PMID: 3790632

> ➤ The unexpected finding in this two-phase study is that seven of eight manic patients fell asleep during negative ion exposure and that six of them had to be awakened after the session was over. The short-lived calm behavior and sense of well-being following awakening may have been as much a function of sleep as of any direct effect benefit of negative ions. It is unlikely that medications accounted for the decrease in agitation.

Sleep

Forced Bed Rest for Treatment of Rapid Cycling Bipolar Disorder May Help Prevent Mania and Rapid Cycling

> **Wehr, T. A.,** et al., "Treatment of Rapidly Cycling Bipolar Patient by Using Extended Bed Rest and Darkness to Stabilize the Timing and Duration of Sleep." *Biological Psychiatry* 43, no. 11 (June 1, 1998): 822–28., Publisher: ELSEVIER INC; PMID: 9611672

> ➤ "Fostering sleep and stabilizing its timing by scheduling regular nightly periods of enforced bed rest in the dark may help prevent mania and rapid cycling in bipolar patients."

Sleep Deprivation

Sleep Restriction and Stimulus Control are Efficacious Procedures for treating insomnia in Bipolar Disorder

> **Kaplan, Katherine A.,** et al., "Behavioral Treatment of Insomnia in Bipolar Disorder." *The American Journal of Psychiatry* 170, no. 7 (July 1, 2013): 716–20. Publisher: AM PSYCHIATRIC ASSN; doi:10.1176/appi.ajp.2013.12050708., PMID: 23820830

> ➤ Sleep restriction and stimulus control appear to be safe and efficacious procedures for treating insomnia in patients with bipolar disorder. Practitioners should encourage regularity in bedtimes and rise times as a first step in treatment, and carefully monitor changes in mood and daytime sleepiness throughout the intervention.

CODEX ALTERNUS

Sleep Deprivation Provides a Positive Antidepressant Response in Rapid Cycling Bipolar Disorder

> **Gill, D. S.,** et al., "Antidepressant Response to Sleep Deprivation as a Function of Time into Depressive Episode in Rapidly Cycling Bipolar Patients." *Acta Psychiatrica Scandinavica* 87, no. 2 (February 1993): 102–9., Publisher: BLACKWELL MUNKSGAARD ; PMID: 8447235

> ➤ Three patients with treatment-resistant rapidly cycling bipolar disorder were studied with multiple sleep deprivations (SD) during several depressive episodes to assess the effect of phase or duration of a depressive episode on SD response. There was little response to SD early in a depressive episode, but responses were often robust late in an episode, sometimes triggering its termination. In 2 subjects, the duration of antidepressant response to SD increased linearly as time into episode increased. Neither the number of SD given in an episode nor the medication status of the patients appeared to account for the observed increases in antidepressant response. These results suggest that the neurobiological substrates underlying depression may change over the course of an episode, resulting in an increased responsivity to sleep deprivation later compared with earlier in the course of an episode in rapidly cycling patients. The generalizability of these findings to unipolar patients remains to be explored.

Sleep Deprivation Shortened Mood Cycle of Manic Depressive Female Patient

> **Lovett Doust, J. W.,** et al.,"Repeated Sleep Deprivation as a Therapeutic Zeitgeber for Circular Type Manic Depressive Disturbance." *Chronobiologia* 7, no. 4 (December 1980): 505–11., Publisher: CASA EDITRICE IL/PONTE; PMID: 7449580

> ➤ A post-menopausal woman suffering from a circular type manic depressive psychosis who had been treated by drugs was followed for 8 months on a self-reporting mood rating scale. The drug regimen was continued over a further 8 months but with the addition of 5 nights of sleep deprivation at the depth of her recurrent depressed moods. Time series analyses of the subject's longitudinal mood scores revealed a persistent cycle of 32 days. After 5 sleep deprivation treatments this cycle shortened to 28 days which endured at least for the ensuing 8 months. After sleep deprivation and decrease of the amplitude, an improvement of mood was obtained. It is suggested that the increased LD ratio obtained in sleep deprivation may be as therapeutic as the actual loss of sleep itself.

Sunshine

Sunny Hospital Rooms Expedite Recovery

> **Beauchemin, K. M.,** et al., "Sunny Hospital Rooms Expedite Recovery from Severe and Refractory Depressions." *Journal of Affective Disorders* 40, no. 1–2 (September 9, 1996): 49–51. PMID: 8882914

> The rooms in our psychiatric inpatient unit are so placed that half are bright and sunny and the rest are not. Reasoning that some patients were getting light therapy inadvertently, we compared the lengths of stay of depressed patients in sunny rooms with those of patients in dull rooms. Those in sunny rooms had an average stay of 16.9 days compared to 19.5 days for those in dull rooms, a difference of 2.6 days (15%): P < 0.05.

More Sunshine May Protect Against Suicide

Vyssoki, Benjamin, et al., "Direct Effect of Sunshine on Suicide." *JAMA Psychiatry* 71, no. 11 (November 2014): 1231–37. doi:10.1001/jamapsychiatry.2014.1198., PMID: 25208208

> More daily sunshine 14 to 60 days previously is associated with low rates of suicide. Our study also suggests that sunshine during this period may protect against suicide.

Combined Sensory Therapies

Combined Total Sleep Deprivation and Light Therapy is Useful in Triggering an Acute Response in Drug-resistant Bipolar Depressed Patients

Benedetti, Francesco, et al., "Combined Total Sleep Deprivation and Light Therapy in the Treatment of Drug-Resistant Bipolar Depression: Acute Response and Long-Term Remission Rates." *The Journal of Clinical Psychiatry* 66, no. 12 (December 2005): 1535–40., ublisher: PHYSICIANS POSTGRADUATE PRESS, INC.; PMID: 16401154

> "The combination of repeated TSD and LT in drug-resistant patients was useful in triggering an acute response. Further clinical research is needed to optimize this treatment option for drug-resistant patients in the long term."

Combination of Sleep Deprivation, Sleep Phase Advance, and Bright Light Therapy use in Bipolar Disorder

Gottlieb, John F., et al., "Outpatient Triple Chronotherapy for Bipolar Depression: Case Report." *Journal of Psychiatric Practice* 18, no. 5 (September 2012): 373–80. Publisher: LIPPINCOTT WILLIAMS & WILKINS; doi:10.1097/01.pra.0000419822.69914.8e., PMID: 22995965

> There is an urgent need for rapid, effective, and safe treatments for bipolar depression. Triple chronotherapy is a combination of sleep deprivation, sleep phase advance, and bright light therapy that has been shown to induce accelerated and sustained remissions in bipolar depression. This case report describes the first outpatient program designed to

administer triple chronotherapy and reviews the organizational and clinical requirements for providing such care.

Total Sleep Deprivation Combined with Lithium and Light Therapy Obtains a Sustained Antidepressant Response in Bipolar Patients

> **Colombo, C.** et al.,"Total Sleep Deprivation Combined with Lithium and Light Therapy in the Treatment of Bipolar Depression: Replication of Main Effects and Interaction." *Psychiatry Research* 95, no. 1 (July 24, 2000): 43–53., Publisher: ELSEVIER IRELAND LTD; PMID: 10904122

> ➤ The results showed that both light therapy and ongoing lithium treatment significantly enhanced the effects of TSD on the perceived mood, with no additional benefit when the two treatments were combined. Subjective sleepiness during TSD, as rated by the self-administered Stanford Sleepiness Scale, was significantly reduced by light exposure, and was correlated with the outcome. This study confirms the possibility of obtaining a sustained antidepressant response to TSD in bipolar patients.

Long Nights, Bedrest, Light Therapy for Rapid Cycling Bipolar Disorder

> **Wirz-Justice, A.,** et al., "A Rapid-Cycling Bipolar Patient Treated with Long Nights, Bedrest, and Light." *Biological Psychiatry* 45, no. 8 (April 15, 1999): 1075–77., Publisher: ELSEVIER INC; PMID: 10386196

> ➤ A previous study using morning light therapy in rapid-cycling bipolar patients worsened clinical state (Leibenluft et al 1995), but was not, as here, administered in combination with long nights and extended sleep. Our independent replication of dark/rest treatment strategy (Wehr et al 1998) indicates that chronobiologic protocols may be used as valuable adjunctive treatments to psychopharmacology, in particular, to interrupt rapid cycling.

Chronotherapeutics Rapidly Decreases Depressive Suicidality in Drug-resistant Bipolar Disorder

> **Benedetti, Francesco,** et al., "Rapid Treatment Response of Suicidal Symptoms to Lithium, Sleep Deprivation, and Light Therapy (chronotherapeutics) in Drug-Resistant Bipolar Depression." *The Journal of Clinical Psychiatry* 75, no. 2 (February 2014): 133–40. Publisher: PHYSICIANS POSTGRADUATE PRESS, INC. doi:10.4088/JCP.13m08455., PMID: 24345382

> ➤ "The combination of total sleep deprivation, light therapy, and lithium is able to rapidly decrease depressive suicidality and prompt antidepressant response in drug-resistant major depression in the course of bipolar disorder."

CODEX ALTERNUS

Exercise and Movement

Aerobic Exercise

Aerobic Exercise is a Possible Treatment for Cognitive Dysfunction in Bipolar Disorder

Kucyi, Aaron, et al., "Aerobic Physical Exercise as a Possible Treatment for Neurocognitive Dysfunction in Bipolar Disorder." *Postgraduate Medicine* 122, no. 6 (November 2010): 107–16. Publisher: JTE Multimedia Company ; doi:10.3810/pgm.2010.11.2228., PMID: 21084787

> ➤ Available studies have documented an array of persisting neurocognitive deficits across disparate bipolar populations. Abnormalities in verbal working memory are highly replicated; deficits in executive function, learning, attention, and processing speed are also a consistent abnormality. The effect sizes of neurocognitive deficits in BD are intermediate between those reported in schizophrenia and major depressive disorder. Several original reports and reviews have documented the neurocognitive-enhancing effects of aerobic exercise in the general population as well as across diverse medical populations and ages. Proposed mechanisms involve nonexclusive effects on neurogenesis, neurotrophism, immunoinflammatory systems, insulin sensitivity, and neurotransmitter systems. Each of these effector systems are implicated in both normal and abnormal neurocognitive processes in BD.

Chiropractic Care

Chiropractic Care Reduces Symptoms in Bipolar Patient

Elster, Erin L., et al., "Treatment of Bipolar, Seizure, and Sleep Disorders and Migraine Headaches Utilizing a Chiropractic Technique." *Journal of Manipulative and Physiological Therapeutics* 27, no. 3 (April 2004): E5. Publisher: MOSBY, INC. doi:10.1016/j.jmpt.2003.12.027., PMID: 15129207

> ➤ At initial examination, evidence of a subluxation stemming from the upper cervical spine was found through thermography and radiography. Chiropractic care using an upper cervical technique was administered to correct and stabilize the patient's upper neck injury. Assessments at baseline, 2 months, and 4 months were conducted by the patient's neurologist. After 1 month of care, the patient reported an absence of seizures and manic episodes and improved sleep patterns. After 4 months of care, seizures and manic episodes remained absent and migraine headaches were reduced from 3 per week to 2 per month. After 7 months of care, the patient reported the complete absence of symptoms. Eighteen months later, the patient remains asymptomatic.

Deep Touch Pressure

CODEX ALTERNUS

Deep Touch Pressure May Be Helpful for Some Patients with Bipolar Disorder in Stressful Situations

Sylvia, Louisa Grandin, et al., "Adjunctive Deep Touch Pressure for Comorbid Anxiety in Bipolar Disorder: Mediated by Control of Sensory Input?" *Journal of Psychiatric Practice* 20, no. 1 (January 2014): 71–77. doi:10.1097/01.pra.0000442942.01479.ce., PMID: 24419314

> ➤ A patient presenting with bipolar I disorder and comorbid anxiety, ADHD, and dyslexia was taught deep touch pressure strategies to alleviate severe symptoms of sensory over-responsivity and anxiety. The patient reported that the techniques were helpful as they allowed her to cope with potentially overwhelming situations in her environment. Clinician-rated functioning also improved over the course of treatment. This case study suggests that deep touch pressure may be useful in patients with bipolar disorder who have SOR and anxiety as comorbid conditions.

Physical Activity

Physical Activity has A Therapeutic Role in Bipolar Disorder

Ng, Felicity, et al., "The Effects of Physical Activity in the Acute Treatment of Bipolar Disorder: A Pilot Study." *Journal of Affective Disorders* 101, no. 1–3 (August 2007): 259–62. Publisher: ELSEVIER BV; doi:10.1016/j.jad.2006.11.014., PMID: 17182104

> ➤ "The results of this trial provide preliminary support for a therapeutic role of physical activity in bipolar disorder, and warrant further investigation with randomised controlled trials."

Yoga

Yoga Exercises Improved Positive State and Lowered Negative Emotion in Bipolar Disorder

Upmesh K. Talwar* et al., "Role of Yogic Exercises in Bipolar Affective Disorder and Schizophrenia" APRIL 2010, *DELHI PSYCHIATRY JOURNAL* Vol. 13 No.1

> ➤ In personal interview, the patients with Bipolar Disorders revealed enhancement in their positive emotional state and lowering of negative emotion. They subjectively reported improvement and control over their physical energy. Marked improvement was noticed in psychopathology among the patients of the study group in specific areas like anxiety, hostility, and excitement. In a pre-conclusive way, it can be said that yogic exercise therapy proved efficacious in the improvement and psychological wellbeing of the patients in the present study.

CODEX ALTERNUS

Mindfulness, Hypnosis and Meditation

Hypnosis

Hypnosis in Regulating Bipolar Affective Disorders

> **Feinstein, A. D.,** et al., "Hypnosis in Regulating Bipolar Affective Disorders." *The American Journal of Clinical Hypnosis* 29, no. 1 (July 1986): 29–38., Publisher: THE SOCIETY; PMID: 3739960

> ➤ A hypnotic procedure is presented for treating bipolar patients in instances where problems encountered in maintaining the patient on pharmacotherapy. Recent studies revealing electrochemical hemispheric asymmetry in manic-depressive illness, in the action of lithium, and in the effects of hypnosis led to speculation of hemispheric electrochemical activity. Advances allowing increased specificity in the regulation of physiological conditions through the use of hypnosis, biofeedback, meditation, and guided imagery provide a plausible rationale for this experimental technique. The procedure includes 1) determining relevant medical and psychosocial parameters, 2) establishing rapport and a positive response set for the therapy, 3) formulating suggestions for electrochemical regulation during heterohypnosis, 4) introducing self-hypnosis, and 5) addressing self-concept issues regarding the role of the illness in the patient's identity. The course of treatment of five bipolar patients is described.

Meditation

Meditation Practice Lowers Depression and Anxiety Symptoms in those with Bipolar Disorder

> **Perich, Tania,** et al., "The Association between Meditation Practice and Treatment Outcome in Mindfulness-Based Cognitive Therapy for Bipolar Disorder." *Behaviour Research and Therapy* 51, no. 7 (July 2013): 338–43. Publisher: PERGAMON doi:10.1016/j.brat.2013.03.006., PMID: 23639299

> ➤ There were significant differences found between those who meditated for 3 days a week or more and those who meditated less often on trait anxiety post-treatment and clinician-rated depression at 12-month follow-up whilst trends were noted for self-reported depression. A greater number of days meditated during the 8-week MBCT program was related to lower depression scores at 12-month follow-up, and there was evidence to suggest that mindfulness meditation practice was associated with improvements in depression and anxiety symptoms if a certain minimum amount (3 times a week or more) was practiced weekly throughout the 8-week MBCT program.

Mindfulness

Mindfulness for Bipolar Disorder is Associated with Changes in Depressive Symptoms

Weber, B., et al., "Mindfulness-Based Cognitive Therapy for Bipolar Disorder: A Feasibility Trial." *European Psychiatry: The Journal of the Association of European Psychiatrists* 25, no. 6 (October 2010): 334–37. Publisher: ELSEVIER FRANCE; doi:10.1016/j.eurpsy.2010.03.007., PMID: 20561769

➢ "Most participants reported having durably, moderately to very much benefited from the program, although mindfulness practice decreased over time. ….change of mindfulness skills was significantly associated with change in depressive symptoms between pre- and post-MBCT assessments."

Deckersbach, Thilo, et al., "Mindfulness-Based Cognitive Therapy for Nonremitted Patients with Bipolar Disorder." *CNS Neuroscience & Therapeutics* 18, no. 2 (February 2012): 133–41. Publisher: BLACKWELL PUBLISHING; doi:10.1111/j.1755-5949.2011.00236.x. PMID: 22070469

➢ "These findings suggest that treating residual mood symptoms with MBCT may be another avenue to improving mood, emotion regulation, well being, and functioning in individuals with bipolar disorder."

Novel Allopathic Therapies

Stellate Ganglion Block

Stellate Ganglion Block Provides Temporary Relief from Depression

Karnosh, L. J., et al., "The Effects of Bilateral Stellate Ganglion Block on Mental Depression; Report of 3 Cases." *Cleveland Clinic Quarterly* 14, no. 3 (July 1947): 133–38.

➢ Temporary block of sympathetic impulses to the brain by procaine injection of both stellate ganglia in 3 patients suffering with endogenous mental depression induced a heightening affect, a relative euphoria, and transitory relief from morbid ideation and psychomotor retardation. The effect of stellate ganglion block on depressed mood suggests that the sympathetic outflow to the brain plays a role in contributing to the cenesthetic or mood level of consciousness. Amplified studies are indicted in order to determine whether sympathetic interruption to the brain through surgery will permanently modify the cyclic behavior of the affective reaction psychoses and whether it can in some cases replace prefrontal lobotomy in the treatment of chronic depression which has proved refractory to shock therapy.

Electric Stimulation

CODEX ALTERNUS

Nonconvulsive Electrotherapy

Nonconvulsive Electrotherapy has High Remission Rates and is Safer Than ECT

Regenold, William T., et al., "Nonconvulsive Electrotherapy for Treatment Resistant Unipolar and Bipolar Major Depressive Disorder: A Proof-of-Concept Trial." *Brain Stimulation*. Accessed July 6, 2015. doi:10.1016/j.brs.2015.06.011.

> ➢ Seizure-free data were obtained from 11 of 13 subjects. Group mean Hamilton Depression Rating Scale 17-item version scores declined significantly ($P = 0.001$) from 20.3 to 8.6. Response and remission rates were 73% (8) and 55% (6), respectively. Cognitive testing using the Mini-Mental State Exam and the Autobiographical Memory Inventory-Short Form did not show declines typically observed with ECT.

Transcranial Direct Current Stimulation

Transcranial Direct Current Stimulation is Effective in Bipolar Depressive Disorder

Brunoni, A. R., et al., "Transcranial Direct Current Stimulation (tDCS) in Unipolar vs. Bipolar Depressive Disorder." *Progress in Neuro-Psychopharmacology & Biological Psychiatry* 35, no. 1 (January 15, 2011): 96–101. Publisher: ELSEVIER INC. doi:10.1016/j.pnpbp.2010.09.010., PMID: 20854868

> ➢ Transcranial direct current stimulation (tDCS) is a non-invasive method for brain stimulation. Although pilot trials have shown that tDCS yields promising results for major depressive disorder (MDD), its efficacy for bipolar depressive disorder (BDD), a condition with high prevalence and poor treatment outcomes, is unknown. In a previous study we explored the effectiveness of tDCS for MDD. Here, we expanded our research, recruiting patients with MDD and BDD. We enrolled 31 hospitalized patients (24 women) aged 30-70 years 17 with MDD and 14 with BDD (n = 14). All patients received stable drug regimens for at least two weeks before enrollment and drug dosages remained unchanged throughout the study. We applied tDCS over the dorsolateral prefrontal cortex (anodal electrode on the left and cathodal on the right) using a 2 mA-current for 20 min, twice-daily, for 5 consecutive days. Depression was measured at baseline, after 5 tDCS sessions, one week later, and one month after treatment onset. We used the scales of Beck (BDI) and Hamilton-21 items (HDRS). All patients tolerated treatment well without adverse effects. After the fifth tDCS session, depressive symptoms in both study groups diminished, and the beneficial effect persisted at one week and one month. In conclusion, our preliminary study suggests that tDCS is a promising treatment for patients with MDD and BDD.

CODEX ALTERNUS

Cranial Electrotherapy Stimulation

Cranial Electrotherapy Stimulation Has Modest Improvement of Patients with Bipolar Disorder

Amr, Mostafa, et al., "Cranial Electrotherapy Stimulation for the Treatment of Chronically Symptomatic Bipolar Patients." *The Journal of ECT* 29, no. 2 (June 2013): e31–32. Publisher: International Society for ECT and Neurostimulation doi:10.1097/YCT.0b013e31828a344d., PMID: 20854868

> ➤ "The Clinical Global Impression improved significantly [mean (SD), 2.7 (0.6) at baseline vs 2.0 (0.0), t = 0, P < 0.001], but mood symptoms change minimally. There were very few adverse effects of CES. Patients with CSBP continue to experience symptoms with CES but also are modestly improved."

Radioelectric Asymmetric Conveyor

Treatment with a Radioelectric Asymmetric Conveyor Shows Good Efficacy in Treating Both Manic and Depressive Phases in Bipolar Disorder

Mannu, Piero, et al., "Long-Term Treatment of Bipolar Disorder with a Radioelectric Asymmetric Conveyor." *Neuropsychiatric Disease and Treatment* 7 (2011): 373–79. Publisher: DOVE MEDICAL PRESS LTD. doi:10.2147/NDT.S22007., PMID: 21822388

> ➤ "REAC showed good efficacy in treating both the manic and depressive phases of bipolar disorder, and the prevention of recurrences/relapses."

Vestibular Stimulation

Caloric Vestibular Stimulation Has a Modulating Effect on Mood and Affective Control

Preuss, Nora, et al., "Caloric Vestibular Stimulation Modulates Affective Control and Mood." *Brain Stimulation* 7, no. 1 (February 2014): 133–40. Publisher: ELSEVIER doi:10.1016/j.brs.2013.09.003., PMID: 24139868

> ➤ The sensitivity index d' (hits - false alarms) was used to measure affective control. Affective control improved during right ear CVS when viewing positive stimuli (P = .005), but decreased during left ear CVS when compared to sham stimulation (P = .009). CVS had a similar effect on positive mood ratings (Positive and Negative Affect Schedule). Positive mood ratings decreased during left ear CVS when compared to sham stimulation, but there was no effect after right ear CVS. The results suggest that CVS, depending on side of stimulation, has a modulating effect on mood and affective control. The results complement previous findings in manic patients and provide new evidence for the clinical potential of CVS.

CODEX ALTERNUS

Left Ear Caloric Vestibular Stimulation is Effective for Short Term Reduction of Manic Delusions

---

Levine, Joseph, et al., "Beneficial Effects of Caloric Vestibular Stimulation on Denial of Illness and Manic Delusions in Schizoaffective Disorder: A Case Report." *Brain Stimulation* 5, no. 3 (July 2012): 267–73. Publisher: ELSEVIER; doi:10.1016/j.brs.2011.03.004., PMID: 21783454

➢ All three patients showed a difference favoring left versus right ear CVS that was maintained for 20 minutes, and diminished over a 60 minute period. EEG analyses showed a numerically non-significant increase in bilateral frontal and central alpha EEG band activation (more pronounced in the right hemisphere) with left but not right ear CVS 5 minutes after the CVS, and that diminished after 20 minutes. The results suggest that left versus right CVS may have a short lived beneficial effect on manic delusions and insight of illness that seem to appear in other types of psychoses (i.e., schizophrenia). These preliminary results suggest that single session CVS may have short lived beneficial effects in mania and perhaps in other types of psychoses. Further research is mandatory.

Caloric Vestibular Stimulation is a Novel Approach for Treatment of Mania

---

Dodson, M. J., et al., "Vestibular Stimulation in Mania: A Case Report." *Journal of Neurology, Neurosurgery, and Psychiatry* 75, no. 1 (January 2004): 168–69., Publisher: B M J PUBLISHING GROUP; PMID: 14707337

➢ "This case describes an impressive and relatively sustained improvement in manic symptoms following left caloric vestibular stimulation. Caloric vestibular stimulation represents a novel approach to the treatment of mania."

CODEX ALTERNUS™

SECTION THREE

Medication-Induced Side Effect Treatments

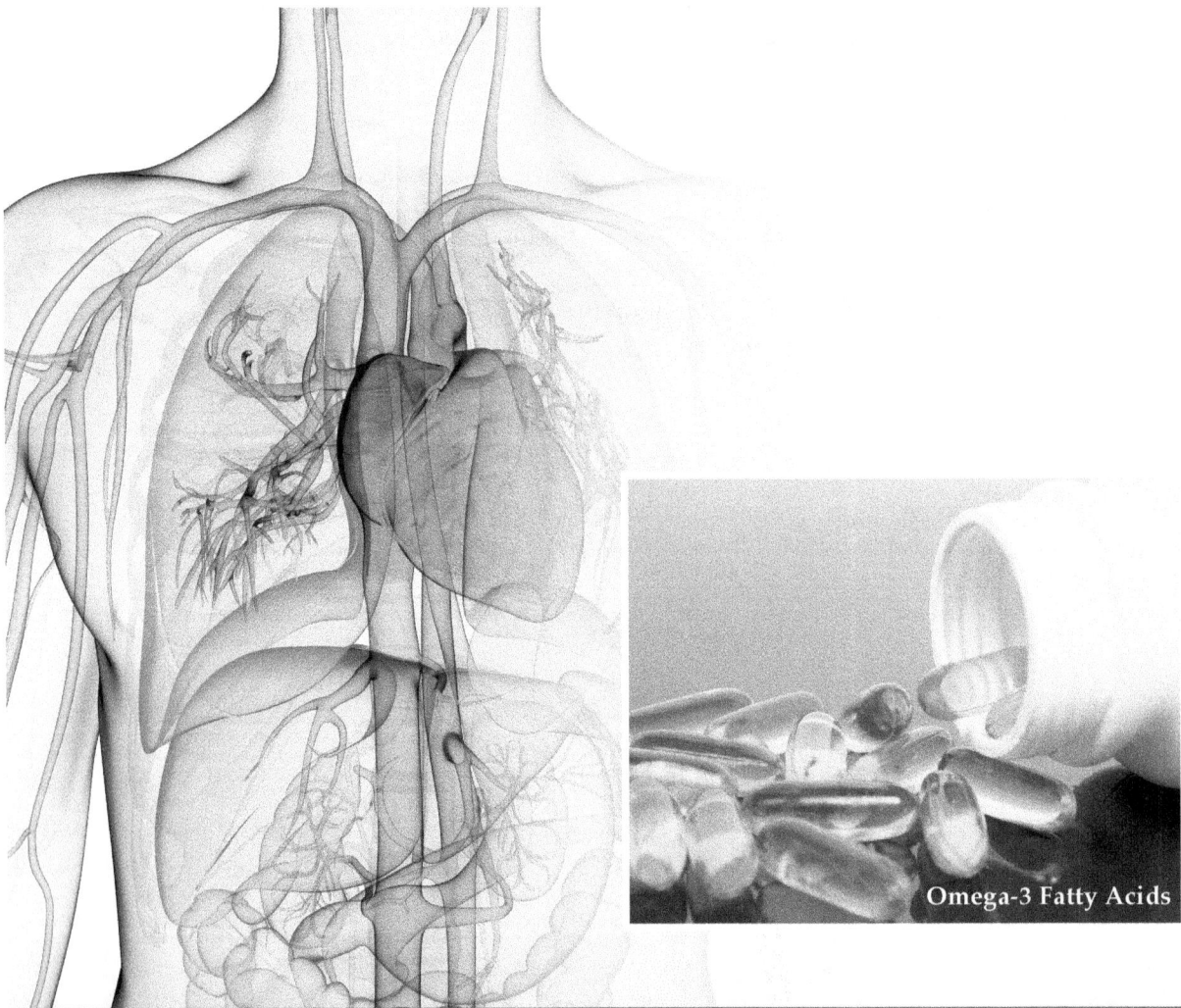

Omega-3 Fatty Acids

CODEX ALTERNUS

Neuroprotection from Neuroleptics

Alpha Lipoic Acid

Alpha Lipoic Acid Down Regulates Antipsychotic-induced DRD2 Upregulation

Deslauriers, Jessica, et al., "Antipsychotic-Induced DRD2 Upregulation and Its Prevention by A-Lipoic Acid in SH-SY5Y Neuroblastoma Cells." *Synapse (New York, N.Y.)* 65, no. 4 (April 2011): 321–31. Publisher: JOHN WILEY & SONS, INC. doi:10.1002/syn.20851., PMID: 20730801

> ➤ "Our results suggest that haloperidol-induced DRD2 upregulation is linked to oxidative stress and provide potential mechanisms by which (±)-α-lipoic acid can be considered as a therapeutic agent to prevent and treat side effects related to the use of first-generation APs."

Alpha Lipoic Acid Significantly Reduces Haldol-induced Neuronal Damage

Perera, Joachim, et al., "Neuroprotective Effects of Alpha Lipoic Acid on Haloperidol-Induced Oxidative Stress in the Rat Brain." *Cell & Bioscience* 1, no. 1 (2011): 12. Publisher: BioMed Central; doi:10.1186/2045-3701-1-12., PMID: 21711768

> ➤ In the present study, we evaluate the protective effect of alpha lipoic acid against haloperidol-induced oxidative stress in the rat brain. Sprague Dawley rats were divided into control, alpha lipoic acid alone (100 mg/kg p.o for 21 days), haloperidol alone (2 mg/kg i.p for 21 days), and haloperidol with alpha lipoic acid groups (for 21 days). Haloperidol treatment significantly decreased levels of the brain antioxidant enzymes super oxide dismutase and glutathione peroxidase and concurrent treatment with alpha lipoic acid significantly reversed the oxidative effects of haloperidol. Histopathological changes revealed significant haloperidol-induced damage in the cerebral cortex, internal capsule, and substantia nigra. Alpha lipoic acid significantly reduced this damage and there were very little neuronal atrophy. Areas of angiogenesis were also seen in the alpha lipoic acid-treated group. In conclusion, the study proves that alpha lipoic acid treatment significantly reduces haloperidol-induced neuronal damage.

Antioxidants

Antioxidants as Potential Therapeutics in Neuropsychiatric Disorders

Pandya, Chirayu D., et al., "Antioxidants as Potential Therapeutics for Neuropsychiatric Disorders." *Progress in Neuro-Psychopharmacology & Biological Psychiatry* 46 (October 1, 2013): 214–23. Publisher: ELSEVIER INC. doi:10.1016/j.pnpbp.2012.10.017., PMID: 23123357

> ➤ "The present article will give an overview of the potential strategies and outcomes of using antioxidants as therapeutics in psychiatric disorders."

Antioxidant Vitamin C is Recommended as Co-Administration with Neuroleptics

Besret, L., et al., "Antioxidant Strategy to Counteract the Side Effects of Antipsychotic Therapy: An in Vivo Study in Rats." *European Journal of Pharmacology* 408, no. 1 (November 10, 2000): 35–39.

> ➤ As ascorbate is a modulator of dopamine transmission in the striatum by enhancing the ability of haloperidol to induce catalepsy in this study, in view of that negative effect, could not promote vitamin C to prevent antipsychotic-induced extrapyramidal symptoms. However, the possibility that the ascorbate effects on dopamine neurons are mediated by antioxidative damage to dopamine neurons must be considered for the concomitant use of an antioxidant when neuroleptics are administered to patients.

Beta-glucan

Beta-glucan has Protective Effects against Lipid Peroxidation Induced by Haldol

Dietrich-Muszalska, Anna, et al., "Beta-Glucan from Saccharomyces Cerevisiae Reduces Plasma Lipid Peroxidation Induced by Haloperidol." *International Journal of Biological Macromolecules* 49, no. 1 (July 1, 2011): 113–16. Publisher: ELSEVIER BV doi:10.1016/j.ijbiomac.2011.03.007., PMID: 21421004

> ➤ "The presented results indicate that beta-glucan seems to have distinctly protective effects against the impairment of plasma lipid molecules induced by haloperidol."

Camel's Urine, Nigella Sativa & Ginger Mixture

Camel's Milk and Urine and Herbal Mixtrure is Efficient at Reducing Toxic Effects of Haldol

Bawazeer, Fayza AA., et al., "Effect of Camel's Urine and Milk, Honey with Nigella Sativa Mixture and Ginger on Haloperidol-induced Histological Alterations in Duodenum of Albino Rats." *Egypt J Exp. Biol (Zool)* 6(1): 1-7 (2010)

> ➤ "In conclusion, the results revealed the toxic effect of haloperidol on duodenum tissue. The mixture of camel's milk and urine is more efficiency in decreasing the toxic effects produced by the drug."

CODEX ALTERNUS

Choke Berries

Polyphenols from Choke Berries Reduce Lipid Peroxidation Caused by Geodon

Dietrich-Muszalska, Anna, et al., "Polyphenols from Berries of Aronia Melanocarpa Reduce the Plasma Lipid Peroxidation Induced by Ziprasidone." *Schizophrenia Research and Treatment* 2014 (2014): 602390. Publisher: Hindawi Publishing Corporation doi:10.1155/2014/602390., PMID: 25061527

> ➤ "Conclusion. Aronox causes a distinct reduction of lipid peroxidation induced by ziprasidone."

Curcumin

Curcumin Has a Protective Effect against the Neurochemical Changes Associated with Haldol Administration

Bishnoi, Mahendra, et al., "Protective Effect of Curcumin, the Active Principle of Turmeric (Curcuma Longa) in Haloperidol-Induced Orofacial Dyskinesia and Associated Behavioural, Biochemical and Neurochemical Changes in Rat Brain." *Pharmacology, Biochemistry, and Behavior* 88, no. 4 (February 2008): 511–22. Publisher: ELSEVIER INC. doi:10.1016/j.pbb.2007.10.009., PMID: 18022680

> ➤ "Interestingly, co-administration of curcumin (25 and 50mg/kg, i.p., 21 days) dose dependently prevented all behavioral, cellular, and neurochemical changes associated with administration of haloperidol."

Dragon-pearl Tea

Dragon-pearl Tea was Shown to Reduce to Reduce Reserpine-induced Gastric Ulcers with a Inhibitory Rate of 73%

Yi, Ruokun, et al., "Antioxidant-Mediated Preventative Effect of Dragon-Pearl Tea Crude Polyphenol Extract on Reserpine-Induced Gastric Ulcers." *Experimental and Therapeutic Medicine* 10, no. 1 (July 2015): 338–44. doi:10.3892/etm.2015.2473., PMID: 26170959

> ➤ Dragon-pearl tea is a type of green tea commonly consumed in Southwest China. In the present study, the antioxidative and anti-gastric ulcer effects of Dragon-pearl tea crude polyphenols (DTCP) were determined in vitro and in vivo. Treatment with 25, 50 or 100 μg/ml DTCP resulted in notable antioxidant effects in vitro, which manifested as 2,2-diphenyl-1-picrylhydrazyl and OH radical-scavenging activity. Furthermore, using an in vivo mouse model, DTCP was shown to reduce the gastric ulcer area in the stomach, in which the 200 mg/kg DTCP dose exhibited the most marked effect, with a gastric ulcer index inhibitory rate of 72.63%. Therefore, the

CODEX ALTERNUS

results indicated that DTCP induced a marked preventative effect on reserpine-induced gastric ulcers in vivo, as a result of its antioxidative capacity.

Fire Brush

Fire Brush Methanolic Extract has a Neuroprotective and Hepatopotective Effect on Haldol induced Toxicities

> **Abdel-Sattar, Essam A.**, et al., "Protective Effect of Calligonum Comosum on Haloperidol-Induced Oxidative Stress in Rat." *Toxicology and Industrial Health* 30, no. 2 (March 2014): 147–53. doi:10.1177/0748233712452601., PMID: 22773435

> ➤ The results showed that the antioxidant activity of the methanolic extract was higher than the aqueous one. HL significantly reduced GSH and increased MDA in brain and liver tissues. These values were nearly normalized, in the examined tissues, on concomitant administration of C. comosum methanolic extract with HL. Superoxide dismutase activity in the examined tissues was significantly decreased by HL administration that was normalized by the coadministration of the methanolic extract and, to a less extent, the water extract. Determination of the brain neurotransmitter contents revealed a marked decrease in norepinephrine, dopamine and serotonin, which were restored to near control values by concomitant administration of both C. comosum extracts with HL. The results of this study showed that C. comosum methanolic and aqueous extracts ameliorated HL-induced neuro- and hepatotoxicities in rats.

Green Tea Epicatechin

Green Tea Epicatechin Significantly Reduces the Lipid Peroxidation of Haldol

> **Dietrich-Muszalska, Anna**, et al., "Epicatechin Inhibits Human Plasma Lipid Peroxidation Caused by Haloperidol in Vitro." *Neurochemical Research* 37, no. 3 (March 2012): 557–62. Publisher: SPRINGER NEW YORK LLC; doi:10.1007/s11064-011-0642-8., PMID: 22076501

> ➤ "'In conclusion, the presented results indicate that epicatechin-the major polyphenolic component of green tea reduced significantly human plasma lipid peroxidation caused by haloperidol. Moreover, epicatechin was found to be more effective antioxidant, than the solution of pure resveratrol or quercetin."

Green Tea Extract Revived Liver Cells from Hepatic Damage Induced by Reserpine

> **Al-Bloushi, S.**, et al., "Green Tea Modulates Reserpine Toxicity in Animal Models." *The Journal of Toxicological Sciences* 34, no. 1 (February 2009): 77–87., PMID: 19182437

> ➤ This study investigated the merits of administering green tea concurrently with reserpine to prevent oxidative hepatic damage with elevated levels of oxidative stress markers, such as Thiobarbituric Acid Reactive Substance (TBARS),

transaminies and cholesterol. Reserpine also induced hepatic ultra-structural damage in the cytoplasmic reticulum (rER), ribosomal stripping and mitochondria elctrtron microscopy examination showed revival of liver cells as a result of green tea extract administration to experimental rats.

Green Tea Extract Produced Reversal of Despair in Normal, Reserpined and Diabetic Mice, Showing an Antidepressant Effect

Singal, Anjali, et al., "Green Tea [Camellia Sinensis (L.) O. Kuntze] Extract Reverses the Despair Behaviour in Reserpinised and Diabetic Mice." *Indian Journal of Experimental Biology* 44, no. 11 (November 2006): 913–17., PMID: 17205714

➢ Green tea (C. sinensis) extract (GTE) dose dependently produced reversal of despair in normal, reserpinised and diabetic mice, thereby demonstrating an antidepressant effect. Although the exact mechanism is yet to be explored, the possible inhibition of catechol-o-methyl transferase and monoamine oxidase enzymes may be responsible for antidepressant activity of GTE.

Green Tea Extract Reduces Oxidative Damage and Protects Kidney from Reserpine-induced Toxicity

Abdel-Majeed, Safer, et al., "Inhibition Property of Green Tea Extract in Relation to Reserpine-Induced Ribosomal Strips of Rough Endoplasmic Reticulum (rER) of the Rat Kidney Proximal Tubule Cells." *The Journal of Toxicological Sciences* 34, no. 6 (December 2009): 637–45., PMID: 19952499

➢ Reserpine was found to cause kidney proximal tubule damage, such as stripping and clustering of ribosomes from the rough endoplasmic reticulum (rER) and demolishing of mitochondrial christae with elevated level of oxidative stress markers, such as TBARS. While the ultrastructural study showed a revival of kidney proximal tubule cells as a result of the administration of green tea extract to rats. We suggest that green tea might elevate antioxidant defense system, clean up free radicals, lessen oxidative damages and protect kidney against reserpine-induced toxicity and thus had a potential protective effect.

Phytochemicals

Phytochemicals Have Neuroprotective Effects in Neuropsychiatric Diseases

Kumar, G. Phani, et al., "Neuroprotective Potential of Phytochemicals." *Pharmacognosy Reviews* 6, no. 12 (July 2012): 81–90. Publisher: Pharmacognosy Network Worldwide doi:10.4103/0973-7847.99898., PMID: 23055633

➢ In this review, we briefly deal with some medicinal herbs focusing on their neuroprotective active phytochemical substances like fatty acids, phenols, alkaloids, flavonoids, saponins, terpenes etc. The resistance of neurons to various stressors by activating specific signal transduction pathways and transcription factors are also discussed. It was observed in the review that a number of herbal medicines used in Ayurvedic practices as well Chinese medicines contain multiple compounds and phytochemicals that may have a neuroprotective effect which may prove beneficial in different neuropsychiatric and neurodegenerative disorders. Though the presence of receptors or transporters for polyphenols or other phytochemicals of the herbal preparations, in brain tissues remains to be ascertained, compounds with multiple targets appear as a potential and promising class of therapeutics for the treatment of diseases with a multifactorial etiology.

Resveratrol and Quercetin

Resveratrol and Quercetin Decrease Lipid Peroxidation Caused by Antipsychotics

Dietrich-Muszalska, Anna, et al., "Inhibitory Effects of Polyphenol Compounds on Lipid Peroxidation Caused by Antipsychotics (haloperidol and Amisulpride) in Human Plasma in Vitro." *The World Journal of Biological Psychiatry: The Official Journal of the World Federation of Societies of Biological Psychiatry* 11, no. 2 Pt 2 (March 2010): 276–81. Publisher: WORLD FEDERATION OF THE SOCIETIES OF BIOLOGICAL PSYCHIATRY doi:10.1080/15622970902718790., PMID: 19225991

> ➤ "We showed that in the presence of polyphenols: resveratrol and quercetin, lipid peroxidation in plasma samples treated with tested drugs was significantly decreased."

Sulforaphane

Broccoli Sprouts Exract Sulforaphane Protects Against Antipsychotic Drug-induced Oxidative Stress

Mas, Sergi, et al., "Sulforaphane Protects SK-N-SH Cells against Antipsychotic-Induced Oxidative Stress." *Fundamental & Clinical Pharmacology* 26, no. 6 (December 2012): 712–21. Publisher: BLACKWELL PUBLISHING LTD. doi:10.1111/j.1472-8206.2011.00988.x., PMID: 21923690

> ➤ "Our results indicate that SF increases GSH levels and induces NQO1 activity and the removal of electrophilic quinones and radical oxygen species. Furthermore, SF could provide protective effects against AP-induced toxicity in dopaminergic cells."

Vitamin C

Vitamin C Reduces the Production of Reactive Oxygen Species from Antipsychotics

CODEX ALTERNUS

Heiser, P., et al., "Effects of Antipsychotics and Vitamin C on the Formation of Reactive Oxygen Species." *Journal of Psychopharmacology (Oxford, England)* 24, no. 10 (October 2010): 1499–1504. ublisher: SAGE SCIENCE PRESS (UK) doi:10.1177/0269881109102538., PMID: 19282419

> "Vitamin C reduced the ROS production of all drugs tested and for haloperidol and clozapine the level of significance was reached. Our study demonstrated that induce the formation of ROS in whole blood of rats, which can be reduced by application of vitamin C."

Vitamin E

Vitamin E Has Plasma Membrane Stabalazation Properties that are compromised by Antipsychotics

Maruoka, Nobuyuki, et al., "Effects of Vitamin E Supplementation on Plasma Membrane Permeabilization and Fluidization Induced by Chlorpromazine in the Rat Brain." *Journal of Psychopharmacology (Oxford, England)* 22, no. 2 (March 2008): 119–27. Publisher: SAGE SCIENCE PRESS (UK); doi:10.1177/0269881107078487., PMID: 18208929

> "CPZ can reduce plasma membrane integrity in the brain, and this reduction can be prevented by vitamin E via its membrane-stabilizing properties, not via its antioxidant activity."

Vitamin E May Be Protective form Haldol-associated Neurotoxicity

Post, Anke, et al., "Mechanisms Underlying the Protective Potential of Alpha-Tocopherol (vitamin E) against Haloperidol-Associated Neurotoxicity." *Neuropsychopharmacology: Official Publication of the American College of Neuropsychopharmacology* 26, no. 3 (March 2002): 397–407. Publisher: NATURE PUBLISHING GROUP; doi:10.1016/S0893-133X(01)00364-5., PMID: 11850154

> "…the present study shows that pre- and co-treatment with vitamin E interferes with the stimulation of apoptotic cascades by haloperidol and, in addition, attenuates some of the undesirable behavioral side-effects of the neuroleptic."

Yin-Chen-Hao-Tang

Yin-Chen-Hao-Tang Exerted a Protective Effect on Thorazine-induced Cholestasis Liver Injury

Yang, Qiaoling, et al. "Chlorpromazine-Induced Perturbations of Bile Acids and Free Fatty Acids in Cholestatic Liver Injury Prevented by the Chinese Herbal Compound Yin-Chen-Hao-Tang." *BMC Complementary and Alternative Medicine* 15, no. 1 (April 16, 2015): 122. doi:10.1186/s12906-015-0627-2., PMID: 25887351

> Obtained data showed that YCHT attenuated the effect of CPZ-induced cholestatic liver injury, which was manifested by the serum biochemical parameters and histopathology of the liver tissue. YCHT regulated the lipid levels as indicated by the reversed serum levels of TC, TG, and LDL-C. YCHT also regulated the disorder of BA and FFA metabolism by CPZ induction. Results indicated that YCHT exerted a protective effect on CPZ-induced cholestasis liver injury. The variance of BA and FFA concentrations can be used to evaluate the cholestatic liver injury caused by CPZ and the hepatoprotective effect of YCHT.

Reversal of Cerebral Atrophy

Exercise

Cardiorespiratory Fitness Increases Brain Volume in Schizophrenic Patients

Scheewe, Thomas W., et al., "Exercise Therapy, Cardiorespiratory Fitness and Their Effect on Brain Volumes: A Randomised Controlled Trial in Patients with Schizophrenia and Healthy Controls." *European Neuropsychopharmacology: The Journal of the European College of Neuropsychopharmacology* 23, no. 7 (July 2013): 675–85. Publisher: ELSEVIER BV doi:10.1016/j.euroneuro.2012.08.008., PMID: 22981376

> The objective of this study was to examine exercise effects on global brain volume, hippocampal volume, and cortical thickness in schizophrenia patients and healthy controls. Irrespective of diagnosis and intervention, associations between brain changes and cardiorespiratory fitness improvement were examined. Sixty-three schizophrenia patients and fifty-five healthy controls participated in this randomised controlled trial. Global brain volumes, hippocampal volume, and cortical thickness were estimated from 3-Tesla MRI scans. Cardiorespiratory fitness was assessed with a cardiopulmonary ergometer test. Subjects were assigned exercise therapy or occupational therapy (patients) and exercise therapy or life-as-usual (healthy controls) for six months 2h weekly. Exercise therapy effects were analysed for subjects who were compliant at least 50% of sessions offered. Significantly smaller baseline cerebral (grey) matter, and larger third ventricle volumes, and thinner cortex in most areas of the brain were found in patients versus controls. Exercise therapy did not affect global brain and hippocampal volume or cortical thickness in patients and controls. Cardiorespiratory fitness improvement was related to increased cerebral matter volume and lateral and third ventricle volume decrease in patients and to thickening in the left hemisphere in large areas of the frontal, temporal and cingulate cortex irrespective of diagnosis. One to 2h of exercise therapy did not elicit significant brain volume changes in patients or controls. However, cardiorespiratory fitness improvement attenuated brain volume changes in schizophrenia patients and

increased thickness in large areas of the left cortex in both schizophrenia patients and healthy controls.

Omega-3 Fatty Acid EPA

Omega-3 Fatty Acid EPA can Reverse Both Phospholipid Abnormalities and Cerebral Atrophy

> **Puri, B. K.**, et al., "Eicosapentaenoic Acid Treatment in Schizophrenia Associated with Symptom Remission, Normalisation of Blood Fatty Acids, Reduced Neuronal Membrane Phospholipid Turnover and Structural Brain Changes." *International Journal of Clinical Practice* 54, no. 1 (February 2000): 57–63., Publisher: MEDICOM INTL INC; PMID: 10750263

> ➤ "These results demonstrate that EPA can reverse both the phospholipid abnormalities previously described in schizophrenia and cerebral atrophy."

Omega-3 Fatty Acid EPA Reveresed Cerebral Atrophy in Schizophrenic Patient

> **Puri, Basant K.**, et al., "High-Resolution Magnetic Resonance Imaging Sinc-Interpolation-Based Subvoxel Registration and Semi-Automated Quantitative Lateral Ventricular Morphology Employing Threshold Computation and Binary Image Creation in the Study of Fatty Acid Interventions in Schizophrenia, Depression, Chronic Fatigue Syndrome and Huntington's Disease." *International Review of Psychiatry (Abingdon, England)* 18, no. 2 (April 2006): 149–54. Publisher: ROUTLEDGE doi:10.1080/09540260600583015., PMID: 16777669

> ➤ The first patient with schizophrenia to be treated solely with the n-3 long-chain polyunsaturated fatty acid eicosapentaenoic acid (EPA) showed a remark- able and sustained remission of positive and negative symptoms starting within a month of this intervention (Puri & Richardson, 1998). His brain was scanned with high-resolution MRI both at one year and six months before starting the EPA, while he remained antipsychotic drug-free. He underwent MRI brain scanning again at baseline (on starting the EPA), and then after taking the fatty acid daily for six months. Using the two techniques described in the previous section, it was found that cerebral atrophy had been taking place during the year before taking the EPA, with an increase in lateral ventricular volume occur- ring from 18,750mm3 (at minus one year with respect to EPA treatment), through 19,440mm3 (at minus six months) to 19,800mm3 at baseline. Normalizing these volumes to the total brain volume at each scan gave corresponding values of the ventricle-to-brain ratios (VBRs) of 0.0147, 0.0153 and 0.0155 (Puri et al., 2000; Puri & Richardson, 2003). After six months of taking EPA (and no other medication), there was a reversal of this cerebral atrophy, with the lateral ventricular volume being 18,850mm3 and the corresponding VBR falling back to 0.0148. These results were the first to indicate that EPA might be able to reverse cerebral atrophy, at least in schizo- phrenia, as well as to treat positive and negative symptoms in this disorder.

CODEX ALTERNUS

Vitamin A

Vitamin A Supplementation May Reverse Loss of Hippocampal Long Term Synaptic Plasticity

> **Misner, D. L.,** et al., "Vitamin A Deprivation Results in Reversible Loss of Hippocampal Long-Term Synaptic Plasticity." *Proceedings of the National Academy of Sciences of the United States of America* 98, no. 20 (September 25, 2001): 11714–19. doi:10.1073/pnas.191369798., Publisher: NATIONAL ACADEMY OF SCIENCES - BIACTIVE WORK; PMID: 11553775

> ➢ Despite its long history, the central effects of progressive depletion of vitamin A in adult mice has not been previously described. An examination of vitamin-deprived animals revealed a progressive and ultimately profound impairment of hippocampal CA1 long-term potentiation and a virtual abolishment of long-term depression. Importantly, these losses are fully reversible by dietary vitamin A replenishment in vivo or direct application of all trans-retinoic acid to acute hippocampal slices. We find retinoid responsive transgenes to be highly active in the hippocampus, and by using dissected explants, we show the hippocampus to be a site of robust synthesis of bioactive retinoids. In aggregate, these results demonstrate that vitamin A and its active derivatives function as essential competence factors for long-term synaptic plasticity within the adult brain, and suggest that key genes required for long-term potentiation and long-term depression are retinoid dependent. These data suggest a major mental consequence for the hundreds of millions of adults and children who are vitamin A deficient.

Weight Gain Side Effect Treatments

Alpha Lipoic Acid

Alpha Lipoic Acid is Effective for Weight loss in Patients with Schizophrenia without Diabetes

> **Ratliff, Joseph C.,** et al., "An Open-Label Pilot Trial of Alpha-Lipoic Acid for Weight Loss in Patients with Schizophrenia without Diabetes." *Clinical Schizophrenia & Related Psychoses*, March 7, 2013, 1–13. Publisher: WALSH MEDICAL MEDIA doi:10.3371/CSRP.RAPA.030113., PMID: 23471087

> ➢ A possible mechanism of antipsychotic-induced weight gain is activation of hypothalamic monophosphate-dependent kinase (AMPK) mediated by histamine 1 receptors. Alpha-lipoic acid (ALA), a potent antioxidant, counteracts this effect and may be helpful in reducing weight for patients taking antipsychotics. The objective of this open label study was to assess the efficacy of ALA (1200mg) on 12 non-diabetic schizophrenia patients over ten weeks. Participants lost significant weight during the intervention (-2.2 kg ± 2.5 kg). ALA was well tolerated and was particularly effective

for individuals taking strongly antihistaminic antipsychotics (-2.9 kg ± 2.6 kg vs. -0.5 kg ± 1.0 kg).

Alpha Lipoic Acid is effective Treatment of Antipsychotic-induced Weight Gain and Improves Metabolic Abnormalities

> **Kim, Eosu,** et al., "A Preliminary Investigation of Alpha-Lipoic Acid Treatment of Antipsychotic Drug-Induced Weight Gain in Patients with Schizophrenia." *Journal of Clinical Psychopharmacology* 28, no. 2 (April 2008): 138–46. Publisher: LIPPINCOTT WILLIAMS & WILKINS; doi:10.1097/JCP.0b013e31816777f7., PMID: 18344723

> ➢ The mean (SD) weight loss was 3.16 (3.20) kg (P = 0.043, last observation carried forward; median, 3.03 kg; range, 0-8.85 kg). On average, body mass index showed a significant reduction (P = 0.028) over the 12 weeks. During the same period, a statistically significant reduction was also observed in total cholesterol levels (P = 0.042), and there was a weak trend toward the reduction in insulin resistance (homeostasis model assessment of insulin resistance) (P = 0.080). Three subjects reported increased energy subjectively. The total scores on the Brief Psychiatric Rating Scale and the Montgomery-Asberg Depression Rating Scale did not vary significantly during the study. These preliminary data suggest the possibility that ALA can ameliorate the adverse metabolic effects induced by AAPDs. To confirm the benefits of ALA, more extended study is warranted.

Alpha Lipoic Acid Prevented Olanzapine-induced Weight Gain in Mice

> **Kim, Hyunjeong,** et al., "Phosphorylation of Hypothalamic AMPK on serine(485/491) Related to Sustained Weight Loss by Alpha-Lipoic Acid in Mice Treated with Olanzapine." *Psychopharmacology,* April 15, 2014. Publisher: SPRINGER-VERLAG ;doi:10.1007/s00213-014-3540-3., PMID: 24733236

> ➢ Body weights were increased by olanzapine in parallel with increased levels of Thr172 phosphorylation of hypothalamic AMPK. Initially increased rate of weight gain was diminished as Thr172 phosphorylation levels were decreased to control levels after 10 days of olanzapine treatment. ALA successfully not only prevented olanzapine-induced weight gain but also induced additional weight loss even relative to control levels throughout the treatment period. During the initial stage, ALA's action was indicated by both suppression of olanzapine-induced Thr172 phosphorylation and an increase in Ser485/491 phosphorylation levels. However, in the later stage when no more increases in Thr172 phosphorylation and weight gain by olanzapine were observed, ALA's action was only indicated by increased levels of Ser485/491 phosphorylation. Our data suggest that anti-obesity effects of ALA may be related to modulation of both Ser485/491 phosphorylation and Thr172 phosphorylation of hypothalamic AMPK, while olanzapine-induced weight gain

may be only associated with increase in Thr172 phosphorylation. This might be an important mechanistic clue for the future development of anti-obesity drugs beyond control of AAPD-induced weight gain.

Behavioral Intervention

A Behavioral Weight Loss Intervention Significantly Reduced Weight Over a Period of 18 Months

Daumit, Gail L., et al., "A Behavioral Weight-Loss Intervention in Persons with Serious Mental Illness." *The New England Journal of Medicine* 368, no. 17 (April 25, 2013): 1594–1602. Publisher: MASSACHUSETTS MEDICAL SOCIETY; doi:10.1056/NEJMoa1214530., PMID: 23517118

➤ A behavioral weight-loss intervention significantly reduced weight over a period of 18 months in overweight and obese adults with serious mental illness. Given the epidemic of obesity and weight-related disease among persons with serious mental illness, our findings support implementation of targeted behavioral weight-loss interventions in this high-risk population.

Dietian Assisted Nutritional Intervention Reduces Weight Gain in Patients on Atypical Antipsychotics

Evans, Sherryn, et al., "Nutritional Intervention to Prevent Weight Gain in Patients Commenced on Olanzapine: A Randomized Controlled Trial." *The Australian and New Zealand Journal of Psychiatry* 39, no. 6 (June 2005): 479–86. Publisher: BLACKWELL PUBLISHING ASIA; doi:10.1111/j.1440-1614.2005.01607.x., PMID: 15943650

➤ After 3 months, the control group had gained significantly more weight than the treatment group (6.0 kg vs 2.0 kg, p < or = 0.002). Weight gain of more than 7% of initial weight occurred in 64% of the control group compared to 13% of the treatment group. The control group's BMI increased significantly more than the treatment group's (2 kg/m(2)vs 0.7 kg/m(2), p < or = 0.03). The treatment group reported significantly greater improvements in moderate exercise levels, quality of life, health and body image compared to the controls. At 6 months, the control group continued to show significantly more weight gain since baseline than the treatment group (9.9 kg vs 2.0 kg, p < or = 0.013) and consequently had significantly greater increases in BMI (3.2 kg/m(2)vs 0.8 kg/m(2), p < or = 0.017). Individual nutritional intervention provided by a dietitian is highly successful at preventing olanzapine-induced weight gain.

Berberine

Berberine Prevents Zyprexa-induced Weight Gain in Rats

CODEX ALTERNUS

Hu, Yueshan, et al., "Metformin and Berberine Prevent Olanzapine-Induced Weight Gain in Rats." *PloS One* 9, no. 3 (2014): e93310. doi:10.1371/journal.pone.0093310., Publisher: PUBLIC LIBRARY OF SCIENCE; PMID: 24667776

> Olanzapine is a first line medication for the treatment of schizophrenia, but it is also one of the atypical antipsychotics carrying the highest risk of weight gain. Metformin was reported to produce significant attenuation of antipsychotic-induced weight gain in patients, while the study of preventing olanzapine-induced weight gain in an animal model is absent. Berberine, an herbal alkaloid, was shown in our previous studies to prevent fat accumulation in vitro and in vivo. Utilizing a well-replicated rat model of olanzapine-induced weight gain, here we demonstrated that two weeks of metformin or berberine treatment significantly prevented the olanzapine-induced weight gain and white fat accumulation. Neither metformin nor berberine treatment demonstrated a significant inhibition of olanzapine-increased food intake. But interestingly, a significant loss of brown adipose tissue caused by olanzapine treatment was prevented by the addition of metformin or berberine. Our gene expression analysis also demonstrated that the weight gain prevention efficacy of metformin or berberine treatment was associated with changes in the expression of multiple key genes controlling energy expenditure. This study not only demonstrates a significant preventive efficacy of metformin and berberine treatment on olanzapine-induced weight gain in rats, but also suggests a potential mechanism of action for preventing olanzapine-reduced energy expenditure.

Berberine May Prevent Weight Gain during Use of Second Generation Antipsychotic Medication

Hu, Yueshan, et al., "Berberine Inhibits SREBP-1-Related Clozapine and Risperidone Induced Adipogenesis in 3T3-L1 Cells." *Phytotherapy Research: PTR* 24, no. 12 (December 2010): 1831–38. Publisher: JOHN/WILEY & SONS LTD. doi:10.1002/ptr.3204., PMID: 20564506

> The results showed that neither clozapine nor risperidone, alone or in combination with berberine had significant effects on cell viability. Eight days treatment with 15 µM clozapine increased adipogenesis by 37.4% and 50 µM risperidone increased adipogenesis by 26.5% during 3T3-L1 cell differentiation accompanied by increased SREBP-1, PPARγ, C/EBPα, LDLR and Adiponectin gene expression. More importantly, the addition of 8 µM berberine diminished the induction of adipogenesis almost completely accompanied by down-regulated mRNA and protein expression levels of SREBP-1-related proteins. These encouraging results may lead to the use of berberine as an adjuvant to prevent weight gain during second generation antipsychotic medication.

CODEX ALTERNUS

Bofu-tsusho-san

Bofu-tsusho-san Effectively Attenuates Weight Gain in Woman on Zyprexa

Yamamoto, Nobutomo, et al., "Bofu-Tsusho-San Effectively Attenuates the Weight Gain Observed after Receiving Olanzapine." *Psychiatry and Clinical Neurosciences* 62, no. 6 (December 2008): 747. Publisher: BLACKWELL PUBLISHING ASIA; doi:10.1111/j.1440-1819.2008.01868.x., PMID: 19068015

> ➤ A 20 year old woman with schizophrenia on medication, experiencing weight gain, lost 2.7kg of weight in 6 months with additional use of Bofu-tsusho-san with no changes of food intake . "In study of obese mice, bofu-tsusho-san produced a significant decrease in fat mass and weight compared with placebo, with-out effecting amount of food ingested.

Curcumin and Telmisartin

Curcumin and Telmisartin Prevents Zyprexa-induced Weight Gain in Rats

Ramesh, Petchi R, et al., "Effects of Curcumin and Telmisartan on Olanzapine and High Fructose Diet Induced Metabolic Syndrome in Spraugue Dawly Rats." *Pharmacognosy Journal* 4, no. 30 (July 2012): 25–29. doi:10.5530/pj.2012.30.5.

> ➤ The present study shows that treatment with curcumin and telmisartan prevents increase in body weight response to olanzapine and HFD-induced weight gain in rats. This suggests curcumin and telmisartan inhibited the olanzapine and HFD effects on body weight. According to our study results, it is possible to attenuate that antipsychotic-induced weight gain in SD rats was inhibited by ACE inhibitors and curcumin, a natural antioxidant.

Green Tea and CLA

Green Tea and CLA Decrease Body Fat in Patients Taking Seroquel Antipsychotic

Katzman, Martin A., et al., "Weight Gain and Psychiatric Treatment: Is There a Role for Green Tea and Conjugated Linoleic Acid?" *Lipids in Health and Disease* 6 (2007): 14. Publisher: BIOMED CENTRAL LTD. doi:10.1186/1476-511X-6-14., PMID: 17477874

> ➤ In these four adults who were taking quietiapine, the concurrent self-administration of green tea and conjugated linoleic acid appeared to be protective against gains in body fat. The results were fairly consistent; each had a decrease in body fat percentage and increase in lean body mass.

CODEX ALTERNUS

Kidney Beans

Phaseolus vulgaris Beans Treated Significantly Weight Loss as Well as an Improved Plasma Lipid Profile.

> **Pawar, Amit**, et al. "Herbal Supplement of *Phaseolus Vulgaroius* L. Beans in Metabolic Abnormalities Induced by Atypical Antipsychotics: A Review." *International Journal of Pharmaceutical and Biological Archives* 2013: 4(4); 620-622

> ➤ Based on all above literature review, Phaseolus vulgaris looks like a perfect herbal supplement to take care of metabolic abnormalities induced by atypical antipsychotics in Schizophrenic patient. Further research is required to be conducted in animals and humans to know the effect of Phaseolus vulgaris supplement.

Ling Gui Zhu Gan Tang

Ling Gui Zhu Gan Tang Mixture is Effective for Psychotropic Drug-Induced Obesity

> **Ding, Guo'an,** et al.,"The Therapeutic Effects of Ling Gui Zhu Gan Tang Mixture in 50 Psychotic Patients with Obesity Induced by the Psychoactive Drugs." *Journal of Traditional Chinese Medicine = Chung I Tsa Chih Ying Wen Pan / Sponsored by All-China Association of Traditional Chinese Medicine, Academy of Traditional Chinese* Medicine 25, no. 1 (March 2005): 25–28., Publisher: JOURNAL OF TRADITIONAL CHINESE MEDICINE PMID: 15889518

> ➤ In order to observe the therapeutic effects of Ling Gui Zhu Gan Tang Mixture (苓桂术甘汤) on obesity induced by psychoactive drugs, 100 psychotics with obesity induced by psychoactive drugs were randomly divided into a treatment group (50 cases) and acontrolgroup (50 cases) for a 8-week treatment. The changes were determined by means of the Brief Psychiatric Rating Scale (BPRS) and the Treatment Emergent Symptom Scale (TESS) with the body weight recorded before and after treatment. The results showed that the total effective rate was 72%in the treatment group, and 14% in the control group, with the former obviously superior to the latter ($P <0.01$). The BPRS scores were 33.02 ± 7.34 in the treatment group and 32.39 ± 3.51 in the control group before treatment; and 20.38 ± 5.10 in the treatment group and 20.82 ± 1.75 in the control group after treatment. The BPRS scores were obviously reduced after treatment in the two groups (both $P <0.01$), but with no significant difference between the two groups ($P >0.05$). This indicates that the Ling Gui Zhu Gan Tang Mixture does not influence the curative effect of the psychoactive drugs while showing the body weight-reducing effect. Therefore, the Ling Gui Zhu Gan Tang Mixture can be used for those psychotic patients with obesity induced by the psychoactive drugs (the incidence is 10-25%) in their continuous course of treatment with the latter drugs.

CODEX ALTERNUS

Meal Replacements

Meal Replacement Shakes or Bars Can Be an Effective Tool for Managing Weight and Improve Metabolic Factors in Patients with Severe Mental Illness

Gelberg, Hollie A., et al., "Meal Replacements as a Weight Loss Tool in a Population with Severe Mental Illness." *Eating Behaviors.* Accessed July 7, 2015. doi:10.1016/j.eatbeh.2015.06.009.

> ➤ While the use of meal replacement shakes or bars may be challenging for some participants with SMI, these case reports illustrate that one daily meal replacement can be an effective tool for successful weight loss and improved metabolic factors in this population. Our experience suggests that participants who did best with meal replacement options were motivated and able to follow the requirements of the protocol.

Melatonin

Melatonin Attenuates Weight Gain, Abdominal Obesity and Hypertriglycerdemia in Schizophrenic Patients on Zyprexa

Modabbernia, Amirhossein, et al., "Melatonin for Prevention of Metabolic Side-Effects of Olanzapine in Patients with First-Episode Schizophrenia: Randomized Double-Blind Placebo-Controlled Study." *Journal of Psychiatric Research* 53 (June 2014): 133–40. Publisher: PERGAMON; doi:10.1016/j.jpsychires.2014.02.013., PMID: 24607293

> ➤ "To summarize, in patients treated with olanzapine, short-term melatonin treatment attenuates weight gain, abdominal obesity, and hypertriglyceridemia. It might also provide additional benefit for treatment of psychosis."

Zyprexa-induced Weight Gain is blocked by Melatonin Replacement Therapy in Rats

Raskind, Murray A., et al., "Olanzapine-Induced Weight Gain and Increased Visceral Adiposity Is Blocked by Melatonin Replacement Therapy in Rats." *Neuropsychopharmacology: Official Publication of the American College of Neuropsychopharmacology* 32, no. 2 (February 2007): 284–88. Publisher: NATURE PUBLISHING GROUP; doi:10.1038/sj.npp.1301093., PMID: 16710316

> ➤ Olanzapine treatment reduced nocturnal plasma melatonin by 55% (p<0.001), which was restored to control levels by olanzapine+melatonin. Body weight increased 18% in rats treated with olanzapine alone, but only 10% with olanzapine+melatonin, 5% with melatonin alone, and 7% with vehicle control. Body weight and visceral fat pad weight increases in rats treated with olanzapine alone were greater than in each of the other three groups (all p<0.01), which were not significantly different. These results suggest that olanzapine-induced increases in body weight and visceral

adiposity may be at least in part secondary to olanzapine-induced reduction of plasma melatonin levels, and that melatonin may be useful for the management of olanzapine-induced weight gain in humans.

Sports

Sports Activity May Help Reduce Weight and Improve Symptoms for Schizophrenics

Soundy, Andrew, et al., "Investigating the Benefits of Sport Participation for Individuals with Schizophrenia: A Systematic Review." *Psychiatria Danubina* 27, no. 1 (March 2015): 2–13., PMID: 25751427

> ➢ This review demonstrates that participation in sports may, at least in the short term, result in small reductions in weight and psychiatric symptoms, and possibly have wider health benefits. Notwithstanding the limitations of the examined studies, sports participation should be considered as an option to improve the physical and mental health of people with schizophrenia. However, further well-designed, adequately-powered studies are needed to confirm the benefits of sport participation in schizophrenia.

Tamarindus Indica

Tamarindus Indica Fruit Pulp Showed Significant Weight Reducing and Hypolipidemic Acitivity in Antipsychotic-induced Obese Rats

Jindal, Vaneeta, et al., "Hypolipidemic and Weight Reducing Activity of the Ethanolic Extract of Tamarindus Indica Fruit Pulp in Cafeteria Diet- and Sulpiride-Induced Obese Rats." *Journal of Pharmacology & Pharmacotherapeutics* 2, no. 2 (2011): 80–84. Publisher: Medknow Publications; doi:10.4103/0976-500X.81896., PMCID:PMC3127355

> ➢ "Thus, the ethanolic extract of Tamarindus indica fruit pulp showed a significant weight-reducing and hypolipidemic activity in cafeteria diet- and sulpiride-induced obese rats."

Vitamin D

Vitamin D May Be a Possible Candidate for Weight Loss from Second Generation Antipsychotics

Nwosu, Benjamin U., et al., "A Potential Role for Adjunctive Vitamin D Therapy in the Management of Weight Gain and Metabolic Side Effects of Second-Generation Antipsychotics." *Journal of Pediatric Endocrinology & Metabolism: JPEM* 24, no. 9–10 (2011): 619–26., Publisher: FREUND PUB. HOUSE, PMID: 22145446

> In summary, SGA medications are increasingly being prescribed to treat psychiatric illnesses in children and adolescents. However, the use of these agents is limited by their severe metabolic side effects. The mechanism(s) of these adverse events are unknown, and there is a lack of consensus on the best approach to address these problems. In conclusion, adjunctive vitamin D therapy may play a role in counteracting the adipogenic effects of SGA agents.

Diabetes Side Effect Treatments

Antipsychotic Withdrawal

Diabetes is Reversible in Some Cases after Antipsychotic Withdrawal

Dibben, C. R. M., et al., "Diabetes Associated with Atypical Antipsychotic Treatment May Be Severe but Reversible: Case Report." *International Journal of Psychiatry in Medicine* 35, no. 3 (2005): 307–11., PMID: 16480245

> Although the presentation of atypical neuroleptic-associated diabetes described here is not widely recognized, some of its elements have previously been documented in the literature. Thus, after reviewing 45 published reports, Jin et al. concluded that 42% of patients with atypical antipsychotic-associated diabetes developed DKA . They also noted that 50% manifested no weight gain during atypical antipsychotic treatment. Sobel et al. and Wilson et al. have also described improvement in diabetes in three patients to the point that insulin was no longer required. Our patients no longer require a hypoglycemic agent or adhere to a diabetic diet. It appears that their diabetes, although severe, was reversible on stopping the antipsychotic medication. All clinicians should be made aware of the need to monitor their patients on atypical antipsychotic agents for hyperglycemia. This article emphasizes the potential risks for such patients who may present for the first time in DKA and who do not follow the classical type 2 diabetes presentation. It also highlights the possibility of a complete recovery from diabetes in these patients once the offending neuroleptic is discontinued.

Berberine

Berberine is Superior to Metformin in the Management of Diabetes

Patil, Tatyasaheb, et al. "Is Berberine Superior to Metformin in Management of Diabetes Mellitus and Its Complications?" *International Journal of Pharmacognosy and Phytochemical Research.* 2105; 7(3);543-553

> Metformin is considered first line antidiabetic to treat diabetes mellitus type 2. Berberine has been used since many years as antidiabetic in Chinese herbal medicine. Regarding Glucose reducing capacity metformin and berberine share few common

pharmacological actions hence berberine could be called as herbal metformin. But berberine scores over metformin as an antidiabetic by certain additional pharmacological mechanism like alpha glucosidase enzyme inhibition, release of GLP 1, modification of gut microbiota, inhibition of enzyme dipeptidyl pepetidase 4 and as a insulin mimetic. Lipid lowering action and effect on polycystic ovarian disease is more superior in berberine than metformin. Cardiovascular protection, prevention of athesclerosis, survival in CHF, inhibition of arrhythmias and antiplatelet action are more profound with berberine as against metformin which needs to be used with lots of caution in diabetics with CHF as it might precipitate lactic acidosis. Minor beneficial effects of metformin on cardiovascular system may get nullified by metformin induced decrease in intestinal Vit B 12 absorption causing hyper homocystenemia and progression of atherosclerosis and endothelial dysfunction. Berberine has neuroprotective action in Alzhmiers and also has antidepressant property. But metformin when used alone without insulin deteriorates Alzhmiers. Though berberine and metformin share anticancer potential, metformin lacks antimicrobial property of berberine. Inhibition of aldose reductase and prevention of complication of diabetes mellitus arising out of accumulation of sorbitol like cataract formation diabetic neuropathy and nephropathy are only reduced by berberine. Berberine has nephroprotective action by different mechanism and also bears anti-urolithic potential. Thus it can be concluded that berberine can be considered to be superior to metformin in management of diabetes and in prevention of its complications.

Vitamin E

Vitamin E Restores Diabetic Schizophrenic Patients on Antipsychotics Circulation in Extremities

Antonio J. DeLiz, M.D., Ph.D., "Administration of Massive Doses of Vitamin E to Diabetic Schizophrenic Patients." *Journal of Orthomolecular Psychiatry*, 1975
http://www.orthomolecular.org/library/jom/1975/pdf/1975-v04n01-p085.pdf

> Dr. Shute states, "Gangrenous areas in the extremities of small size may often be salvaged by this agent (Alpha-Tocopherol or vitamin E) notably in diabetics... We have many colour photographs of such patients, patients who had been advised by the ablest surgeons to have amputation." Dr. Shute states, on the basis of clinical evidence, that the healing of these areas of gangrene by Alpha-Tocopherol was achieved by mobilizing collateral circulation and by locally improved tissue oxygenation. This news came to the author when this paper was already being edited. The author states, therefore, "My paper cannot claim the originality that I thought it could." (See Totgyes, S., and Shute, E.V.: The Summary, 6-48, 1954; Shute, Evan V., B.A., M.B.. F.R.C.S. [C] , F.R.S.M., Med., Se. D., Director of the Shute

CODEX ALTERNUS

Institute for Clinical and Laboratorial Medicine, London, Canada: Alpha-Tocopherol [Vitamin E] in Cardiovascular Disease. The Summary, p. 6, December, 1973.)

Zinc

Maternal Zinc Deficiency May Be the Cause of Diabetes in Some Schizophrenics

Andrews, R. C., et al., "Diabetes and Schizophrenia: Genes or Zinc Deficiency?" *Lancet (London, England)* 340, no. 8828 (November 7, 1992): 1160., PMID: 1359228

> ➤ Findings of Hales et al. strongly support the recent claim some cases of diabetes are caused by gestational zinc deficiency. They suggested that the association was caused by an unspecified maternal dietary deficiency and, on these grounds challenge the dogma of genetic control of twin concordance differences in diabetes. In both schizophrenia and non-insulin-dependent diabetes differences in concordance rates of monozygotic and dizygotic twins are regarded as evidence for genetic aetiology. If one accepts the arguments of Hales et al. that twin concordance differences can be explained by environmental factors acting antenatally or perinatially, then the notion of schizophrenia as a genetic disorder is equally open to challenge.

Polydipsia-Hyponatremia Side Effect Treatments

Behavioral Intervention

Behavioral Intervention for Polydipsia in Schizophrenia Incorporates Self-monintoring, Stimulus Control, Coping Skills Training and Reinforement Components

Costanzo, Erin S., et al., "Behavioral and Medical Treatment of Chronic Polydipsia in a Patient with Schizophrenia and Diabetes Insipidus." *Psychosomatic Medicine* 66, no. 2 (April 2004): 283–86., Publisher: American Psychomatic Society; PMID: 15039516

> ➤ The 12-session individual behavioral intervention incorporated self-monitoring, stimulus control, coping skills training, and reinforcement components. The patient engaged fully in the treatment program, and she successfully restricted her fluid intake. Her diabetes insipidus could therefore be treated with desmopressin, a medication that requires fluid restriction, and she experienced a concomitant reduction in polyuria and urinary incontinence. The outpatient behavioral intervention demonstrated promising outcomes in a chronically mentally ill patient whose polydipsia had underlying psychogenic and physiological components. This case highlights the efficacy of combining behavioral and medical interventions.

CODEX ALTERNUS

Biofeedback is Effective for the Treatment of Polydipsia in Schizophrenia

> **Waller, G.,** et al., "A 'Biofeedback' Approach to the Treatment of Chronic Polydipsia." *Journal of Behavior Therapy and Experimental Psychiatry* 24, no. 3 (September 1993): 255–59., Publisher: PERGAMON; PMID: 8188850

> ➤ "The patient showed substantially increased sodium concentration, which was maintained despite the withdrawal of feedback. This behavioral method appears promising in settings where restriction of fluid intake is not practical or ethical."

Behavioral Treatment of Polydipsia is Effecive in After Hospital Discharge

> **Bowen, L.,** et al., "Successful Behavioral Treatment of Polydipsia in a Schizophrenic Patient." *Journal of Behavior Therapy and Experimental Psychiatry* 21, no. 1 (March 1990): 53–61., Publisher: PERGAMON; PMID: 2372769

> ➤ Behavioral treatment of a 35 year old female with chronic schizophrenia and water intoxication with seizures was conducted on an inpatient psychiatric unit. Treatment included frequent daily weights, restricted fluid intake, positive reinforcement for program compliance, and time-out from reinforcement following significant weight gain or other specified program violations. The final 6 months of the 30 month treatment program were a maintenance phase during which most contingencies were faded and all fluid restrictions were removed. There was no reported recurrence of polydipsia after 18 months of community placement.

Behavioral Intervention to Reduce Water Intake Reduces Hyponatremia in Schizophrenic Patient

> **Pavalonis, D.,** et al., "Behavioral Intervention to Reduce Water Intake in the Syndrome of Psychosis, Intermittent Hyponatremia, and Polydipsia." *Journal of Behavior Therapy and Experimental Psychiatry* 23, no. 1 (March 1992): 51–57., Publisher: PERGAMON; PMID: 1430251

> ➤ We describe a non-intensive behavioral intervention using an A-B design with extended follow-up on an open psychiatric unit to reduce water intake in a 52-year-old man with the syndrome of psychosis, intermittent hyponatremia, and polydipsia. A reinforcement schedule contingent upon weight gain secondary to water intake was employed. Mean diurnal weight gain was 7.1 pounds during a 23-week baseline which dropped to 4.1 pounds following 23 weeks of treatment and at a 1-year follow-up. Estimated fluid consumption dropped from 10 liters to 4 liters daily and incidents of hyponatremia decreased by 62%.

CODEX ALTERNUS

Salt

Salt in the Management of Self-induced Water Intoxication of Schizophrenic Patients

Vieweg, W. V., et al., "Oral Sodium Chloride in the Management of Schizophrenic Patients with Self-Induced Water Intoxication." *The Journal of Clinical Psychiatry* 46, no. 1 (January 1985): 16–19., Publisher: PHYSICIANS POSTGRADUATE PRESS, INC; PMID: 3965438

> ➤ Hyponatremia is always present in patients with water intoxication and accounts for many of the life-threatening symptoms and signs found in this population. In schizophrenic patients, water restriction, a cornerstone in the treatment of water intoxication, may be impossible to implement over the course of long-term management. The use of oral sodium chloride administration in such patients and its short-term efficacy in preventing major motor seizures are described.

Sports Drink

Electrolyte-Balanced Sports Drink is Effective for Polydipsia-Hyponatremia in Schizophrenia

QUITKIN, FREDERIC M., et al., "Electrolyte-Balanced Sports Drink for Polydipsia-Hyponatremia in Schizophrenia." *American Journal of Psychiatry* 160, no. 2 (February 1, 2003): 385–a. Publisher: AM PSYCHIATRIC ASSN; doi:10.1176/appi.ajp.160.2.385-a., PMID: 12562594

> ➤ One month after discharge, Mr. A's sodium levels were still below normal (127 mmol/liter) and appeared to be life threatening. He did not understand the importance of limiting fluid intake. His elderly mother was unable to monitor his drinking. Mr. A's fluid intake was limited to an electrolyte-balanced sports drink. He took one 19-mg salt pill with each meal. In the past year, his sodium levels have been normal, there have been no seizures, and his mental status has improved. At the time this treatment was initiated, hyponatremia, coma, and death appeared possible. Use of previously recommended behavioral and pharmacological treatments were unsuccessful (1–4). While water restriction of a delusional polydipsic patient outside a hospital may not be feasible, an electrolyte-balanced solution may be lifesaving. This anecdotal observation requires replication. Of note is that this patient's mental status improved, as evidenced by enhanced orientation, with stabilized sodium levels.

Urea

Oral Urea Treatment is Partially Effective for Polydipsia-Hyponatermia Syndrome in Schizophrenic Patients

CODEX ALTERNUS

Kawai, Nobutoshi, et al., "Oral Urea Treatment for Polydipsia-Hyponatremia Syndrome in Patients with Schizophrenia." *Journal of Clinical Psychopharmacology* 29, no. 5 (October 2009): 499–501. Publisher: LIPPINCOTT WILLIAMS & WILKINS doi:10.1097/JCP.0b013e3181b3b38c., PMID: 19745654

> This study has some limitations. The study was designed as an open naturalistic trial without a control group. The sample size was small. The mean sodium concentration with the highest dosage used (67.5 g/d) was still below reference range, suggesting that oral urea treatment would not be an entire solution for PHS. We could not find significant difference between mean serum sodium concentrations with 45- and 67.5-g doses. The optimal urea dosage should be determined in future studies. Neverless, increased serum sodium levels not only in the morning but also in the afternoon in schizophrenic patients with PHS support the notion that the oral urea treatment possibly reduces the risk of severe hyponatremia. Further studies with larger sample sizes and longer-term protocols are required to evaluate beneficial effects and safety of oral urea treatment for schizophrenic patients with PHS.

Urea Appears to Be an Effective Therapeutic Approach for Polydisia-Hyponatermia Syndrome

Verhoeven, Anne, et al., "Treatment of the Polydipsia-Hyponatremia Syndrome with Urea." *The Journal of Clinical Psychiatry* 66, no. 11 (November 2005): 1372–75., Publisher: PHYSICIANS POSTGRADUATE PRESS, INC; PMID: 16420073

> "These preliminary data show that urea appears to be an effective therapeutic approach for the polydipsiahyponatremia syndrome."

Group Psychotherapy

Group Psychotherapy for Polydipsia Reduces Self-Induced Water Intoxication in Schizophrenic Patients

Millson, R. C., et al., "Self-Induced Water Intoxication Treated with Group Psychotherapy." *The American Journal of Psychiatry* 150, no. 5 (May 1993): 825–26., Publisher: AM PSYCHIATRIC ASSN; PMID: 8480834

> The authors conducted a controlled, prospective 4-month study of 10 male inpatients with chronic schizophrenia and polydipsia. The five men who were treated with group psychotherapy drank significantly less fluid than the five men not given this therapy. The effect of group psychotherapy quickly dissipated in the follow-up period, indicating the need for ongoing treatment.

CODEX ALTERNUS

Cardiac and Blood Disorder Side Effect Treatments

Aspirin

Aspirin appears to be the Molecule of Choice for Cardiovascular Disease Prevention in Bipolar Disorders

Fond, Guillaume, et al.,"Aspirin for Prevention of Cardiovascular Events in Bipolar Disorders." *Psychiatry Research* 219, no. 1 (September 30, 2014): 238–39. Publisher: ELSEVIER IRELAND LTD; doi:10.1016/j.psychres.2014.05.011., PMID: 24913832

> "The burden of CVD among patients with bipolar disorders is thus substantial. Aspirin appears as a molecule of choice to be tested in CVD prevention in bipolar disorders."

Aspirin is Doubly Helpful in Bipolar Disorder for Prevention of Cardiovascular Events

Fond, Guillaume, et al., "Recently Discovered Properties of Aspirin May Be Doubly Helpful in Bipolar Disorders." *Medical Hypotheses* 82, no. 5 (May 2014): 640–41. Publisher: CHURCHILL LIVINGSTONE; doi:10.1016/j.mehy.2014.02.028., PMID: 24650419

> "Aspirin may be doubly helpful in bipolar disorders, for prevention of cardiovascular events as well as an anti-inflammatory drug that may influence and protest the central nervous system."

B Vitamin and Omega 3

Correction of Omega-3 EFA Deficiency and B Vitamin Status Reduces the Risk of Cardiovascular Disease

Kemperman, R. F. J., et al., "Low Essential Fatty Acid and B-Vitamin Status in a Subgroup of Patients with Schizophrenia and Its Response to Dietary Supplementation." *Prostaglandins, Leukotrienes, and Essential Fatty Acids* 74, no. 2 (February 2006): 75–85. Publisher: CHURCHILL LIVINGSTONE; doi:10.1016/j.plefa.2005.11.004., PMID: 16384692

> We conclude that a subgroup of patients with schizophrenia has biochemical EFA deficiency, omega3/DHA marginality, moderate hyperhomocysteinemia, or combinations. Correction seems indicated in view of the possible relation of poor EFA and B-vitamin status with some of their psychiatric symptoms, but notably to reduce their high risk of cardiovascular disease.

CODEX ALTERNUS

Coenzyme Q10

Coenzyme Q10 is Protective for Neuroleptic-induced Cell Damage in Rat Myocardial Cells

> **Chiba, M.**, et al., "A Protective Action of Coenzyme Q10 on Chlorpromazine-Induced Cell Damage in the Cultured Rat Myocardial Cells." *Japanese Heart Journal* 25, no. 1 (January 1984): 127–37., Publisher: NANKODO CO. LTD. PMID: 6737696

> ➢ "These findings suggest that CoQ may protect myocardial cells from CPZ-induced injury, and that prostaglandins may play an important role in the action of CoQ."

Curcumin

Curcumin Could Be a Protective Agent for Thorazine-induced Heart Injury

> **Bashandy, Manar A.**, et al., "Cardiotoxic Effect of Chloropromazine in Adult Male Albino Rats and the Possible Curcumin Cardioprotection" *Journal of American Science* 2012; 8(8)

> ➢ Chlorpromazin causes myocardial damage in experimental rats. Curcumin could be used as protective agents against long term use of chlorpromazine to ameliorate damaging effects on myocardial muscles as it has positive contribution as a dietary supplement for the prevention of myocardial injury and heart disease.

Gamma-oryzanol

Gamma-oryzanol is Safe and Effective in the Treatment of Dyslipidemia in Schizophrenic Patients on Neuroleptics

> **Sasaki, J.**, et al., "Effects of Gamma-Oryzanol on Serum Lipids and Apolipoproteins in Dyslipidemic Schizophrenics Receiving Major Tranquilizers." *Clinical Therapeutics* 12, no. 3 (June 1990): 263–68., PMID: 1974170

> ➢ The subjects were 20 chronic schizophrenic patients with dyslipidemia (total cholesterol levels greater than or equal to 220 mg/dl, triglycerides greater than or equal to 150 mg/dl, or high-density lipoprotein cholesterol less than or equal to 40 mg/dl) who had been receiving neuroleptics for a mean of ten years. Each patient was given 100 mg of gamma-oryzanol three times daily for 16 weeks. Total cholesterol and low-density lipoprotein cholesterol levels, respectively, decreased significantly, from 204 and 124 mg/dl at baseline to 176 and 101 mg/dl at week 12. High-density lipoprotein cholesterol levels were 36.1 mg/dl at baseline and 35.9 mg/dl at week 12. Apolipoprotein (apo) B levels decreased significantly from 116 mg/dl to 101 mg/dl at week 16; apo A-II levels increased significantly from 31.7 mg/dl to 34.7 mg/dl; and the apo B/apo A-I ratio declined significantly from 0.99 to

CODEX ALTERNUS

0.84. No treatment side effects were recorded. It is concluded that gamma-oryzanol is safe and effective in the treatment of dyslipidemia.

Magnesium Sulphate and Potassium

Infusion of Epsom Salt, Potassium and Mellaril Discontinuation was Effective Management with Polymorphic Ventricular Tachycardia of torsade de piontes.

> **Sinkiewicz, Władysław,** et al., "[Polymorphic ventricular tachycardia of torsade de pointes type in patient with schizophrenia treated with thioridazine]." *Polskie Archiwum Medycyny Wewnętrznej* 116, no. 6 (December 2006): 1188–91., PMID: 18634530

> ➤ A case of 82 year-old female with schizophrenia treated with thioridazine with a long QT syndrome and polymorphic ventricular tachycardia of torsade de pointes type was presented. Additional predisposing factor for cardiac arrhythmia was diarrhea with subsequent hypokalemia. Infusion of magnesium sulphate, potassium supplementation and thioridazine discontinuation was effective management of the pathient.

Omega-3

Omega-3 Fatty Acids Have a Significant Reduction on Triglyceride Levels in Patients Using Clozapine

> **Caniato, Riccardo N.,** et al., "Effect of Omega-3 Fatty Acids on the Lipid Profile of Patients Taking Clozapine." *The Australian and New Zealand Journal of Psychiatry* 40, no. 8 (August 2006): 691–97. Publisher: BLACKWELL PUBLISHING ASIA; doi:10.1111/j.1440-1614.2006.01869.x., PMID: 16866765

> ➤ This study demonstrated high rates of lipid abnormalities in the participants. Participants taking omega-3 fatty acids demonstrated a statistically significant reduction in mean serum triglyceride levels of 22%. There was an associated increase in total cholesterol (6.6%) and low-density lipoprotein cholesterol (22%). Common side-effects included fishy burps or breath, but no serious side-effects or interactions where observed. Omega-3 fatty acids may be of value in patients taking clozapine and who have elevated serum triglyceride levels. Limitations of the study, practical implications and directions for future research are discussed.

CODEX ALTERNUS

Omega-3 Fatty Acids Decrease Fasting Insulin Levels in Patients on Zyprexa, Depakote or Lithium Combination

> **Toktam, Faghihi,** et al., "Effect of Early Intervention with Omega-3 on Insulin Resistance in Patients Initiated on Olanzapine with Either Sodium Valproate or Lithium: A Randomized, Double-Blind, Placebo-Controlled Trial." *Iranian Journal of Psychiatry* 5, no. 1 (2010): 18–22., Publisher: Psychiatry & Psychology Research Center, Tehran University of Medical Sciences; PMID: 22952485

> ➤ At the end of the study, no significant difference was observed between the two arms in terms of FBS, fasting insulin, HbA(1c) and HOMA-IR. However, trends toward decreasing both fasting insulin levels (p=0.06) and HOMA-IR (p=0.07) were noted in the group receiving omega-3. No significant changes in the outcome variables were observed from the baseline to the final measurements in both groups. This study noted that adding omega-3 fatty acids at the commencement of olanzapine combination therapy with valproate or lithium could not favorably influence glucose-insulin homeostasis. However, trends toward a decrease in insulin levels (p=0.06) and HOMA-IR (p=0.07) observed in patients receiving omega-3 suggest a possible beneficial role of this supplement.

Omega-3 Fatty Acids are Promising Treatments for Antipsychotic-induced Dyslipidemia

> **Pisano, Simone,** et al., "Antipsychotic-Induced Dyslipidemia Treated with Omega 3 Fatty Acid Supplement in an 11-Year-Old Psychotic Child: A 1-Year Follow-Up." *Journal of Child and Adolescent Psychopharmacology* 23, no. 2 (March 2013): 139–41. Publisher: MARY ANN/LIEBERT, INC. PUBLISHERS; doi:10.1089/cap.2012.0060., PMID: 23480323

> ➤ This case report represents the first example of treatment strategy of antipsychotic-induced dyslipidemia in children, on the basis of evidence that omega 3 is effective in the treatment of dyslipidemia in general medicine (Balk et al. 2006). Although considering all limitations of a single case report, the degree of reduction of TC, LDL, and TG, as well as the increase of HDL, the long period of follow-up and the stopping–reintroducing strategy provide some evidence of the direct effect of omega 3 supplement on metabolic changes. We have to highlight that non-significant changes of lifestyle or diet were reported by parents during the treatment. The data on weight need clarification. Weight seems to be independent of omega 3 supplement but we report a slight stabilization effect at beginning of treatment. On the basis of this report, a possible role of omega 3 fatty acid supplement in the treatment of antipsychotic-induced dyslipidemia could be hypothesized. We suggest that omega 3 supplement treatment, associated with physical exercise and balanced diet, could be a good strategy to moderate antipsychotic-induced dyslipidemia, and a short trial of this strategy can avoid sudden switches of antipsychotic drug. Our group is planning a trial to test the possible preventive role of omega 3 fatty acid

supplement in antipsychotic-induced metabolic syndrome in children and adolescents.

Omega-3 Fatty Acids Are Associated With Improvements in Triglyceride and HDL Cholesterol Levels in Patients Taking Atypical Antipsychotics

Fetter, Jeffrey Charles, et al., "N-3 Fatty Acids for Hypertriglyceridemia in Patients Taking Second-Generation Antipsychotics." *Clinical Schizophrenia & Related Psychoses* 7, no. 2 (2013): 73–77A. Publisher: WALSH MEDICAL MEDIA ; doi:10.3371/CSRP.FEBR.012513., PMID: 23367502

> ➢ In this pilot study, treatment with N-3 FA was associated with improvements in triglyceride and HDL levels. Further study is warranted to assess more completely whether this prescription dietary supplement can reduce triglycerides in patients taking second-generation antipsychotics.

Omega-3 Consumption and Supplementation May Protect Against Sudden Cardiac Death in Schizophrenia

Scorza, Fulvio A., et al., "Omega-3 Consumption and Sudden Cardiac Death in Schizophrenia." *Prostaglandins, Leukotrienes, and Essential Fatty Acids* 81, no. 4 (October 2009): 241–45. Publisher: CHURCHILL LIVINGSTONE; doi:10.1016/j.plefa.2009.06.008., PMID: 19628381

> ➢ As omega-3 fatty acids have been considered a cardioprotector agent, reducing cardiac arrhythmias and hence sudden cardiac deaths and given their relative safety and general health benefits, our update article summarizes the knowledge by the possible positive effects of omega-3 supplementation and fish consumption against sudden cardiac death in patients with schizophrenia. However, fish species should be selected with caution due to contamination with toxic methylmercury.

Omega-3 Fatty Acids for Hypertriglycerdemia in Patients Taking Second Generation Antipsychotics

Caniato, Riccardo N., et al., "Effect of Omega-3 Fatty Acids on the Lipid Profile of Patients Taking Clozapine." *The Australian and New Zealand Journal of Psychiatry* 40, no. 8 (August 2006): 691–97. Publisher: BLACKWELL PUBLISHING ASIA; doi:10.1111/j.1440-1614.2006.01869.x., PMID: 16866765

> ➢ Participants taking omega-3 fatty acids demonstrated a statistically significant reduction in mean serum triglyceride levels of 22%. There was an associated increase in total cholesterol (6'6%) and low-density lipoprotein cholesterol (22%). Common side-effects included fishy burps or breath, but no serious side effects or interactions were observed.Omega-3 fatty acids may be of value in patients taking clozapine and who have elevated serum triglyceride levels.

CODEX ALTERNUS

Potassium

Lithium Related Cardiac Events May Be Treatable By Potassium Chloride

Kast, R., et al., "Reversal of Lithium-Related Cardiac Repolarization Delay by Potassium." *Journal of Clinical Psychopharmacology* 10, no. 4 (August 1990): 304–5.; PMID: 2126792

> ➤ "Sinus node dysfunction and cardiac repolarization delays might also be lithium-related adverse effects treatable by oral potassium chloride."

Withania somnifera

Hypolipidemic and Hypoglycemic Actions of Withania somnifera for Treatment in Schizophrenia

Agnihotri, Akshay P., et al., "Effects of Withania Somnifera in Patients of Schizophrenia: A Randomized, Double Blind, Placebo Controlled Pilot Trial Study." *Indian Journal of Pharmacology* 45, no. 4 (August 2013): 417–18. Publisher: MEDKNOW PUBLICATIONS PVT LTD. doi:10.4103/0253-7613.115012., PMID: 24014929

> ➤ "No change in all three biochemical parameters was found after 1 month of treatment in the placebo group. However, a statistically significant (p<0.05) reduction in serum triglycerides and FBG was observed after 1 month of WS treatment compared to the placebo group."

Vitamin B

B Vitamin Therapy Causes a Decline in Symptoms of Schizophrenia and Homocysteine Levels to Decline

Levine, Joseph, et al., "Homocysteine-Reducing Strategies Improve Symptoms in Chronic Schizophrenic Patients with Hyperhomocysteinemia." *Biological Psychiatry* 60, no. 3 (August 1, 2006): 265–69. Publisher: ELSEVIER INC. doi:10.1016/j.biopsych.2005.10.009., PMID: 16412989

> ➤ Homocysteine levels declined with vitamin therapy compared with placebo in all patients except for one noncompliant subject. Clinical symptoms of schizophrenia as measured by the Positive and Negative Syndrome Scale declined significantly with active treatment compared with placebo. Neuropsychological test results overall, and Wisconsin Card Sort (Categories Completed) test results in particular, were significantly better after vitamin treatment than after placebo. A subgroup of schizophrenic patients with hyperhomocysteinemia might benefit from the simple addition of B vitamins.

CODEX ALTERNUS

High-dose Vitamin B6 Decreases Homocysteine Levels in Patients with Schizophrenia

> **Miodownik, Chanoch,** et al., "High-Dose Vitamin B6 Decreases Homocysteine Serum Levels in Patients with Schizophrenia and Schizoaffective Disorders: A Preliminary Study." *Clinical Neuropharmacology* 30, no. 1 (February 2007): 13–17. Publisher: LIPPINCOTT WILLIAMS & WILKINS; doi:10.1097/01.WNF.0000236770.38903.AF., PMID: 17272965

> ➤ Age was significantly positively correlated with Hcy levels at baseline (r = 0.392, P = 0.004). All other parameters, including diagnosis, disease duration, and pyridoxal-5-phosphate serum level, were not correlated with Hcy serum levels at baseline. After vitamin B6 treatment, Hcy serum levels significantly decreased (14.2 +/- 3.4 vs. 11.8 +/- 2.0 micromol/L, respectively, t = 2.679, P = 0.023); this decrease being statistically significant in men but not in women. High doses of vitamin B6 lead to a decrease in Hcy serum level in male patients with schizophrenia or schizoaffective disorder.

Vitamin D

Patients with Greater Vitamin D Levels have Significant Decrease in Total Cholesterol Levels

> **Thakurathi, Neelam,** et al., "Open-Label Pilot Study on Vitamin D$_3$ Supplementation for Antipsychotic-Associated Metabolic Anomalies." *International Clinical Psychopharmacology* 28, no. 5 (September 2013): 275–82. Publisher: LIPPINCOTT WILLIAMS & WILKINS; doi:10.1097/YIC.0b013e3283628f98., PMID: 23694999

> ➤ Previous studies have linked vitamin D deficiency to hypertension, dyslipidemia, diabetes mellitus, and cardiovascular disease. The aim of this study was to investigate the short-term effects of vitamin D$_3$ supplementation on weight and glucose and lipid metabolism in antipsychotic-treated patients. A total of 19 schizophrenic or schizoaffective patients (BMI>27 kg/m^2) taking atypical antipsychotics were recruited and dispensed a 2000 IU daily dose of vitamin D$_3$. On comparing baseline with week 8 (study end) results, we found a statistically significant increase in vitamin D$_3$ and total vitamin D levels but no statistically significant changes in weight, glucose, or lipids measurements. Patients whose vitamin D$_3$ level at week 8 was 30 ng/ml or more achieved a significantly greater decrease in total cholesterol levels compared with those whose week 8 vitamin D$_3$ measurement was less than 30 ng/ml. These results suggest that a randomized trial with a longer follow-up period would be helpful in further evaluating the effects of vitamin D$_3$ on weight, lipid metabolism, and on components of metabolic syndrome in antipsychotic-treated patients.

CODEX ALTERNUS

Drug-induced Sexual Dysfunction Treatments

Acupuncture

Acupuncture is Effective Treatment for Sexual Dysfunction Secondary to Antidepressants

Khamba, Baljit, et al., "Efficacy of Acupuncture Treatment of Sexual Dysfunction Secondary to Antidepressants." *Journal of Alternative and Complementary Medicine (New York, N.Y.)* 19, no. 11 (November 2013): 862–69. Publisher: REASONHOLD LTD doi:10.1089/acm.2012.0751., PMID: 23790229

> ➤ "This study suggests a potential role for acupuncture in the treatment of sexual side effects of SSRIs and SNRIs as well for a potential benefit of integrating medical and complementary and alternative practitioners."

Ginkgo Biloba

Prozac-Induced Genital Anesthesia Relieved by Ginkgo Biloba Extract

Ellison, J. M., et al., "Fluoxetine-Induced Genital Anesthesia Relieved by Ginkgo Biloba Extract." *The Journal of Clinical Psychiatry* 59, no. 4 (April 1998): 199–200., Publisher: PHYSICIANS POSTGRADUATE PRESS, INC. PMID: 9590676

> ➤ The improvement in this patient's genital anesthesia appears temporally associated with use of EGb, but this uncontrolled case report cannot refute with certainty the possibility that she improved spontaneously. Because antidepressant-induced sexual dysfunctions impair patients' quality of life and reduce compliance with treatment, more rigorously controlled double- blind investigation of EGb and other potential remedies for anti- depressant-induced sexual dysfunctions is desired.

Maca Root

Maca Root May Alleviate SSRI-induced Sexual Dysfunction

Dording, Christina M., et al., "A Double-Blind, Randomized, Pilot Dose-Finding Study of Maca Root (L. Meyenii) for the Management of SSRI-Induced Sexual Dysfunction." *CNS Neuroscience & Therapeutics* 14, no. 3 (2008): 182–91. Publisher: BLACKWELL PUBLISHING; doi:10.1111/j.1755-5949.2008.00052.x., PMID: 18801111

> ➤ "Maca was well tolerated. Maca root may alleviate SSRI-induced sexual dysfunction, and there may be a dose-related effect. Maca may also have a beneficial effect on libido."

CODEX ALTERNUS

Saffron

Saffron is Efficacious Treatment for Prozac Related Erectile Dysfunction

Modabbernia, Amirhossein, et al., "Effect of Saffron on Fluoxetine-Induced Sexual Impairment in Men: Randomized Double-Blind Placebo-Controlled Trial." *Psychopharmacology* 223, no. 4 (October 2012): 381–88. Publisher: SPRINGER-VERLAG doi:10.1007/s00213-012-2729-6., PMID: 22552758

> Nine patients (60%) in the saffron group and one patient (7%) in the placebo group achieved normal erectile function (score > 25 on erectile function domain) at the end of the study (P value of Fisher's exact test = 0.005). Frequency of side effects were similar between the two groups. Saffron is a tolerable and efficacious treatment for fluoxetine-related erectile dysfunction.

Saikokaryukotsuboreito

Saikokaryukotsuboreito Herbal Medicine is Effective for Antipsychotic Induced Sexual Dysfunction in Men

Takashi, Tsuboi, et al., "Effectiveness of Saikokaryukotsuboreito (herbal Medicine) for Antipsychotic-Induced Sexual Dysfunction in Male Patients with Schizophrenia: A Description of Two Cases." *Case Reports in Psychiatry* 2014 (2014): 784671. Publisher: Hindawi Publishimg Corporation; doi:10.1155/2014/784671., PMID: 24587934

> Antipsychotics sometimes cause sexual dysfunction in people with schizophrenia. The authors report the effectiveness of Saikokaryukotsuboreito (Japanese traditional herbal medicine, Chai-Hu-Jia-Long-Gu-Mu-Li-Tang in Chinese) for antipsychotic-induced sexual dysfunction in two male patients with schizophrenia. The first patient was a 28-year-old man with schizophrenia who suffered erectile dysfunction induced by olanzapine 10 mg/day; the erectile dysfunction significantly improved following the treatment of Saikokaryukotsuboreito 7.5 g/day. The other case was a 43-year-old man with schizophrenia who was receiving fluphenazine decanoate at 50 mg/month and had difficulties in ejaculation; add-on of Saikokaryukotsuboreito 7.5 g/day recovered his ejaculatory function. There has been no report on the effectiveness of Japanese herbal medicine formulations for antipsychotic-induced sexual dysfunction. Although the effectiveness of Saikokaryukotsuboreito needs to be tested in systematic clinical trials, this herbal medicine may be a treatment option to consider for this annoying side effect.

CODEX ALTERNUS

Hypersalvation Side Effect Treatments

Suoquan Pill

Suoquan Pill May Be Effective for Reducing Clozapine-induced Salvation

Kang, B., et al., "[Effect of suo quan pill for reducing clozapine induced salivation]." *Zhongguo Zhong Xi Yi Jie He Za Zhi Zhongguo Zhongxiyi Jiehe Zazhi = Chinese Journal of Integrated Traditional and Western Medicine / Zhongguo Zhong Xi Yi Jie He Xue Hui, Zhongguo Zhong Yi Yan Jiu Yuan Zhu Ban* 13, no. 6 (June 1993): 347–48, 325., Publisher: Chinese Association of the Integration of Traditional and Western Medicine; PMID: 8257839

> "There was a significant difference in effect on salvation between the therapeutic group (21 cases) and the controlled group (19 cases), P<0.01."

Wuling Powder

Suoquan Pill and Wuling Powder May Be Natural Treatments for Hypersalivation in Schizophrenia

Hung, Chia-Chun, et al., "Treatment Effects of Traditional Chinese Medicines Suoquan Pill and Wuling Powder on Clozapine-Induced Hypersalivation in Patients with Schizophrenia: Study Protocol of a Randomized, Placebo-Controlled Trial." *Zhong Xi Yi Jie He Xue Bao = Journal of Chinese Integrative Medicine* 9, no. 5 (May 2011): 495–502., Publisher: SPRINGER-VERLAG BERLIN-HEIDELBERG; PMID: 21565135

> "It is hypothesized that SQP and WLP will have a beneficial effect in controlling clonzapine-induced hypersalivation symptoms."

Urinary Incontinence Side Effect Treatments

Ephedrine

Ephedrine is a Safe and Effective Treatment for Clozapine-Associated Urinary Incontinence

Fuller, M. A., et al., "Clozapine-Induced Urinary Incontinence: Incidence and Treatment with Ephedrine." *The Journal of Clinical Psychiatry* 57, no. 11 (November 1996): 514–18., PMID: 8968299

> "Ephedrine appears to be a safe and effective treatment clozapine-associated UI. By inference, it is likely that clozapine may cause UI via its anti-alpha-adrenergic properties."

CODEX ALTERNUS

Metabolic Syndrome Side Effect Treatments

DHEA

DHEA is Effective at Maintaining Body Mass Index and Waist Circumference Compared to Monotherapy and Decreased Glucose Levels

Holka-Pokorska, J.A., et al., "The Stabilizing Effect of Dehydroepiandrosterone on Clinical Parameters of Metabolic Syndrome in Patients with Schizophrenia Treated with Olanzapine - a Randomized, Double-Blind Trial." *Psychiatria Polska* 49, no. 2 (2015): 363–76. doi:10.12740/PP/30180., PMID: 26093599

> ➢ It resulted in a statistically significant decrease in the fasting blood glucose level. It resulted in stabilization of anthropometric parameters related to the diagnosis of metabolic syndrome, i.e. waist circumference and BMI (the parameters remained constant in the DHEA subgroup though they increased in the placebo subgroup).

Diet and Exercise

Healthy Diet and Exercise are Interventions for Metabolic Syndrome in Bipolar Disorder Treated with Atypical Antipsychotics

Bell, Paul F., et al., "Treatment of Bipolar Disorders and Metabolic Syndrome: Implications for Primary Care." *Postgraduate Medicine* 121, no. 5 (September 2009): 140–44. Publisher: JTE Multimedia Company; doi:10.3810/pgm.2009.09.2060., PMID: 19820282

> ➢ Recognition of the prevalence of mood disorders and increased availability of medication options have led to calls for treating bipolar disorders in the primary care setting. Second-generation antipsychotic medications (SGAs) were initially lauded for treating bipolar disorders because of their efficacy and perceived safety relative to first-generation antipsychotic medications. Metabolic syndrome is a constellation of risk factors for cardiovascular disease and type 2 diabetes mellitus, which may emerge when treating bipolar disorders with SGAs. We conducted a search of the research literature examining the association between different SGAs and metabolic syndrome. Based on our review, we offer guidelines for monitoring patient status regarding metabolic syndrome and for providing interventions to promote healthy diet and exercise.

Healthy Eating and Physical Activity Communicated in Writing and Verbally with Social Support and Lifestyle Changes May Prevent the Development of Metabolic Syndrome in Psychotic Disorders

Bergqvist, Anette, et al., "Preventing the Development of Metabolic Syndrome in People with Psychotic Disorders--Difficult, but Possible: Experiences of Staff Working in Psychosis Outpatient Care in Sweden." *Issues in Mental Health Nursing* 34, no. 5 (May 2013): 350–58. Publisher: TAYLOR & FRANCIS INC. doi:10.3109/01612840.2013.771234.; PMID: 23663022

> ➢ Nursing interventions focusing on organising daily routines before conducting a more active prevention of metabolic syndrome, including information and practical support, were experienced as necessary. The importance of healthy eating and physical activity needs to be communicated in such a way that it is adjusted to the person's cognitive ability, and should be repeated over time, both verbally and in writing. Such efforts, in combination with empathic and seriously committed community-based social support, were experienced as having the best effect over time. Permanent lifestyle changes were experienced as having to be carried out on the patient's terms and in his or her home environment.

Melatonin

Melatonin Decreases Rise in Cholesterol and Systolic Blood Pressure in Bipolar Children

Mostafavi, Ali, et al., "Melatonin Decreases Olanzapine Induced Metabolic Side-Effects in Adolescents with Bipolar Disorder: A Randomized Double-Blind Placebo-Controlled Trial." *Acta Medica Iranica* 52, no. 10 (October 2014): 734–39., Publisher: Tehran University of Medical Sciences, the Faculty of Medicine; PMID: 25369006

> ➢ Administration of melatonin along with olanzapine and lithium carbonate could significantly inhibit the rise in cholesterol level and SBP compared to placebo. The effect of melatonin on TG was more obvious in boys. Melatonin was more effective in prevention of SBP rise.

Melatonin is Effective and Attenuates Antipsychotics Adverse Metabolic Effects in Bipolar Disorder

Romo-Nava, Francisco, et al., "Melatonin Attenuates Antipsychotic Metabolic Effects: An Eight-Week Randomized, Double-Blind, Parallel-Group, Placebo-Controlled Clinical Trial." *Bipolar Disorders* 16, no. 4 (June 2014): 410–21. Publisher: BLACKWELL MUNKSGAARD; doi:10.1111/bdi.12196., PMID: 24636483

> ➢ Our results show that melatonin is effective in attenuating SGAs' adverse metabolic effects, particularly in bipolar disorder. The clinical findings allow us to propose that SGAs may disturb a centrally mediated metabolic balance that causes adverse

metabolic effects and that nightly administration of melatonin helps to restore. Melatonin could become a safe and cost-effective therapeutic option to attenuate or prevent SGA metabolic effects.

Saffron

Saffron Extract Prevents Metabolic Syndrome in Patients with Schizophrenia

Fadai, F., et al., "Saffron Aqueous Extract Prevents Metabolic Syndrome in Patients with Schizophrenia on Olanzapine Treatment: A Randomized Triple Blind Placebo Controlled Study." *Pharmacopsychiatry* 47, no. 4–5 (July 2014): 156–61. Publisher: GEORG/THIEME VERLAG; doi:10.1055/s-0034-1382001.. PMID: 24955550

➤ "SAE could prevent metabolic syndrome compared to crocin and placebo. Furthermore, both SAE and crocin prevented increases in blood glucose during the study."

Vitamin D

Vitamin D Supplementation Can Alleviate Antipsychotic-induced Metabolic Disturbances in Vitamin D Deficient States

Dang, Ruili, et al., "Vitamin D Deficiency Exacerbates Atypical Antipsychotic-Induced Metabolic Side Effects in Rats: Involvement of the INSIG/SREBP Pathway." *European Neuropsychopharmacology: The Journal of the European College of Neuropsychopharmacology*, May 9, 2015. doi:10.1016/j.euroneuro.2015.04.028.

➤ Thus, the present study aimed to evaluate the effects of VD deficiency and VD supplementation on antipsychotic-induced metabolic changes in rats. After 4-week administration, clozapine (10mg/kg/d) and risperidone (1mg/kg/d) both caused glucose intolerance and insulin resistance in VD deficient rats, but not in rats with sufficient VD status. Antipsychotic treatments, especially clozapine, elevated serum lipid levels, which were most apparent in VD deficient rats, but alleviated in VD-supplemented rats. Additionally, antipsychotic treatments down-regulated INSIGs and up-regulated SREBPs expression in VD deficient rats, and these effects were attenuated when VD status was more sufficient. Collectively, this study disclose the novel findings that antipsychotic-induced metabolic disturbances is exacerbated by VD deficiency and can be alleviated by VD supplementation, providing new evidence for the promising role of VD in prevention and treatment of metabolic disorders caused by antipsychotic medications. Furthermore, our data also suggest the involvement of INSIG/SREBP pathway in the antipsychotic-induced hyperlipidemia and beneficial effects of VD on lipid profile.

CODEX ALTERNUS

Hyperprolactinemia and Amenorrhea Side Effect Treatments

Peony-Glycyrrhiza

Peony-Glycyrrhiza Decoction May Be a Natural Treatment for Hyperprolactinemia in Schizophrenia

Yuan, Hai-Ning, et al., "A Randomized, Crossover Comparison of Herbal Medicine and Bromocriptine against Risperidone-Induced Hyperprolactinemia in Patients with Schizophrenia." *Journal of Clinical Psychopharmacology* 28, no. 3 (June 2008): 264–370. Publisher: LIPPINCOTT WILLIAMS & WILKINS; doi:10.1097/JCP.0b013e318172473c., PMID: 18480682

> "Peony-Glycyrrhiza Decoction treatment produced a significant baseline-endpoint decrease in serum PRL levels, without exacerbating psychosis and changing other hormones, and decreased the amplitudes were similar to those of BMT (24% vs 21%-38%)."

> "These results suggest that herbal therapy can yield additional benefits while having comparable efficacy in treating antipsychotic-induced hyperprolactinemia in individuals with schizophrenia."

Shakuyaku-kanzo-to

Shakuyaku-kanzo-to is Effective for Treatment of Neuroleptic-induced Hyperprolactinemia

Yamanda K. , et al.,"Effectiveness of Herbal Medicine (Shakuyaku-kanzo-to) for Neuroleptic_Induced Hyperprolactinemia." *J Clin Psychopharmacol* Vol 17/No 3 June 1997, Publisher: LIPPINCOTT WILLIAMS & WILKINS

> There were statistically significant changes in p-PRL levels from 26.6 (SD 10.8) ng/mL at baseline to 20.8 (SD 11.2) mg/mL at 4 weeks and 24.0 (SD 11.4) ng/mL at 8 weeks (F=8.408, df=2,38,p= 0.0009). Post hoc analysis demonstrated statistically significant differences between p-PRL levels at 4 and 8 weeks (p< 0.01) and between p-PRL levels at 4 and 8 weeks (p<0.05). Plasma PRL levels at 8 weeks were not significantly different from those at baseline. In five patients, the p-PRL levels decreased by more than 50% with TJ-68 treatment. Three of 10 patients, who had complained of reduced sexual desire, experienced subjective improvement. Potassium levels and other laboratory data showed no significant changes with TJ-68 administration. Neither exacerbation of psychosis nor other adverse effects occurred.

CODEX ALTERNUS

Hori, Hikaru, et al., "Herbal Medicine (Shakuyaku-Kanzo-To) Improves Olanzapine-Associated Hyperprolactinemia: A Case Report." *Journal of Clinical Psychopharmacology* 33, no. 1 (February 2013): 122–23. Publisher: LIPPINCOTT WILLIAMS & WILKINS doi:10.1097/01.jcp.0000426177.36207.da., PMID: 23288231

> ➢ "In conclusion, shakuyaku-kanzo-to might be useful for treating amenorrhea without worsening psychotic symptoms in patients with schizophrenia."

Shakuyaku-kanzo-to is Effective in Correcting Neuroleptic-induced Amenorrhea

Yamanda K., et al., "Herbal Medicine (Shakuyaku-kanzo-to) in the Treatment of Risperidone-induced Amenorrhea." *J Clin Psychopharmacol*, Vol. 19/No.1 August 1999, Publisher: LIPPINCOTT WILLIAMS & WILKINS

> ➢ This report demonstrates TJ-68 to be effective in correcting neuroleptic-induced amenorrhea and hyperprolactinemia. Addition of TJ-68 lowered the p-PRL level from 22 to 9.5ng/mL, and menstruation recovered after 3 weeks of administration. Discontinuation of this compound resulted in the return of irregularity of menstruation and hyperprolactinemia.

Tongdatang

Tongdatang Serial Recipe May Be an Effective Natural Treatment of Antipsychotic-induced Glactorrhea-Amenorrhea Syndrome

Ding, Ying, et al., "[Effect of Tongdatang Serial Recipe on antipsychotic drug-induced galactorrhea-amenorrhea syndrome]." *Zhongguo Zhong Xi Yi Jie He Za Zhi Zhongguo Zhongxiyi Jiehe Zazhi = Chinese Journal of Integrated Traditional and Western Medicine / Zhongguo Zhong Xi Yi Jie He Xue Hui, Zhongguo Zhong Yi Yan Jiu Yuan Zhu Ban* 28, no. 3 (March 2008): 263–65., Publisher: Chinese Association of the Integration of Traditional and Western Medicine; PMID: 18476433

> ➢ Therapeutic efficacy on the 49 patients of the treatment group was cured in 31 (63.3%), markedly effective in 11 (22.4%), effective in 4 (8.2%) and ineffective in 3 (6.1%), with a total effective rate of 93.9%, while in 47 patients of the control group, the corresponding cases (%) was 0, 3(6.4%), 7(14.9%) and 37 (78.7%), respectively, with the total effective rate of 21.3%.

Vitamin C

Vitamin C May Obviate the Negative Effects of Neuroleptics Have on Menstruation

Kanofsky, J. D., et al., "Ascorbic Acid Action in Neuroleptic-Associated Amenorrhea." *Journal of Clinical Psychopharmacology* 9, no. 5 (October 1989): 388–89., Publisher: LIPPINCOTT WILLIAMS & WILKINS; PMID: 2571621

> The above cases suggest that ascorbic acid at the dose of 2 g orally three times a day may obviate the negative effect neuroleptics can have on menstruation. Given, the wide array of suggestive evidence, we believe that ascorbic acid supplementation should be systematically studied in women who are amenorrheic secondary to neuroleptic use.

Gastrointestinal Disorder Side Effect Treatments

Acidophilus

Acidophilus is Effective for Zoloft-induced Diarrhea

Kline, M. D., et al., "Acidophilus for Sertraline-Induced Diarrhea." *The American Journal of Psychiatry* 151, no. 10 (October 1994): 1521–22., Publisher: AM PSYCHIATRIC ASSN; PMID: 8092348

> The mechanism by which selective serotonin reuptake inhibitor antidepressants cause gastrointestinal side effects, including· diarrhea, is unknown. Orally administered Lactobacillus acidophilus has· been reported to he helpful for maldigestion secondary to lactose intolerance and also helpful for symptoms of irritable bowel syndrome (2). Orally administered acidophilus can ·apparently survive gastric acidity and alter intestinal flora and has been reported to inhibit same enteropathogens (3). Live acidophilus is available in capsule and tablet form in health food stores; both patients reported here took acidophil us capsules labeled to contain 500 million ·organisms per capsule. An open trial is planned to confirm the potential benefits of acidophilus for diarrhea induced by selective serotonin reuptake inhibitors.

Dai-kenchu-to

Herbal Dai-kenchu-to Treatment Improves Antipsychotic –induced Hypoperistalsis

Satoh, Kazuko, et al., "Effect of Dai-Kenchu-to (Da-Jian-Zhong-Tang) on the Delayed Intestinal Propulsion Induced by Chlorpromazine in Mice." *Journal of Ethnopharmacology* 86, no. 1 (May 2003): 37–44., Publisher: ELSEVIER IRELAND LTD; PMID: 12686439

> "These results demonstrated that Dai-kenchu-to improves chlorpromazine-induced hypoperistalsis via cholinergic systems and that Zanthoxylum Fruit is the main contributor to this action of Dai-kenchu-to."

Gorei-san

Gorei-san Herbal Treatment May Be Effective for SSRI-induced Nausea and Dyspepsia

CODEX ALTERNUS

Yamada K., et al., "Herbal Medicine in the Treatment of Fluvoxamine-induced Nausea and Dyspepsia." *Psychiatry and Clinical Neurosciences* (1999), 53, 681, Publisher: BLACKWELL PUBLISHING ASIA

> ➢ In summary, our results suggest that a herbal medicine, Gorei-san, may be effective for fluvoxamine-induced nausea and dyspepsia, without severe adverse events. Further studies are needed to confirm our results."

Yamada K., et al., "Effectiveness of Gorei-san (TJ-17) for the Treatment of SSRI-induced Nausea and Dyspepsia: Preliminary Observations." *Clin Neuropharmacol* 2003 May-Jun;26(3):112-4, Publisher: LIPPINCOTT WILLIAMS & WILKINS

> ➢ Gorei-san (TJ-17), which is composed of five herbs (Alismatis rhizome, Atractylodis lanceae rhizome, Polyporus, Hoelen, and Cinnamomi cortex), is a Japenses herbal medicine that has been used to treat nausea, dry mouth, edema, headache, and dizziness. The authors investigated the efficiency of TJ-17 for patients who experienced nausea or dyspepsia induced by SSRIs. Twenty outpatients who experienced nausea or dyspepsia induced by SSRIs were recruited for the study. Seventeen patients were female, three were male, and patient age ranged from 21 to 74 years (49.8 +/- 17.0 years). TJ-17 was added to the previous regimen. Nausea and dyspepsia disappeared completely in nine patients, decreased in four patients, decreased slightly in two, and did not change in five patients. No adverse events were associated with the addition of TJ-17 in any patient.

Probiotics

Probiotic Supplementation May Prevent Somatic Symptoms Associated with Schizophrenia

Dickerson, Faith B., et al., "Effect of Probiotic Supplementation on Schizophrenia Symptoms and Association with Gastrointestinal Functioning: A Randomized, Placebo-Controlled Trial." *The Primary Care Companion to CNS Disorders* 16, no. 1 (2014). Publisher: Physicians Postgraduate Press; doi:10.4088/PCC.13m01579., PMID: 24940526

> ➢ Repeated-measures analysis of variance showed no significant differences in the PANSS total score between probiotic and placebo supplementation (F = 1.28, P = .25). However, patients in the probiotic group were less likely to develop severe bowel difficulty over the course of the trial (hazard ratio = 0.23; 95% CI, 0.09-0.61, P = .003). Conclusions: Probiotic supplementation may help prevent a common somatic symptom associated with schizophrenia.

Rikkunshi

Herbal Rikkunshi Treatment Reduces Nausea and Vomiting Associated with SSRIs

CODEX ALTERNUS

Oka, Takakazu, et al., "Rikkunshi-to Attenuates Adverse Gastrointestinal Symptoms Induced by Fluvoxamine." *BioPsychoSocial Medicine* 1 (2007): 21. Publisher: BIOMED CENTRAL LTD. doi:10.1186/1751-0759-1-21., PMID: 18001480

> "This study suggests that Rikkunshi-to reduces FLV-induced adverse events, especially nausea, and improves QOL related to GI symptoms without affecting the antidepressant effect of FLV."

Lithium Side Effect Treatments

Aspirin

Aspirin Reduces Clinical Deterioration in Subjects on Lithium

Stolk, Pieter , et al., "Is Aspirin Useful in Patients on Lithium? A Pharmacoepidemiological Study Related to Bipolar Disorder." *Prostaglandins, Leukotrienes, and Essential Fatty Acids* 82, no. 1 (January 2010): 9–14. Publisher: CHURCHILL LIVINGSTONE doi:10.1016/j.plefa.2009.10.007., PMID: 19939659

> "Low dose aspirin produced a statistically significant duration-independent reduction in relative risk of clinical deterioration in subjects on lithium, whereas other NSAIDs and glucocorticoids did not."

Aspirin for Treatment of Lithium-associated Sexual Dysfunction in Men

Saroukhani, Sepideh, et al., "Aspirin for Treatment of Lithium-Associated Sexual Dysfunction in Men: Randomized Double-Blind Placebo-Controlled Study." *Bipolar Disorders* 15, no. 6 (September 2013): 650–56. Publisher: BLACKWELL MUNKSGAARD doi:10.1111/bdi.12108., PMID: 23924261

> By week 6, patients in the aspirin group showed significantly greater improvement in the total (63.9% improvement from baseline) and erectile function domain (85.4% improvement from baseline) scores than the placebo group (14.4% and 19.7% improvement from baseline, p-values=0.002 and 0.001, respectively). By week 6, 12 (80%) patients in aspirin group and three (20%) patients in placebo group met the criteria of minimal clinically important change [x(2) (1)=10.800, p=0.001]. Other IIEF domains also showed significant improvement at end of trial.

Food

Administration of Food with Lithium Reduces Side Effects

Jeppsson, J., et al.,"The Influence of Food on Side Effects and Absorption of Lithium." *Acta Psychiatrica Scandinavica* 51, no. 4 (May 1975): 285–88., PMID: 1096537

> From this investigation, it may be concluded that food does not impair the absorption of lithium from this type of tablet. Administration on an empty stomach may give purgative side effects, and the resultant rapid passage through the intestine may lead to reduced absorption. On the basis of these results, we recommend that lithium tablets of slow relase type be administered with meals.

Potassium

Supplementary Potassium Intake May be of Benefit to Lithium-treated Patients

Unknown Author, "Effects of Potassium Against the Toxicity of Lithium" *Danish Medical Bulletin*, Volume 31, No.4, August 1984

> The influence of dietary potassium content on some toxic actions of lithium in rats given lithium in the food for prolonged time has been studied. A high potassium intake diminished gastrointestinal disturbances and growth retardation. The impaired ability of the kidneys to retain sodium and water and to secrete potassium and hydrogen ion was improved. The lithium-induced epithelial and enzyme histochemical changes of the distal convoluted tubules and cortical and medullary collecting ducts were diminished. The mechanisms underlying these effects of potassium are unknown, but presumably they are not due to replacement of a lithium-induced potassium depletion. Measurements of lithium clearance in awake unoperated animals indicate that high potassium intake increases the fractional delivery of tubular fluid to the distal parts of the nephron and increases the reabsorption of sodium and water in the distal tubules. Some effects similar to those of potassium could also be found in rats given other natriuretic drugs; this indicates that some of the effects of potassium are not due to specific interactions between potassium and lithium. The results indicate that a supplementary potassium intake may be part of the benefit to lithium-treated patients.

Sodium and Potassium

Using Both Sodium and Potassium is Suggested to Maintain Therapeutic Effectiveness and Reduce Toxicity of Lithium

Cater, R. E. "The Use of Sodium and Potassium to Reduce Toxicity and Toxic Side Effects from Lithium." *Medical Hypotheses* 20, no. 4 (August 1986): 359–83; PMID: 3639285

> Studies in rats find that animals develop toxic side effects at serum levels which are therapeutic for man. Most of the toxic effects were prevented by feeding sodium and

potassium. The rats must ingest and excrete comparatively higher amounts of lithium than humans to maintain these levels. Sodium used alone has been shown to reduce side effects in man, but was found to reduce therapeutic effectiveness at fixed lithium dosages. Evidence is presented to suggest that therapeutic effectiveness can be maintained and toxicity reduced, by using both sodium and potassium, and by modestly raising the dosage of lithium.

Essential Fatty Acids

Safflower Oil, or Evening Promise Oil Combined with Vitamins C, B6, and Zinc May be an Effective way to Treat Lithium-Induced Tremor

Lieb, J., et al., "Treatment of Lithium-Induced Tremor and Familial Essential Tremor with Essential Fatty Acids." *Progress in Lipid Research* 20 (1981): 535–37; PMID: 7394066

> ➢ Irrespective of whether the underlying theory is correct, there can be no dout that the treatment with essential fatty acids is successful in controlling tremors caused by lithium, alcohol withdrawal and familial essential tremor. In about half of the patients, the resolution of tremor is complete and in about half, it is substantial but not complete. Other nutritional factors include vitamin C, pryridoxine and zinc. We are currently exploring the possibility that adding these nutrients to the essential fatty acids may enhance the effectiveness of the therapy.

Caffeine Intake

Caffeine Intake May Have a Paradoxical Response in Some Patients, In Some Cases Caffeine May Steady the Nerves for Patients on Lithium

Jefferson, J. W. "Lithium Tremor and Caffeine Intake: Two Cases of Drinking Less and Shaking More." *The Journal of Clinical Psychiatry* 49, no. 2 (February 1988): 72–73; PMID: 3338980

> ➢ Most patients troubled by lithium tremor will find caffeine reduction beneficial, but some patients may experience a paradoxical response, especially if their caffeine intake was quite high when they were stabilized on therapeutic doses of lithium. In such cases, patients may find that resumption of coffee intake might actually steady the nerves. However, the more sensible treatment approach would be to continue with little or no caffeine intake and reduce lithium dosage with little of no caffeine intake and reduce lithium dosage accordidly to reestablish an appropriate therapeutic serum level.

Vitamin B6

Vitamin B6 Shows Impressive Improvement for Lithium-induced Tremor

CODEX ALTERNUS

> **Miodownik, Chanoch**, et al., "Lithium-Induced Tremor Treated with Vitamin B6: A Preliminary Case Series." *International Journal of Psychiatry in Medicine* 32, no. 1 (2002): 103–8., Publisher: BAYWOOD PUBLISHING CO., INC. PMID: 12075913

> ➢ After the addition of vitamin B6 to their treatment, according to their SAS scores four patients showed impressive improvement until total disappearance of their tremor. The subjective scale, on which the patients scored their impression of clinical improvement, showed similar results.

Table Salt

Salt Supplements Reduce the Side-effects of Lithium Treatment

> **Bleiweiss, H.**, et al., "Salts Supplements with Lithium." *Lancet* 1, no. 7643 (February 21, 1970): 416., Publisher: LANCET PUBLISHING GROUP; PMID: 4189720

> ➢ Unintentionally, two experiments were performed. One woman, had been doing very well on the above combination, discontinued the salt supplement while remaining on the maintenance dose of lithium carbonate. 4 weeks later she became nauseated and dizzy and complained of strange ill-defined feelings and general weakness shortly after taking each dose. A second patient was started on lithium carbonate without salt supplements and had similar symptoms 1 ½ weeks after treatment was started. These side-effects disappeared when sodium chloride supplements were started. We conclude that sodium chloride supplements may diminish the side effects frequently reported with lithium carbonate treatment. Further investigations are indicated.

> ➢ "Treatment initially consisted of 600mg. lithium carbonate thrice daily, and the dose was gradually increased to up to 2.7 g daily, together with sodium chloride, 0.5−1.0 g thrice daily. Peak plasma-lithium levels ranged from 0.55 to 1.03 meq. Per litre. "

Table Salt May Prevent Lithium Toxicity and Mania in Patients on a Low Sodium Diet

> **Burton, H. B.** "Do You Use Salt?" *The American Journal of Psychiatry* 128, no. 2 (August 1971): 238–39., PMID: 5112958

> ➢ Case report of a patient on a low sodium diet who became manic from lithium toxicity and responded to the addition of non-iodized table salt added to her diet on a daily basis. The author recommended all patients on lithium use salt to reduce spikes increases in plasma levels of lithium.

CODEX ALTERNUS

Inositol

Inositol was Effective Monotherapy for Both Bipolar Symptoms and Psoriasis in this Woman's Case

Kontoangelos, Konstantinos, et al., "Administration of Inositol to a Patient with Bipolar Disorder and Psoriasis: A Case Report." *Cases Journal* 3 (2010): 69. doi:10.1186/1757-1626-3-69., PMID: 20178574

> ➢ A 62-year-old female Caucasian patient suffering from bipolar disorder, since the age of 32, presenting manic episodes when without lithium treatment. Lithium treatment caused severe exacerbation of psoriasis and was discontinued while anti-psoriatic treatment had no effect. The last 4 years the patient receives 3 gr per day of inositol alone and her mood has been stabilized while there is also a remarkable improvement on her psoriatic lesions. Taking into consideration the course of her bipolar disorder when lithium was discontinued previously we consider that the 4 years of follow up assessments of this patient as a satisfactory time period for concluding that inositol has been a very effective treatment, replacing lithium, for mood stabilization and psoriasis.

Inositol has a Significant Effect on Psoriasis with Patients on Lithium

Allan, S. J. R., et al., "The Effect of Inositol Supplements on the Psoriasis of Patients Taking Lithium: A Randomized, Placebo-Controlled Trial." *The British Journal of Dermatology* 150, no. 5 (May 2004): 966–69. doi:10.1111/j.1365-2133.2004.05822.x. , PMID: 15149510

> ➢ The inositol supplements had a significantly beneficial effect on the psoriasis of patients taking lithium. No such effect was detected on the psoriasis of patients not on lithium.

Safflower Oil

Safflower Oil was Effective in Remitting Symptoms of Lithium Neurotoxicity

Lieb, J. "Linoleic Acid in the Treatment of Lithium Toxicity and Familial Tremor." *Prostaglandins and Medicine* 4, no. 4 (April 1980): 275–79., PMID: 7394066

> ➢ Lithium inhibits the synthesis of prostaglandin (PG) El by blocking the mobilization of dihomogammalinolenic acid (DGLA). Toxicity due to lithium might be related to reduced PGEl formation. In five patients who developed toxic effects on low doses of lithium, linoleic acid in the form of safflower oil was given in an attempt to raise levels of the linoleic acid metabolite, DGLA. In all five patients the safflower oil was

effective in remitting the symptoms of neurotoxicity. Safflower oil was also effective in a patient with familial tremor.

Omega-3 Fatty Acids

Akkerhuis, Grad W., et al., "Lithium-Associated Psoriasis and Omega-3 Fatty Acids." *The American Journal of Psychiatry* 160, no. 7 (July 2003): 1355., PMID: 12832259

> ➤ Our positive findings regarding 4–6 g/day (but not 2 g/day) of omega-3 fatty acids in these two patients with lithium-associated psoriasis are in line with the positive results from recent studies of infusions of omega-3 fatty acids in patients with acute psoriasis (3). In addition to studies in patients with bipolar disorder, we suggest further studies of omega-3 fatty acids in patients with (lithium-associated) psoriasis.

Selenium

Selenium May Restore Lithium Plasma Micronutrient and Glucose Levels to Control Conditions

Kiełczykowska, Małgorzata, et al., "Could Selenium Administration Alleviate the Disturbances of Blood Parameters Caused by Lithium Administration in Rats?" *Biological Trace Element Research* 158, no. 3 (June 2014): 359–64. doi:10.1007/s12011-014-9952-4., PMID: 24676629

> ➤ Lithium is widely used in medicine, but its administration can cause numerous side effects. The present study aimed at the evaluation of the possible application of selenium, an essential and antioxidant element, as a protective agent against lithium toxicity. The experiment was performed on four groups of Wistar rats: I (control)—treated with saline, II (Li)—treated with lithium (Li_2CO_3), III (Se)—treated with selenium (Na_2SeO_3) and IV (Li+Se)—treated with lithium and selenium (Li_2CO_3 and Na_2SeO_3) in the form of water solutions by stomach tube for 6 weeks. The following biochemical parameters were measured: concentrations of sodium, potassium, calcium, magnesium, phosphorus, iron, urea, creatinine, cholesterol, glucose, total protein and albumin and activities of alkaline phosphatase, aspartate aminotransferase and alanine aminotransferase in serum as well as whole blood superoxide dismutase and glutathione peroxidase. Morphological parameters such as red blood cells, haemoglobin, haematocrit, mean corpuscular volume, mean corpuscular haemoglobin, mean corpuscular haemoglobin concentration, platelets, white blood cells, neutrophils as well as lymphocytes were determined. Lithium significantly increased serum calcium and glucose (2.65±0.17 vs. 2.43± 0.11; 162±31 vs. 121±14, respectively), whereas magnesium and albumin were decreased (1.05±0.08 vs. 1.21±0.15; 3.85. ±0.12 vs. 4.02±0.08, respectively). Selenium given with lithium restored these parameters to values similar to those observed in the control (Ca—

2.49±0.08, glucose—113±26, Mg—1.28±0.09, albumin—4.07±0.11). Se alone or coadministered with Li significantly increased aspartate aminotransferase and glutathione peroxidase. The obtained outcomes let us suggest that the continuation of research on the application of selenium as an adjuvant in lithium therapy seems warranted.

Valproic Acid–induced Toxicity Side Effect Treatments

Carnitine

Carnitine is an Effective Treatment for Valproic Acid-induced Toxicity

> **Lheureux, Philippe E. R.,** et al., "Science Review: Carnitine in the Treatment of Valproic Acid-Induced Toxicity - What Is the Evidence?" *Critical Care (London, England)* 9, no. 5 (October 5, 2005): 431–40. Publisher: BIOMED CENTRAL LTD. doi:10.1186/cc3742., PMID: 16277730

> ➤ Valproic acid (VPA) is a broad-spectrum antiepileptic drug and is usually well tolerated, but rare serious complications may occur in some patients receiving VPA chronically, including haemorrhagic pancreatitis, bone marrow suppression, VPA-induced hepatotoxicity (VHT) and VPA-induced hyperammonaemic encephalopathy (VHE). Some data suggest that VHT and VHE may be promoted by carnitine deficiency. Acute VPA intoxication also occurs as a consequence of intentional or accidental overdose and its incidence is increasing, because of use of VPA in psychiatric disorders. Although it usually results in mild central nervous system depression, serious toxicity and even fatal cases have been reported. Several studies or isolated clinical observations have suggested the potential value of oral L-carnitine in reversing carnitine deficiency or preventing its development as well as some adverse effects due to VPA. Carnitine supplementation during VPA therapy in high-risk patients is now recommended by some scientific committees and textbooks, especially paediatricians. L-carnitine therapy could also be valuable in those patients who develop VHT or VHE. A few isolated observations also suggest that L-carnitine may be useful in patients with coma or in preventing hepatic dysfunction after acute VPA overdose. However, these issues deserve further investigation in controlled, randomized and probably multicentre trials to evaluate the clinical value and the appropriate dosage of L-carnitine in each of these conditions.

Carnitine-pantothenic Acid Has Protective Effect on Valproic Acid-induced Hepatotoxicity

> **Felker, Dana,** et al., "Evidence for a Potential Protective Effect of Carnitine-Pantothenic Acid Co-Treatment on Valproic Acid-Induced Hepatotoxicity." *Expert Review of Clinical Pharmacology* 7, no. 2 (March 2014): 211–18. Publisher: FUTURE DRUGS LTD. doi:10.1586/17512433.2014.871202., PMID: 24450420

> ➤ Valproic acid is approved for treatment of seizures and manic episodes of bipolar disorder, and continues to be one of the most commonly prescribed antiepileptic drugs in the world. Hepatotoxicity is a rare but serious side effect resulting from its use, particularly in young patients. This adverse effect does not display normal dose-response curves and can be lethal in children. A review of the purported mechanisms of action suggest hepatotoxicity results from increased oxidative stress, caused by a reduction in beta-oxidation and an increase in activation of certain metabolizing enzymes. There is also evidence that both carnitine and pantothenic acid are involved in the regulation of valproic acid-induced hepatotoxic processes, and clinical evidence has shown that treatment with either compound shows protective effects against hepatotoxicity. These results suggest a potential increase in protective effects with cotreatment of carnitine and pantothenic acid.

Levocarnitine

Levocarnitine Supplementation May Enhance Recovery from Hypocarnitinemia in Psychiatric Patients

Cuturic, Miroslav, et al., "Clinical Outcomes and Low-Dose Levocarnitine Supplementation in Psychiatric Inpatients with Documented Hypocarnitinemia: A Retrospective Chart Review." *Journal of Psychiatric Practice* 16, no. 1 (January 2010): 5–14. Publisher: LIPPINCOTT WILLIAMS & WILKINS; doi:10.1097/01.pra.0000367773.03636.d1., PMID: 20098226

> ➤ We hypothesize that correction of carnitine depletion, either by levocarnitine supplementation or by valproate dose reduction, may enhance recovery from hypocarnitinemia-associated encephalopathy in psychiatric patients. Our findings also suggest that ethnic traits may affect carnitine bioavailability as well as cognitive outcomes in this clinical context. Further studies of carnitine metabolism and supplementation in psychiatric patients are warranted.

CODEX ALTERNUS™

Extrapyramidal Symptoms Side Effect Treatments

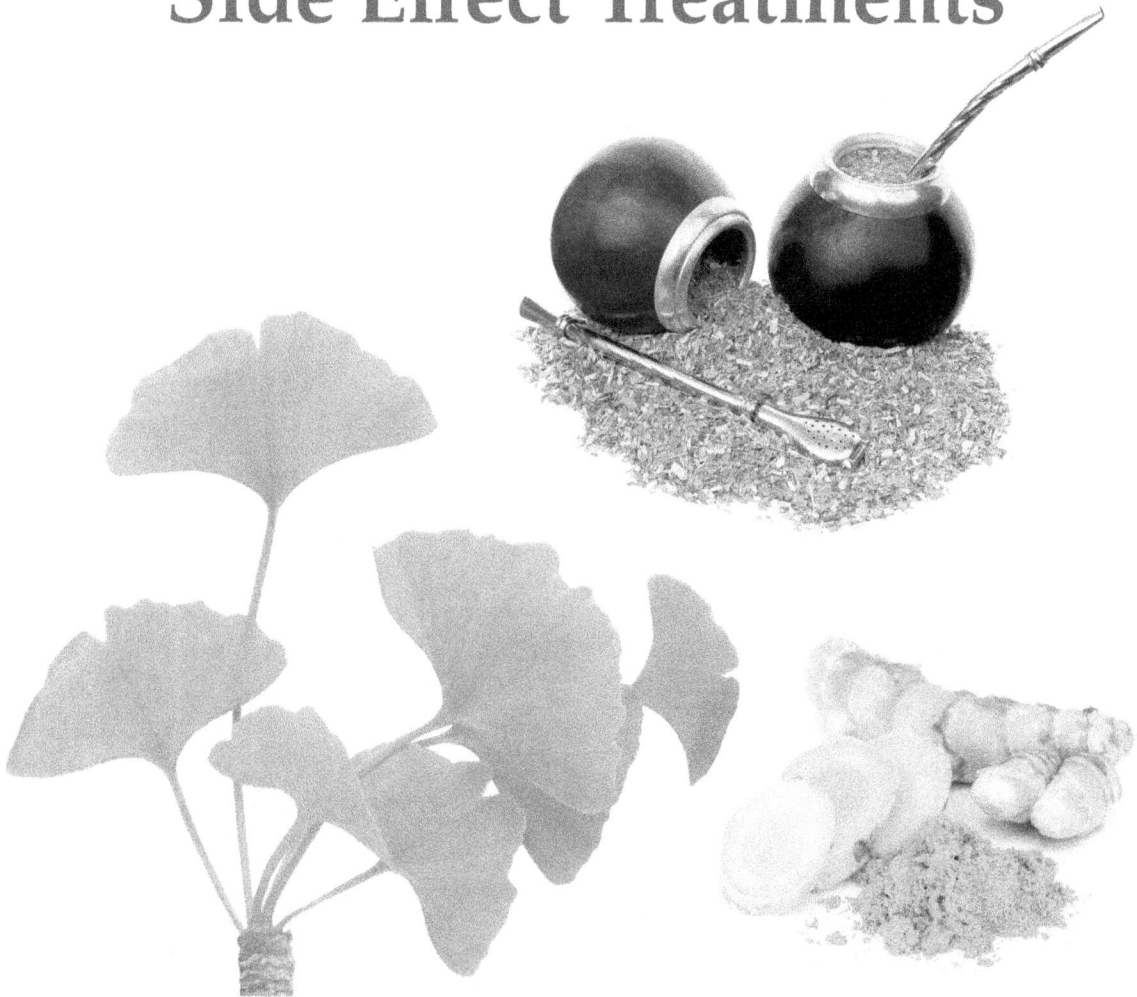

Antioxidants (clockwise from bottom left): Ginkgo biloba, Yerba mate, Curcumin

CODEX ALTERNUS

Tardive Dyskinesia Side Effect Treatments

Alpha Lipoic Acid

Alpha Lipoic Acid Improves Tardive Dyskinesia

> **Thaakur, Santhrani,** et al., "Effect of Alpha Lipoic Acid on the Tardive Dyskinesia and Oxidative Stress Induced by Haloperidol in Rats." *Journal of Neural Transmission (Vienna, Austria: 1996)* 116, no. 7 (July 2009): 807–14. Publisher: SPRINGER-VERLAG WIEN doi:10.1007/s00702-009-0232-y., PMID: 19444377

> ➢ "In conclusion, ALA improves TD and catalepsy by scavenging hydroxyl radicals, singlet oxygen hypochlorous acid, and regenerating other antioxidants such as glutathione, vitamin C, ubiquinol (coenzyme Q 10) an indirectly vitamin E...."

Amino Acids

Branched Chained Amino Acids Decrease Tardive Dyskinesia Symptoms

> **Richardson, M. A.,** et al., "Branched Chain Amino Acids Decrease Tardive Dyskinesia Symptoms." *Psychopharmacology* 143, no. 4 (April 1999): 358–64., Publisher: SPRINGER-VERLAG; PMID: 10367552

> ➢ "The BCAA show promise as a treatment for TD. The decrease in TD symptoms seen in the trial may have been modulated by the BCAA treatment-induced increased availability of the BCAA and decreased availability of Phe to the brain."

> **Richardson, Mary Ann,** et al., "Efficacy of the Branched-Chain Amino Acids in the Treatment of Tardive Dyskinesia in Men." *The American Journal of Psychiatry* 160, no. 6 (June 2003): 1117–24., Publisher: AM PSYCHIATRIC ASSN; PMID: 12777270

> ➢ "Branched-chain amino acids constitute a novel, safe treatment for tardive dyskinesia, with a strong potential for providing significant improvement in the diseased physiognomy of the afflicted person."

> **Richardson, Mary Ann,** et al., "Efficacy of the Branched-Chain Amino Acids in the Treatment of Tardive Dyskinesia in Men." *The American Journal of Psychiatry* 160, no. 6 (June 2003): 1117–24., Publisher: AM PSYCHIATRIC ASSN; PMID: 14744176

> ➢ "The substantial symptom decrease and tolerability observed suggest the use of the BCAA formulation for the treatment of TD in children and adolescents and warrant further large-scale studies."

CODEX ALTERNUS

Ashwagandha

Ashwagandha Prevents Haldol –induced Tardive Dyskinesia

Bhattacharya, Salil K., et al., "Effect of Withania Somnifera Glycowithanolides on a Rat Model of Tardive Dyskinesia." *Phytomedicine: International Journal of Phytotherapy and Phytopharmacology* 9, no. 2 (March 2002): 167–70. Publisher: ELSEVIER GMBH doi:10.1078/0944-7113-00089, PMID: 11995951

> ➢ "The results indicate the reported antioxidant effect of WSG rather than it's GABA-mimetic action , may be responsible for the prevention of haloperidol-induced TD."

Biofeedback

Biofeedback May Be an Effective Treatment for Tardive Dyskinesia

Albanese, H., et al., "Biofeedback Treatment of Tardive Dyskinesia: Two Case Reports." *The American Journal of Psychiatry* 134, no. 10 (October 1977): 1149–50., Publisher: AM PSYCHIATRIC ASSN; PMID: 900274

> ➢ The two patients described were both intelligent people who experienced social embarrassment because of severe mouth movements. The first patient had the movements for 5 months before biofeedback training; the second had the movements for only 1 month. Both had been off medication for 1 month for without change in movements and improved markedly by the 3rd session of biofeedback training. A characteristic of tardive dyskinesia is that voluntary quieting of movement in one part of the body often results in shifting the movement to another part of the body. This did not occur in either patient, despite the already existing foot and finger movements in the first patient described. A general reduction of tension was experienced by both patients, and both gave reports of increased well-being. Since spontaneous remission occurs in tardive dyskinesia, it cannot be proven that the biofeedback treatment was responsible for the marked improvement of these two patients. However, the improvement was first noted within the training sessions and increased progressively with training, later extending to periods out-side the training sessions. Also, in each instance there had been no noticeable improvement before treatment began. We believe this observation warrants further investigation of the treatment approach, and we hope that this report will stimulate others to try similar methods.

Chaihu Taoren

Chaihu Taoren Capsules May Effectively Releive Symptoms of Tardive Dyskinesia

Su, Jian-min, et al., "[Relationship between tardive dyskinesia and the polymorphism of superoxide dismutase val9Ala and efficacy of Chaihu Taoren Capsules on it]." *Zhongguo Zhong Xi Yi Jie He Za Zhi Zhongguo Zhongxiyi Jiehe Zazhi = Chinese Journal of Integrated Traditional and Western Medicine / Zhongguo Zhong Xi Yi Jie He Xue Hui, Zhongguo Zhong Yi Yan Jiu Yuan Zhu Ban* 27, no. 8 (August 2007): 700–703., Publisher: Chinese Association of the Integration of Traditional and Western Medicine; PMID: 17879532

> ➢ "The CTD could effectively relieve the symptoms of TD, its efficacy might be related with the genotype of SOD, and 9Ala is considered to be a protective factor for the susceptibility to TD."

Chiropractic Manipulation

Chiropractic Management of Musculoskeletal Pain Secondary to Tardive Dyskinesia

Schoonderwoerd, Kelly, et al., "Chiropractic Management of Musculoskeletal Pain Secondary to Tardive Dyskinesia." *The Journal of the Canadian Chiropractic Association* 49, no. 2 (June 2005): 92–95., Publisher: THE ASSOCIATION; PMID: 17549198

> ➢ "A case report is presented of a patient affected by TD who suffered mechanical musculoskeletal pain secondary to its effects, and was managed by chiropractic care."

Ceruletide

Ceruletide is a Novel and Practical Treatment for Tardive Dyskinesia

Kojima, T., et al., "Treatment of Tardive Dyskinesia with Ceruletide: A Double-Blind, Placebo-Controlled Study." *Psychiatry Research* 43, no. 2 (August 1992): 129–36., Publisher: ELSEVIER IRELAND LTD; PMID: 1357701

> ➢ The effectiveness of a once-weekly i.m. injection of ceruletide (0.8 microgram/kg) in suppressing the symptoms of neuroleptic-induced tardive dyskinesia (TD) was evaluated in a double-blind, placebo-controlled, matched-pairs study. Global evaluation of the severity of TD symptoms over the 8-week study period revealed a significant improvement with ceruletide as compared with placebo. Analysis of the therapeutic response to ceruletide over the course of treatment revealed a slow, but long-lasting improvement of TD symptoms. Side effects, which were mild and transient, consisted mainly of nausea and epigastric discomfort. The incidence of side effects did not differ between the ceruletide- and placebo-treated groups. Ceruletide appears to be a novel and practical treatment that can substantially alleviate the symptoms of dyskinesia.

Nishikawa, T., et al., "Treatment of Tardive Dyskinesia with Ceruletide." *Progress in Neuro-Psychopharmacology & Biological Psychiatry* 12, no. 5 (1988): 803–12., Publisher: ELSEVIER INC. PMID: 2906160

> Seven patients with TD were treated with a single dose of ceruletide 0.8 microgram/kg i.m. 2. EMG and MV were recorded, and the average power spectrum was computed. 3. Effect of ceruletide on TD within 2 hr after injection was varied (3 cases: inhibitory, 2 cases: facilitatory, 2 cases: no effect). 4. Two patients with severe TD, who showed improvement after a single administration, received repeated administration of ceruletide (0.6 microgram/kg i.m.) and their TD symptoms were recorded on videotape for blind consensus ratings. In both patients ceruletide caused a marked decrease in severity of TD, and the effects lasted for several weeks. 5. The present findings might contribute to further understanding of the role of CCK in the brain and to the treatment of TD.

Choline

Oral Choline is Effective in the Treatment of Tardive Dyskinesia

Growdon, J. H., et al., "Oral Choline Administration to Patients with Tardive Dyskinesia." *The New England Journal of Medicine* 297, no. 10 (September 8, 1977): 524–27. Publisher: MASSACHUSETTS MEDICAL SOCIETY; doi:10.1056/NEJM197709082971002., PMID:887103

> Twenty patients with stable buccal-lingual-masticatory movements took oral doses of choline for two weeks according to a double-blind crossover protocol. Plasma choline levels rose from 12.4 +-1.0 to 33.5+-2.5 nmol per milliliter (mean +- S.E.M.; P<0.001) during this period. Choreic movements decreased in nine patients, worsened in one and were unchanged in 10. Thus, oral doses of choline can be useful in neurologic diseases in which an increase in acetylcholine release is desired.

EMG Feedback

EMG Feedback from the Masseter Muscle was Effective in Controling Tardive Dsykinesia

Sherman, R. A., et al., "Successful Treatment of One Case of Tardive Dyskinesia with Electromyographic Feedback from the Masseter Muscle." *Biofeedback and Self-Regulation* 4, no. 4 (December 1979): 367–70., Publisher: PLENUM PRESS; PMID: 526478

> "Evidence from one case with a 15-month follow-up is presented to support the conclusion that electromyographic (EMG) feedback from the masseter was effective in controlling tardive dyskinesia, while a combination of EMG feedback from the frontalis and verbal muscle relaxation training were not."

Fatty Acids

Fish oil Decreased Motor Disorders, Memory Dysfunction and Neuroleptic-Induced Oxidative Damage

Barcelos, Raquel Cristine Silva, et al., "Effects of Omega-3 Essential Fatty Acids (omega-3 EFAs) on Motor Disorders and Memory Dysfunction Typical Neuroleptic-Induced: Behavioral and Biochemical Parameter." *Neurotoxicity Research* 17, no. 3 (April 2010): 228–37. doi:10.1007/s12640-009-9095-0., Publisher: F P/GRAHAM PUBLISHING COMPANY; PMID: 19644727

> ➢ "The FO decreased the motor disorders, memory dysfunction, and oxidative damage typical neuroleptic-induced"

Essential Fatty Acids LA and GLA Supplementation Delays the Onset of Dyskinesia in Huntington's Disease

Vaddadi, K., et al., "Dyskinesias and Their Treatment with Essential Fatty Acids: A Review." *Prostaglandins, Leukotrienes, and Essential Fatty Acids* 55, no. 1–2 (August 1996): 89–94., Publisher: CHURCHILL LIVINGSTONE; PMID: 8888129

> ➢ Clinical improvement in HD (Huntington's Disease) with LA and GLA supplementation is a novel finding…." It has been suggested that in individuals at early stages of HD, or in individuals at risk of developing HD, if given EFA's probably of both n-6 and n-3 series on long term basis might delay the onset of HD.

EPA Supplementation Produces Significant Improvement in Memory in Patients with Tardive Dyskinesia

Vaddadi, K. S., et al., "A Double-Blind Trial of Essential Fatty Acid Supplementation in Patients with Tardive Dyskinesia." *Psychiatry Research* 27, no. 3 (March 1989): 313–23., Publisher: ELSEVIER IRELAND LTD; PMID: 2565585

> ➢ The antidyskinetic effect of EPA supplementation was marginally significant but not clinically important. However, active treatment produced significant improvements in total psychopathology scores and schizophrenia subscales scores, and significant improvement in memory.

Gingko Biloba

Gingko Biloba is an Effective Treatment for Tardive Dyskinesia

Zhang, Wu-Fang, et al., "Extract of Ginkgo Biloba Treatment for Tardive Dyskinesia in Schizophrenia: A Randomized, Double-Blind, Placebo-Controlled Trial." *The Journal of Clinical Psychiatry* 72, no. 5 (May 2011): 615–21. Publisher: PHYSICIANS POSTGRADUATE PRESS, INC. doi:10.4088/JCP.09m05125yel., PMID: 20868638

> ➢ "EGb-761 appears to be an effective treatment for reducing the symptoms of TD in schizophrenia patient

CODEX ALTERNUS

Indian Gooseberry

Indian Gooseberry Exerts a Prophylactive Effect Against Neuroleptic-induced Tardive Dyskinesia

Bhattachary, S. K., et al., "Effect of Emblica Officinalis Tannoids on a Rat Model of Tardive Dyskinesia." *Indian Journal of Experimental Biology* 38, no. 9 (September 2000): 945–47., Publisher: SCIENTIFIC PUBLISHERS; PMID: 12561957

> ➢ "The results suggest that EOT exerts a prophylactive effect against neuroleptic-induced TD....."

Insulin

Insulin May Decrease the Intensity of Symptoms in Tardive Dykinesia

Mouret, J., et al., "Low Doses of Insulin as a Treatment of Tardive Dyskinesia: Conjuncture or Conjecture?" *European Neurology* 31, no. 4 (1991): 199–203., Publisher: S./KARGER AG PMID: 1868860

> ➢ Twenty chronic schizophrenic outpatients (13 males, 7 females), aged 20-67 (mean: 38.3), accepted to participate in this double-blind, placebo-controlled study. They were randomly assigned to either the insulin treatment group (10 patients) or to the insulin-placebo group (10 patients). They received a subcutaneous injection of 10 units of standard insulin or placebo at 10 a.m. From day 1 to day 15, injections were performed daily and, thereafter, every other week for 5 weeks totalizing 20 injections in 90 days. At day 7, the insulin treatment group showed a sharp decrease in the intensity of TD symptoms which persisted throughout the duration of the study. By contrast, no change in TD symptomatology was observed in the insulin-placebo-treated group. Although a direct effect on DA neurones, or at least the participation of such an effect, cannot be excluded, our data favor a role of decreased glucose availability in reversing receptor hypersensitivity.

Kamisoyosan

Kampo Medicine Kamisoyosan Provides a Meaningful Reduction in Involuntary Movements in Tardive Dyskinesia

Lee, Jung Goo, et al., "Clinical Effectiveness of the Kampo Medicine Kamishoyosan for Adjunctive Treatment of Tardive Dyskinesia in Patients with Schizophrenia: A 16-Week Open Trial." *Psychiatry and Clinical Neurosciences* 61, no. 5 (October 2007): 509–14. Publisher: BLACKWELL PUBLISHING ASIA ; doi:10.1111/j.1440-1819.2007.01700.x., PMID: 17875029

> "A meaningful reduction in total abnormal involuntary movement scale scores was observed in the tardive dyskinesia group"

Lecithin

Lecithin Can Suppress Tardive Dyskinesia

> **Growdon, J. H.,** et al., "Lecithin Can Suppress Tardive Dyskinesia." *The New England Journal of Medicine* 298, no. 18 (May 4, 1978): 1029–30., Publisher: MASSACHUSETTS MEDICAL SOCIETY; PMID: 642995

> The mean number of movements decreased in all patients during lecithin ingestion (Table 1), and serum choline levels rose from a mean +-S.D. of 10.0 +- 2.2 to 22.8+-5.1 nmol per milliliter (P<0.01). Lecithin was as effective as choline chloride: the number of buccal-lingual-masticatory movements decreased as they had during choline administration. In addition, lecithin may be more acceptable to patients, since it does not have a bitter taste of fishy body odor as associated with choline ingestion. These data suggest that lecithin may constitute an effective mode of neurotransmitter precursor therapy for conditions in which physicians wish to increase cholinergic tone.

Melatonin

Melatonin is Beneficial for The Treatment of Antipsychotic –induced Tardive Dyskinesia

> **Shamir, E.,** et al., "Melatonin Treatment for Tardive Dyskinesia: A Double-Blind, Placebo-Controlled, Crossover Study." *Archives of General Psychiatry* 58, no. 11 (November 2001): 1049–52., Publisher: AMERICAN MEDICAL ASSOCIATION; PMID: 11695951

> "In conclusion, the results of the present study demonstrate that melatonin treatment is beneficial for antipsychotic-induced TD."

Morin

Morin (Flavonol) Has Neuroprotective Potential in Haloperidol-induced Tardive Dyskinesia

> **Selvakumar GP.,** et al., "Morin Attenuates Haloperidol-induced Tardive Dyskinesia and Oxidative Stress in Mice." *Journal of Natural Sciences Research* Vol.2, No.8, 2012

> " These results indicate that morin have beneficial role in mitigating HP-induced damage of dopaminergic neurons, possibly via its neuroprotective and its antioxidant potential."

Muscimol

GABA Agonist Muscimol was found to Provide Relief from Tardive Dyskinesia

CODEX ALTERNUS

Tamminga, C. A., et al., "Improvement in Tardive Dyskinesia after Muscimol Therapy." *Archives of General Psychiatry* 36, no. 5 (May 1979): 595–98. Publisher: AMERICAN MEDICAL ASSOCIATION

> ➤ Muscimol, thought to be a agonist of gamma-aminobutyric acid (GABA), was administered to eight neuroleptic-free subjects with tardive dyskinesia. At oral dose levels from 5 to 9 mg, involuntary movements were consistently attenuated, usually in the absence of sedation. These results support the view that pharmacologic attempts to stimulate GABA-mediated synaptic transmission may afford symptomatic relief to patients with tardive dyskinesia.

Osteopathic Manipulation

Osteopathic Management of Tardive Dyskinesia is Beneficial

Reifsnyder, Jeremy W., et al., "Conservative Approach to Tardive Dyskinesia-Induced Neck and Upper Back Pain." *The Journal of the American Osteopathic Association* 113, no. 8 (August 2013): 636–39. Publisher: THE ASSOCIATION; doi:10.7556/jaoa.2013.025., PMID: 23918915

> ➤ Although it is unlikely that spinal manipulation would result in a reversal of tardive dyskinesia, osteopathic physicians should consider the use of OMT to address pain associated with tardive dyskinesia. With relief of pain, patients can have an improved quality of life, with positive changes to their overall mental and physical health. A controlled clinical trial assessing the safety and effectiveness of spinal manipulation over a longer time frame would be helpful to establish further use of OMT in the management of tardive dyskinesia–induced neck and back pain.

Pryidoxal 5 Phosphate (P-5-P)

P-5-P is 40% Effective in the Treatment of Tardive Dyskinesia

Adelufosi, Adegoke Oloruntoba, et al., "Pyridoxal 5 Phosphate for Neuroleptic-Induced Tardive Dyskinesia." *The Cochrane Database of Systematic Reviews* 4 (2015): CD010501. doi:10.1002/14651858.CD010501.pub2., PMID: 25866243

> ➤ People taking pyridoxal 5 phosphate in these studies experienced more than 40% improvement in their tardive dyskinesia compared to those on placebo, so had less severe tardive dyskinesia. Experience of side effects were similar between treatment groups with participants taking pyridoxal 5 phosphate experiencing nomore or less side effects than participants in the placebo group and they did not experience greater worsening of their psychiatric symptoms than those on placebo. Evidence from the studies is weak, but suggests pyridoxal 5 phosphate may be effective in the treatment of tardive dyskinesia.

CODEX ALTERNUS

Spirulina

Spirulina Decreases Haldol-induced Oxidative Stress and Tardive Dyskinesia

> **Thaakur, S. R.,** et al., "Effect of Spirulina Maxima on the Haloperidol Induced Tardive Dyskinesia and Oxidative Stress in Rats." *Journal of Neural Transmission (Vienna, Austria: 1996)* 114, no. 9 (September 2007): 1217–25. Publisher: SPRINGER-VERLAG doi:10.1007/s00702-007-0744-2., PMID: 17530160

> ➤ Spirulina supplementation at a dose of 180mg/kg significantly improved enzymatic and nonenzymatic antioxidants and decreased tardive dyskinesia induced by haloperidol. In conclusion the results of the present investigation suggest that spirulina decreases haloperidol induced oxidative stress and TD by many mechanisms as it is a cocktail of antioxidants.

Triiodothyronine

Triiodthyronine May Be Associated with Better Cognitive Function and Less EPS in Schizophrenia

> **Ichioka, Shugo,** et al., "Triiodothyronine May Be Possibly Associated with Better Cognitive Function and Less Extrapyramidal Symptoms in Chronic Schizophrenia." *Progress in Neuro-Psychopharmacology & Biological Psychiatry* 39, no. 1 (October 1, 2012): 170–74. Publisher: ELSEVIER INC. doi:10.1016/j.pnpbp.2012.06.008., PMID: 22750309

> ➤ These findings suggest that BDNF, free T_3, and prolactin may be associated with cognitive function and/or extrapyramidal symptoms in patients with chronic schizophrenia. Notably, free T_3 may be possibly associated with better cognitive function and less extrapyramidal symptoms, although our cross-sectional study could not reveal a causal relationship.

Tryptophan

Tryptophan Supplementation May Ameliorate Neuroleptic-induced Tardive Dyskinesia

> **Ali, Obaid,** et al., "Effects of Tryptophan and Valine Administration on Behavioral Pharmacology of Haloperidol." *Pakistan Journal of Pharmaceutical Sciences* 18, no. 2 (April 2005): 23–28., Publisher: FACULTY OF PHARMACY, UNIVERSITY OF KARACHI ; PMID: 16431394

> ➤ "These findings suggest a possible serotonergic involvement in neuroleptic induced tardive dyskinesia and amelioration of the disorder through TRP supplementation."

Vitamin B₆

Vitamin B6 is Effective in the Treatment of Tardive Dyskinesia

> **Lerner, Vladimir,** et al., "Vitamin B6 Treatment for Tardive Dyskinesia: A Randomized, Double-Blind, Placebo-Controlled, Crossover Study." *The Journal of Clinical Psychiatry* 68, no. 11 (November 2007): 1648–54., Publisher: PHYSICIANS POSTGRADUATE PRESS, INC; PMID: 18052557

> ➢ "Vitamin B6 appears to be effective in reducing symptoms of TD."

Vitamin E and Vitamin C

Vitamin E and C is Efficacious Treatment for Tardive Dyskinesia

> **Michael, Nikolaus,** et al., "Severe Tardive Dyskinesia in Affective Disorders: Treatment with Vitamin E and C." *Neuropsychobiology* 46 Suppl 1 (2002): 28–30. doi:68019., Publisher: S./KARGER AG; PMID: 12571430

> ➢ "…Combining vitamin E with C was a safe and efficacious in the treatment of tardive dyskinesia in affective disorder."

Yi-gan-san

Yi-gan-san resulted in Significant Improvement of Tardive Dyskinesia and Psychotic Symptoms

> **Miyaoka, Tsuyoshi,** et al., "Yi-Gan San for the Treatment of Neuroleptic-Induced Tardive Dyskinesia: An Open-Label Study." *Progress in Neuro-Psychopharmacology & Biological Psychiatry* 32, no. 3 (April 1, 2008): 761–64. Publisher: ELSEVIER INC. doi:10.1016/j.pnpbp.2007.12.003., PMID: 18201810

> ➢ "Administration of YGS resulted in a statistically significant improvement in tardive dyskinesia and psychotic symptoms"

Orofacial Dyskinesia Side Effect Treatments

Ashwagandha

Ashwagandha is Effective at Preventing Haldol-induced Orofacial Dyskinesia

CODEX ALTERNUS

Naidu, Pattipati S., et al., "Effect of Withania Somnifera Root Extract on Haloperidol-Induced Orofacial Dyskinesia: Possible Mechanisms of Action." *Journal of Medicinal Food* 6, no. 2 (2003): 107–14. Publisher: MARY ANN/LIEBERT, INC. PUBLISHERS doi:10.1089/109662003322233503., PMID: 12935321

> ➤ "These findings strongly suggest that oxidative stress plays a significant role in HP-induced orofacial dyskinesia and that Ws could be effective in preventing neuroleptic-induced extrapyramidal side effects."

Brazilian Orchid

Brazilian Orchid Tree Prevents Vacuous Chewing Movements Induced By Haldol

Peroza, Luis Ricardo, et al., "Bauhinia Forficata Prevents Vacuous Chewing Movements Induced by Haloperidol in Rats and Has Antioxidant Potential in Vitro." *Neurochemical Research* 38, no. 4 (April 2013): 789–96. d Publisher: SPRINGER NEW YORK LLC doi:10.1007/s11064-013-0981-8., PMID: 23377855

> ➤ Haloperidol treatment induced VCMs, and co-treatment with B.forficata partially prevented this effect. Haloperidol reduced the locomotor and exploratory activities of animals in the open fields test, which was not modified by B. foficata treatment. Our present data showed that B. forficta has antioxidant potential and partially protects against VCMs induced by haloperidol in rats. Taken together, our data suggest the protection by natural compounds against VCMs induced by Haloperidol in rats.

Ceruletide

Ceruletide is Effective on Severe Orofacial Dyskinesia

Nishikawa, T., et al., "Biphasic and Long-Lasting Effect of Ceruletide on Tardive Dyskinesia." *Psychopharmacology* 86, no. 1–2 (1985): 43–44., Publisher: SPRINGER-VERLAG; PMID: 3927366

> ➤ A 55-year-old schizophrenic inpatient with buccolingual dyskinesia was treated with a single dose of ceruletide 0.8 micrograms/kg IM. Time-course effects of the drug were then followed for up to 6 weeks after injection. To assess changes in severity of bucco-lingual dyskinesia objectively, electromyogram (EMG) and microvibration (MV) were recorded. Simultaneously, bucco-lingual dyskinesias were also evaluated by using a five-point rating scale. Before injection of ceruletide, severity of dyskinesia was "moderate" and 3-4 Hz of dyskinetic oral movements were dominant. "Extremely severe" and repetitious gross oral movements (around 1 Hz) were observed within a few minutes after injection and continued for up to 1 h. Thereafter, oral movements tended to decrease, and they disappeared completely 3 weeks after injection. This biphasic and long-lasting effect of ceruletide on tardive dyskinesia might contribute to further

understanding of the physio-pathophysiological role of cholecystokinin-like peptides in the brain, and provide a basis for practical treatment of tardive dyskinesia.

Curcumin

Curcumin is Able to Reverse Changes Caused by Exposure to Haldol in Orofacial Dyskinesia

Bishnoi, Mahendra, et al., "Protective Effect of Curcumin, the Active Principle of Turmeric (Curcuma Longa) in Haloperidol-Induced Orofacial Dyskinesia and Associated Behavioural, Biochemical and Neurochemical Changes in Rat Brain." *Pharmacology, Biochemistry, and Behavior* 88, no. 4 (February 2008): 511–22. Publisher: ELSEVIER INC. doi:10.1016/j.pbb.2007.10.009., PMID: 18022680

> ➤ "In present study, curcumin was able to reverse the behavioral, biochemical and neurochemical changes caused by exposure to haloperidol possibly by virtue of its antioxidant effect...."

Curcumin Prevents Haldol-induced Orofacial Dyskinesia

Sookram, Christal, et al., "Curcumin Prevents Haloperidol-Induced Development of Abnormal Oro-Facial Movements: Possible Implications of Bcl-XL in Its Mechanism of Action." *Synapse (New York, N.Y.)* 65, no. 8 (August 2011): 788–94. Publisher: JOHN WILEY & SONS, INC. doi:10.1002/syn.20905., PMID: 21218454

> ➤ "These results suggest that curcumin may be a promising treatment to prevent the development of AOFMs and further suggest some therapeutic value in the treatment of movement disorders."

Curry Tree Leaves

Curry Tree Leaves Could be a Potential Drug Candidate for the Prevention of Neuroleptic-induced Orofacial Dyskinesia

Patil, Rupali, et al., "Reversal of Haloperidol-Induced Orofacial Dyskinesia by Murraya Koenigii Leaves in Experimental Animals." *Pharmaceutical Biology* 50, no. 6 (June 2012): 691–97. Publisher: TAYLOR & FRANCIS THE NETHERLANDS doi:10.3109/13880209.2011.618841., PMID: 22136413

> ➤ "The study concludes the M. koenigii could be screened as a potential drug for the prevention or treatment of neuroleptic-induced OD."

CODEX ALTERNUS

Gallic Acid

Gallic Acid May Have a Promissory Use in the Treatment of Involuntary Oral Movements

Reckziegel, Patrícia, et al., "Gallic Acid Decreases Vacuous Chewing Movements Induced by Reserpine in Rats." *Pharmacology, Biochemistry, and Behavior* 104 (March 2013): 132–37. doi:10.1016/j.pbb.2013.01.001., PMID: 23313549

> ➤ As result, reserpine increased the number of VCMs in rats, and this effect was maintained for at least three days after its withdrawal. Gallic acid at two different doses (13.5 and 40.5mg/kg/day) has reduced VCMs in rats previously treated with reserpine. Furthermore, we investigated oxidative stress parameters (DCFH-DA oxidation, TBARS and thiol levels) and Na(+),K(+)-ATPase activity in striatum and cerebral cortex, however, no changes were observed. These findings show that gallic acid may have promissory use in the treatment of involuntary oral movements.

Ginkgo Biloba

Ginkgo Biloba is Equivalent to Vitamin E in Attenuating and Preventing Vacuous Chewing Movements

An, Hui-Mei, et al., "Extract of Ginkgo Biloba Is Equivalent to Vitamin E in Attenuating and Preventing Vacuous Chewing Movements in a Rat Model of Tardive Dyskinesia." *Behavioural Pharmacology*, August 29, 2013. Publisher: LIPPINCOTT WILLIAMS & WILKINS; doi:10.1097/FBP.0b013e3283656d87., PMID: 23994817

> ➤ In study one, EGb761 and vitamin E, administered by an oral gavage for 5 weeks during withdrawal from chronic haloperidol treatment, decreased VCMs significantly, showing 83.8 and 91.0% reduction, respectively, compared with the haloperidol-alone group. In study two, the concomitant administration of EGb761 and vitamin E led to significantly fewer VCMs, by 64.4 and 73.9%, respectively, compared with the haloperidol-alone group. There was no significant difference in either study between EGb761 and vitamin E treatment.

Glycine and D-Cycloserine

Glycine and D-Cycloserine Attenuate Vacuous Chewing Movements in Rats

Shoham, Shai, et al., "Glycine and D-Cycloserine Attenuate Vacuous Chewing Movements in a Rat Model of Tardive Dyskinesia." *Brain Research* 1004, no. 1–2 (April 9, 2004): 142–47. Publisher: ELSEVIER BV; doi:10.1016/j.brainres.2004.01.022., PMID: 15033429

> ➤ High dose DCS significantly reduced VCM without affecting other motor parameters. GLY treatment resulted in significantly less VCM but also reduced rearing, grooming

and mobility. In contrast, low dose DCS and placebo did not significantly affect any of these parameters. These findings indicate that the use of GLY and DCS results in attenuation of VCM in rats and may have an effect on TD in humans. Clinical trials with this type of compounds for patients suffering from TD are warranted.

Ginseng (Korean)

Korean Ginseng Could be Useful in the Treatment of Drug-induced Orofacial Dyskinesia

Sanghavi, Chetankumar R., et al., "Korean Ginseng Extract Attenuates Reserpine-Induced Orofacial Dyskinesia and Improves Cognitive Dysfunction in Rats." *Natural Product Research* 25, no. 7 (April 2011): 704–15. Publisher: Taylor & Francis Health Sciences doi:10.1080/14786410802583031., PMID: 20628966

> ➤ "The present study concludes that oxidative stress might play an important role in reserpine-induced abnormal oral movements and Korean ginseng extract could be useful in the treatment of drug-induced dyskinesia and amnesia."

Hibiscus

Hibiscus has a Protective Effect Against Resperpine-induced Orofacial Dyskinesia

Nade, V. S., et al., "Effect of Hibiscus Rosa Sinensis on Reserpine-Induced Neurobehavioral and Biochemical Alterations in Rats." *Indian Journal of Experimental Biology* 47, no. 7 (July 2009): 559–63., Publisher: SCIENTIFIC PUBLISHERS; PMID: 19761039

> ➤ "The results from the presents study suggested Hibiscus rosa sinensis had a protective role against resperpine-induced orofacial dyskinesia and oxidative stress."

Indian Madder

Indian Madder Has a Protective Effect in Drug-induced Orofacial Dyskinesia

Patil, Rupali A., et al., "Protective Effect of Rubia Cordifolia on Reserpine-Induced Orofacial Dyskinesia." *Natural Product Research* 26, no. 22 (2012): 2159–61. Publisher: Taylor & Francis Health Sciences; doi:10.1080/14786419.2011.635341., PMID: 22092272

> ➤ It is concluded that oxidative stress might play an important role in reserpine-induced abnormal oral movements and MERC significantly protected animals against reserpine-induced orofacial dyskinesia and has great potential in the treatment of neuroleptic induced orofacial dyskinesia.

Melatonin

Melatonin Could Be a Potential Drug for the Prevention of Neuroleptic-induced Orofacial Dyskinesia

Naidu, Pattipati S., et al., "Possible Mechanism of Action in Melatonin Attenuation of Haloperidol-Induced Orofacial Dyskinesia." *Pharmacology, Biochemistry, and Behavior* 74, no. 3 (February 2003): 641–48., Publisher: ELSEVIER INC. PMID: 12543230

> ➤ "In conclusion, melatonin could be screened as a potential drug candidate for the prevention or treatment of neuroleptic-induced orofacial dyskinesia"

Nicotine

Nicotine Reduces Antipsychotic-induced Orofacial Dyskinesia

Bordia, Tanuja, et al., "Nicotine Reduces Antipsychotic-Induced Orofacial Dyskinesia in Rats." *The Journal of Pharmacology and Experimental Therapeutics* 340, no. 3 (March 2012): 612–19. Publisher: AMERICAN SOCIETY FOR PHARMACOLOGY & EXPERIMENTAL THERAPEUTICS; doi:10.1124/jpet.111.189100., PMID: 22144565

> ➤ "The present results are the first to suggest that nicotine may be useful for improving the tardive dyskinesia associated with antipsychotic use."

Nitric Oxide

NO Donors L-arginine May Be a Possible Therapeutic Option for Orofacial Dyskensia

Bishnoi, Mahendra, et al., "Co-Administration of Nitric Oxide (NO) Donors Prevents Haloperidol-Induced Orofacial Dyskinesia, Oxidative Damage and Change in Striatal Dopamine Levels." *Pharmacology, Biochemistry, and Behavior* 91, no. 3 (January 2009): 423–29. Publisher: ELSEVIER INC. doi:10.1016/j.pbb.2008.08.021., PMID: 18789960

> ➤ Besides, haloperidol also increased striatal superoxide anion levels and decreased striatal NO and citrulline levels which were prevented by molsidomine and l-arginine. On chronic administration of haloperidol, there was a decrease in the striatal levels of dopamine, which was again reversed by treatment with NO donors. The findings of the present study suggested for the involvement of NO in the development of neuroleptic-induced TD and indicated the potential of NO donors as a possible therapeutic option. Furthermore, a sub-study on a possible schizophrenic phenotype, i.e. a possible clinical worsening in the animals receiving NO donors and neuroleptics will substantiate the clinical utility of the study.

Pecan Shell

Pecan Shell Extract is Able to Prevent and Reverse Orofacial Dyskinesia

> **Trevizol, Fabiola,** et al., "Comparative Study between Two Animal Models of Extrapyramidal Movement Disorders: Prevention and Reversion by Pecan Nut Shell Aqueous Extract." *Behavioural Brain Research* 221, no. 1 (August 1, 2011): 13–18. Publisher: ELSEVIER BV doi:10.1016/j.bbr.2011.02.026., PMID: 21356248

> ➢ "Comparatively, the pecan shell AE was able to both prevent and reverse OD but only prevent catalepsy."

Quercetin

Quercetin Could Be a Potential Therapeutic Agent for the Treatment of Tardive Dyskinesia

> **Naidu, Pattipati S.**, et al., "Reversal of Reserpine-Induced Orofacial Dyskinesia and Cognitive Dysfunction by Quercetin." *Pharmacology* 70, no. 2 (February 2004): 59–67. Publisher: S./KARGER AG; doi:10.1159/000074669., PMID: 14685008

> ➢ In conclusion, the results of the present study clearly indicated that quercetin has a protective role against reserpine-induced orofacial dyskinesia and associated cognitive dysfunction. Consequently, quercetin could be considered as a potential therapeutic agent for the treatment of TD.

Reveratrol

Reveratrol is a Neuroprotective Agent Reducing Motor Disorders Induced by Antipsychotic Treatment

> **Busanello, Alcindo,** et al., "Resveratrol Reduces Vacuous Chewing Movements Induced by Acute Treatment with Fluphenazine." *Pharmacology, Biochemistry, and Behavior* 101, no. 2 (April 2012): 307–10. Publisher: ELSEVIER INC. doi:10.1016/j.pbb.2012.01.007., PMID: 22266770

> ➢ Fluphenazine treatment produced VCM in 70% of rats and concomitant treatment with resveratrol decreased the prevalence to 30%, but did not modify the intensity of the VCM's. Furthermore, the fluphenazine administration reduced the locomotor and exploratory activity of animals in the open field test. Resveratrol treatment was able to protect the reduction of both parameters. Taken together, our data suggest that resveratrol could be considered a potential neuroprotective agent by reducing motor disorders induced by fluphenzine treatment.

Rubiaceae

Rubiaceae Significantly Inhibits Haldol-induced Orofacial Dyskinesia

CODEX ALTERNUS

Maxia, Andrea, et al., "Ethanolic Extract of Rubia Peregrina L. (Rubiaceae) Inhibits Haloperidol-Induced Catalepsy and Reserpine-Induced Orofacial Dyskinesia." *Natural Product Research* 26, no. 5 (2012): 438–45. Publisher: Taylor & Francis Health Sciences doi:10.1080/14786419.2010.511015., PMID: 22316173

> ➤ "The extract of R. peregrine intraperitoneally significantly inhibited haloperidol-induced catalepsy in mice. In rats, the extract significantly inhibited orofacial dyskinesia induced by reserpine."

Rutin

Rutin is a Possible Therapeutic Option to Treat Orofacial Dyskinesia

Bishnoi, Mahendra, et al., "Protective Effect of Rutin, a Polyphenolic Flavonoid against Haloperidol-Induced Orofacial Dyskinesia and Associated Behavioural, Biochemical and Neurochemical Changes." *Fundamental & Clinical Pharmacology* 21, no. 5 (October 2007): 521–29. Publisher: BLACKWELL PUBLISHING LTD. doi:10.1111/j.1472-8206.2007.00512.x., PMID: 17868205

> ➤ "The findings of the present study suggested the involvement of free radicals in the development of neuroleptic-induced orofacial dyskinesia, a putative model of TD, and rutin as a possible therapeutic option to treat this hyperkinetic movement disorder."

Sea Buckhorn

Sea Buckhorn Extract Has a Protective Role Against Haldol-induced Orofacial Dyskinesia

Batool, Farhat, et al., "Protective Effects of Aqueous Fruit Extract from Sea Buckthorn (Hippophae Rhamnoides L. Spp. Turkestanica) on Haloperidol-Induced Orofacial Dyskinesia and Neuronal Alterations in the Striatum." *Medical Science Monitor: International Medical Journal of Experimental and Clinical Research* 16, no. 8 (August 2010): BR285–92., Publisher: MEDICAL SCIENCE INTERNATIONAL PUBLISHING; PMID: 20671610

> ➤ "Hippophae rhamnoides fruit extract has a protective role against haloperidol-induced orofacial dyskinesia. Consequently, use of Hippophae rhamnoides as a possible therapeutic agent for the treatment of tardive dyskinesia should be considered."

Spikenard

Spikenard Offers Significant Protection Against Drug-induced Orofacial Dyskinesia

Patil, Rupali A., et al., "Reversal of Reserpine-Induced Orofacial Dyskinesia and Catalepsy by Nardostachys Jatamansi." *Indian Journal of Pharmacology* 44, no. 3 (May 2012): 340–44. Publisher: MEDKNOW PUBLICATIONS PVT LTD. doi:10.4103/0253-7613.96307., PMID: 22701243

> "The study concludes that ANJ and TNJ significantly protected animals against reserpine-induced orofacial dyskinesia as well as catalepsy suggesting its potential value in the treatment of neuroleptic-induced orofacial dyskinesia and Parkinson's disease."

Velvet Bean

Velvet Bean Attenuates Haldol-induced Orofacial Dyskinesia

Pathan, Amjadkhan A., et al., "Mucuna Pruriens Attenuates Haloperidol-Induced Orofacial Dyskinesia in Rats." *Natural Product Research* 25, no. 8 (April 2011): 764–71. Publisher: Taylor & Francis Health Sciences; doi:10.1080/14786410902819087., PMID: 20635303

> "The results of the present study suggest thst MEMP by virtue of its free radical scavenging activity prevents neuroleptic-induced TD."

Visual Feedback

TV Monitor Visual Feedback Treatment, Self-Control and DD Promting Behavioral Treatments May Decrease Orofacial Dyskinesia's

Jackson, G. M., et al., "A Comparison of Two Behavioral Treatments in Decreasing the Orofacial Movement of Tardive Dyskinesia." *Biofeedback and Self-Regulation* 8, no. 4 (December 1983): 547–53., Publisher: PLENUM PRESS. PMID: 6675730

> In a study with an elderly female subject, two behavioral treatments were evaluated in terms of their effectiveness in decreasing orofacial movement associated with tardive dyskinesia. Video feedback and discreet-discrete prompting, a self-control procedure using a portable audio signal generator, were compared by means of an alternating treatments experimental design. Video and instructional controls were included in the study. Results indicated that both procedures were effective in decreasing orofacial movement. In addition, during the concluding phase of the study, a prompting card was carried by the subject at all times as a reminder to control mouth movements on an ongoing basis. The concluding phase resulted in generalization of treatment effect to the non-treatment environment. Follow-up sessions indicated maintenance of treatment effects.

Vitamin B

B-vitamins Help Attenuate Haldol-induced Orofacial Dyskinesia

Macêdo, Danielle Silveira, et al., "B Vitamins Attenuate Haloperidol-Induced Orofacial Dyskinesia in Rats: Possible Involvement of Antioxidant Mechanisms." *Behavioural Pharmacology* 22, no. 7 (October 2011): 674–80. Publisher: LIPPINCOTT WILLIAMS & WILKINS; doi:10.1097/FBP.0b013e32834aff6d., PMID: 21918383

> "All groups treated with B vitamins presented a decrease in lipid peroxide formation. The data suggest a promising role for B vitamins in the prevention of OD."

CODEX ALTERNUS

Vitamin C and E

Vitamin C and E have Beneficial Effects against the Development of Orofacial Dyskinesia

> **Faria, Rulian Ricardo,** et al., "Beneficial Effects of Vitamin C and Vitamin E on Reserpine-Induced Oral Dyskinesia in Rats: Critical Role of Striatal Catalase Activity." *Neuropharmacology* 48, no. 7 (June 2005): 993–1001. Publisher: PERGAMON doi:10.1016/j.neuropharm.2005.01.014., PMID: 15857626

> ➤ "These results indicate a beneficial effect of these vitamins and reinforce the critical role of striatal catalase against the development of oral dyskinesia's."

White Mulberry

White Mulberry Leaves Extract Has a Protective Effect Against Haldol-induced Orofacial Dyskinesia

> **Nade, V. S.,** et al., "Protective Effect of Morus Alba Leaves on Haloperidol-Induced Orofacial Dyskinesia and Oxidative Stress." *Pharmaceutical Biology* 48, no. 1 (January 2010): 17–22. Publisher: TAYLOR & FRANCIS THE NETHERLANDS doi:10.3109/13880200903029357., PMID: 20645751

> ➤ "The results suggest a protective effect of Morbus alba extract against haloperidol-induced orofacial dyskinesia and oxidative stress."

Wild Mint

Wild Mint Extract Showed a Beneficiary Effect by Reducing Haldol Induced Adverse Events

> **Basini, Jyothi,** et al., Protective Effect of Methanolic Extract of Metha Arvensis L. Leaves on Haloperidol Induced Extrapyramidal Movement Disorders in Albino Rats." *Pharmanest,* 2251-0541, ISSN 0976-3090

> ➤ High dose of MEMA showed a beneficiary effect by reducing the haloperidol induced adverse effects in albino rats. Thus, supplementation of MEMA along with haloperidol showed a protective effect over oxidative stress induced neuronal damage in albino rats.

Yerba Mate

Yerba Mate Prevents Haldol-induced Orofacial Dyskinesia

Colpo, G., et al., "Ilex Paraguariensis Has Antioxidant Potential and Attenuates Haloperidol-Induced Orofacial Dyskinesia and Memory Dysfunction in Rats." *Neurotoxicity Research* 12, no. 3 (October 2007): 171–80., Publisher: F P/GRAHAM PUBLISHING COMPANY ; PMID: 17967741

> "Rats treated with "mate" did not exhibit an increase in vacuous chewing movements observed in rats treated with haloperidol." The "mate" prevented the effects of haloperidol in this behavioral paradigm."

Yokukansan

Yokukansan is Effective in Reducing Vacuous Chewing Movements in Haldol Treated Rats

Sekiguchi, Kyoji, et al., "Ameliorative Effect of Yokukansan on Vacuous Chewing Movement in Haloperidol-Induced Rat Tardive Dyskinesia Model and Involvement of Glutamatergic System." *Brain Research Bulletin* 89, no. 5–6 (December 1, 2012): 151–58. Publisher: ELSEVIER INC. doi:10.1016/j.brainresbull.2012.08.008., PMID: 22982367

> "Oral administration of YKS (0.1 and 0.5g/kg) once a day for three weeks (21 days) from the 12th week to 15th week ameliorated the haloperidol decanoate-induced increase in VCM in a dose-dependent manner."

Tardive Dystonia Side Effect Treatments

Acupuncture

Acupuncture Has a Positive Effect on Tardive Dystonia

Tani, Makiko, et al., "[Effect of acupuncture treatment for a patient with severe axial dystonia appearing during treatment for schizophrenia]." *Seishin Shinkeigaku Zasshi = Psychiatria Et Neurologia Japonica* 107, no. 8 (2005): 802–10., PMID: 16259404

> "It is suggested that acupuncture treatment has had a positive effect on tardive dystonia including axial dystonia. The patient also achieved improved stability with regards to symptoms of schizophrenia."

Ceruletide

Ceruletide Showed Rapid Amelioration of Tardive Dystonia

Sugawara, M., et al., "Tardive Dystonia and Ceruletide Effects: Case Report." *Progress in Neuro-Psychopharmacology & Biological Psychiatry* 16, no. 1 (January 1992): 127–34., Publisher: ELSEVIER INC. PMID: 1557504

➤ One schizophrenic patient with drug-induced tardive dystonia was treated with ceruletide. After the injection, dystonia showed a tendency toward rapid amelioration in 3 days; meanwhile, however, mental manifestations became exacerbated within 3 weeks. We discuss some aspects of the effects of ceruletide.

Orengedoku-to

Orengedoku-to Augmentation to Yokukan-san Treatment Results in Reduction of Tardive Dystonia

Okamoto, Hideki, et al., "Orengedoku-to Augmentation in Cases Showing Partial Response to Yokukan-San Treatment: A Case Report and Literature Review of the Evidence for Use of These Kampo Herbal Formulae." *Neuropsychiatric Disease and Treatment* 9 (2013): 151–55. Publisher: DOVE MEDICAL PRESS LTD. doi:10.2147/NDT.S38318., PMID: 23378767

➤ A 44-year-old male had started to use methamphetamine at the age of 20. When he was 32 years old, he began to exhibit signs of methamphetamine-induced psychotic disorder accompanied by perceptional delusions and auditory hallucinations and started to take antipsychotic medication irregularly. After twice serving prison time, the patient stopped using methamphetamine and began taking 6mg of risperidone regularly at the age of 42, which caused severe tardive dystonia affecting his whole body. His tardive dystonia was refractory to conventional medications such as the maximum doses of tizanidine—a centrally acting skeletal muscle relaxant—benzodiazepines, and anticholinerigic drugs, as well as other atypical antipsychotics like 10mg of olanzapine or 30mg of aripiprazole. When he arrived at our hospital he was unable to sit still in the waiting room. In addition, he had been irritable and aggressive toward his mother, who lived with him, which often resulted in destruction of property at the home. When yokukan-san (7.5g/day) was added to his conventional medication, his involuntary movements were reduced by 30% after 2 weeks. Then, when orengedoku-to (7.5g/day) augmentation was started after 4 weeks, the tardive dystonia was reduced by 80% after 6 weeks. He was able to sit on the same bench with other patients in the waiting room for the first time in 2 years and property destruction became much less common occurrence, although the attitude toward his mother remained abrupt.

Shakuyaku-Kanzo-to

Shakuyaku-Kanzo-to is as Effective as Drugs in the Treatment of Dystonia

Ota, Takafumi, et al., "Effects of Shakuyaku-Kanzo-to on Extrapyramidal Symptoms During Antipsychotic Treatment: A Randomized, Open-Label Study." *Journal of Clinical Psychopharmacology* 35, no. 3 (June 2015): 304–7. doi:10.1097/JCP.0000000000000312. PMID: 25839338

➤ Twenty of the 22 patients completed the study (10 patients in the shakuyaku-kanzo-to group and 10 patients in the biperiden group). There was a time effect on the Drug-Induced Extrapyramidal Symptom Scale total score ($P < 0.01$), suggesting that both shakuyaku-kanzo-to and biperiden decreased EPS. Notably, there was a time × drug interaction in dystonia, suggesting that shakuyaku-kanzo-to had a greater effect on dystonia compared with biperiden. No significant changes were observed in plasma homovanillic acid or serum prolactin levels after 2 weeks of treatment in either group. The effects of shakuyaku-kanzo-to on abnormal muscle tonus and dopamine D2 receptors may have contributed to improve EPS. These results suggest that shakuyaku-kanzo-to may be useful in decreasing EPS, especially dystonia, in patients undergoing treatment with antipsychotic agents.

Vitamin E

Vitamin E Substantially Improves Tardive Dystonia

Dannon, P. N., et al., "Vitamin E Treatment in Tardive Dystonia." *Clinical Neuropharmacology* 20, no. 5 (October 1997): 434–37., Publisher: LIPPINCOTT WILLIAMS & WILKINS ; PMID: 9331519

> "We present a case of one young man with tardive dystonia secondary to neuroleptic treatment, whose condition substantially improved with treatment by 1200mg/d(IU) of vitamin E."

Parkinsonian Side Effect Treatments

DHEA

DHEA Supplementation is Effective for Parkinsonian Symptoms in Schizophrenics Treated with Antipsychotics

Nachshoni, Tali, et al., "Improvement of Extrapyramidal Symptoms Following Dehydroepiandrosterone (DHEA) Administration in Antipsychotic Treated Schizophrenia Patients: A Randomized, Double-Blind Placebo Controlled Trial." *Schizophrenia Research* 79, no. 2–3 (November 15, 2005): 251–56. Publisher: ELSEVIER BV doi:10.1016/j.schres.2005.07.029., PMID: 16126372

> Recent investigation in schizophrenia indicated dehydroepiandrosterone (DHEA) levels to be inversely correlated with extrapyramidal symptomatology (EPS). This study thus investigates the effect of DHEA administration on medication-induced EPS. Inpatients with schizophrenia or schizoaffective disorder were randomized in double-blind fashion to receive either 100 mg DHEA or placebo in addition to a constant dosage of antipsychotic medication. Parkinsonism showed a favorable effect of DHEA with a significant time effect ($p < 0.0001$), as well as a significant group by time interaction ($p < 0.05$) and with no change noted on akathisia. Change of DHEA blood levels was negatively associated with change of Parkinsonism ($p < 0.05$) as well as with change of

CODEX ALTERNUS

total EPS ratings (p < 0.05). DHEA appears to demonstrate a significant effect on EPS, with improvement observed particularly in Parkinsonian symptoms.

Kami-shoyo-san

Kampo Kami-shoyo-san is Effective for Antipsychotic-induced Parkinsonism

Ishikawa, T., et al., "Effectiveness of the Kampo Kami-Shoyo-San (TJ-24) for Tremor of Antipsychotic-Induced Parkinsonism." *Psychiatry and Clinical Neurosciences* 54, no. 5 (October 2000): 579–82. Publisher: BLACKWELL PUBLISHING ASIA; doi:10.1046/j.1440-1819.2000.00756.x., PMID: 11043809

> "The results showed a statistical significant reduction in tremor after administration of kami-shoyo-san, with 62.5% patients showing improvements of one point or more."

Kava Kava

Kava Kava Extract Attenuates Extrapyramidal Side Effects of Neuroleptic Drugs

Boerner, Reinhard J., et al., "Attenuation of Neuroleptic-Induced Extrapyramidal Side Effects by Kava Special Extract WS 1490." *Wiener Medizinische Wochenschrift (1946)* 154, no. 21–22 (November 2004): 508–10., Publisher: Bei L.W. Seidel & Sohn; PMID: 15638068

> We studied at 42 patients (17 female, 25 male) with different psychiatric diagnoses, who were pretreated by neuroleptics, the efficacy and tolerability of Kava special extract WS 1490 on extrapyramidal side effects. In both patient and physician questionnaires as well as in the physicians global ratings, significant improvements were found for all extrapyramidal signs and symptoms recorded. The concomitant intake of WS 1490 was well tolerated by the patients. The findings of this observational study suggest that extrapyramidal side effects of neuroleptic drugs may be attenuated by Kava special extract WS 1490.

Magnesium-B6

Magnesium-B6 Treatment Results in a Marked Reduction of Extrapyramidal Disorders

Panteleeva, G. P., et al., "[Cerebrolysin and magnesium-B6 in the treatment of side effects of psychotropic drugs]." *Zhurnal Nevrologii I Psikhiatrii Imeni S.S. Korsakova / Ministerstvo Zdravookhraneniia I Meditsinskoĭ Promyshlennosti Rossiĭskoĭ Federatsii, Vserossiĭskoe Obshchestvo Nevrologov [i] Vserossiĭskoe Obshchestvo Psikhiatrov* 99, no. 1 (1999): 37–41., Publisher: Media Sfera; PMID: 11530457

> 51 patients were observed. Schizophrenia was diagnosed in 31 patients and endogenous depression in 20 cases. All the patients had extrapyramidal and somato-vegetative side

effects of neuroleptics and antidepressive drugs, and were resistant to conventional corrective therapy for at least a period of 3 weeks. In addition to current treatment of both basic disease and adverse effects, cerebrolysin was administered (5-10 ml i.v./dr, during 28 days) and magme B6 (20-30 ml per os during 21 days). By the treatment endpoint either moderate or marked reduction of extrapyramidal disorders (according to ESRS) was observed in 74.4% of patients treated by cerebrolysin and in 72.2% treated by magne B6; somato-vegetative adverse effects reduced (by SARS) in 85.8% and in 83.8% respectively. Both drugs showed equally high efficacy against hyperkinetic and cardiovascular side effects (symptoms relief was in 59-62% and 65-69%, respectively). Cerebrolysin is more preferable in cases of side vegetative events, dysomnia and dysuria; magne B6 was more effective in correction of akineto-hypertonic and hyperkinetic-hypertonic syndromes as well as in cholinolytic side effects.

Red Rice Bran Oil

Red Rice Bran Oil Effectivly Attenuates Haldol Induced Parkinsonian Symptoms

Naz, Farah, et al. "Suppression and the Treatment of Haloperidol Induced Extrapyramidal Side Effects and Anxiety Syndrome by the Coadministration of Red Rice Bran Oil in Rats." *International Journal of Endorsing Health Sciences Research*, Volume 2, Issue 2, December 2014

> The present study shows that haloperidol induced parkinsonian like effects following the administration of red rice bran oil were attenuated. This can be explained in terms of positive effects of tocotrienols, tocopherols and omega 3 rich nutrients that are found in red rice bran oil. The present results are consistent with the previous studies which suggest the use of red rice bran oil in nutraceutics as it is thought to be more effective in treating haloperidol induced deficits i.e. parkinsonian like symptoms and tardive dyskinesia. A manifest and remarkable use of red rice bran oil is to treat the haloperidol induced tardive VCMs, thereby attenuating the facial musculature and involuntary movements.

Vitamin B6

Vitamin B6 May Be Efficient as a Treatment for Tardive Dyskinesia and Parkinsonism

Miodownik, Chanoch, et al., "[Vitamin B6 add-on therapy in treatment of schizophrenic patients with psychotic symptoms and movement disorders]." *Harefuah* 142, no. 8–9 (September 2003): 592–96, 647., Publisher: HA-HISTADRUT; PMID: 14518160

> "The authors suggest that vitamin B6 may be efficient as a treatment for tardive dyskinesia and parkinsonism induced by neuroleptic agents."

Vitamin B6 Improves Drug-induced Parkinsonism and Psychosis

Sandyk, R., et al., "Pyridoxine Improves Drug-Induced Parkinsonism and Psychosis in a Schizophrenic Patient." *The International Journal of Neuroscience* 52, no. 3–4 (June 1990): 225–32., Publisher: TAYLOR & FRANCIS INC; PMID: 2269609

> ➢ A schizophrenia patient with severe neuroleptic-induced Parkinsonism and Tardive Dyskinesia is presented in whom administration of pyridoxine (vitamin B6) (100mg/d) resulted in a dramatic and persistant attenuation of the movement disorder as well as a reduction of psychoatic behavior.

Vitamin B12

Acute Onset of Extrapyramidal Symptom Can Be a Manifestation of Vitamin B 12 Deficiency

Joy, M. A., et al., "Vitamin B12 Deficiency Presenting with an Acute Reversible Extrapyramidal Syndrome." *Neurology India* 53, no. 1 (March 2005): 120., Publisher: Medknow Publications and Media Pvt, Ltd. PMID: 15805674

> ➢ In conclusion, acute onset extrapyramidal syndrome can be a rare manifestation of vitamin B12 deficiency, which is reversible with therapy. Serum B12 levels should be checked in patients who do not have an obvious cause for an acute extrapyramidal syndrome.

Vitamin B12 Deficiency Presenting With an Acute Reversible Extrapyramidal Syndrome

Kumar, S., et al., "Vitamin B12 Deficiency Presenting with an Acute Reversible Extrapyramidal Syndrome." *Neurology India* 52, no. 4 (December 2004): 507–9., Publisher: Medknow Publications and Media Pvt, Ltd. PMID: 15626849

> ➢ Vitamin B12 deficiency usually presents with pernicious anemia or various neuropsychiatric manifestations. Commonly seen neuropsychiatric manifestations include large fiber neuropathy, myelopathy, (subacute combined degeneration of the spinal cord), dementia, cerebellar ataxia, optic atrophy, psychosis, and mood disorders. The present report highlights an unusual presentation of vitamin B12 deficiency-acute onset extrapyramidal syndrome in a 55-year-old man. The patient presented with a 10 day history of slowness of all activities including a slow gait, mild tremors of hands and low volume speech. On examination, he had features of mask-like facies, reduced blink rate and cogwheel rigidity. He was investigated for possible causes and was found to have features of vitamin B12 deficiency. Other causes for acute onset parkinsonism were excluded by appropriate investigations. He showed a dramatic improvement following treatment with intramuscular vitamin B12 injections. At five-year follow-up, he was found to be functionally independent with no neurological deficits.

CODEX ALTERNUS

Vitamin B12 and Folate

Vitamin B12 and Folate Deficiency Cause Psychotic Disorder and Extrapyramidal Symptoms in a 12 year-old Boy

> **Dogan, Murat,** et al., "Psychotic Disorder and Extrapyramidal Symptoms Associated with Vitamin B12 and Folate Deficiency." *Journal of Tropical Pediatrics* 55, no. 3 (June 2009): 205–7. Publisher: OXFORD UNIVERSITY PRESS; doi:10.1093/tropej/fmn112., PMID: 19095695

➢ Vitamin B12 and folate deficiency causing neuropsychiatric and thrombotic manifestations, such as peripheral neuropathy, subacute combined degeneration of cord, dementia, ataxia, optic atrophy, catatonia, psychosis, mood disturbances, myocardial infarction and portal vein thrombosis are well known. This present report highlights an unusual presentation of vitamin B12 deficiency-psychotic disorder, extrapyramidal symptoms in a 12-year-old boy. His symptoms responded to parenteral vitamin B12 therapy. So with this report we emphasized that serum vitamin B12 and folate levels should be measured, especially in those patients who present with other known neuropsychiatric features of vitamin B12 and folate deficiency.

Vitamin C and Zinc

Vitamin C and Zinc Deficiency Have Been Known to Cause Parkinsonism and Supplementation May Reverese the Tremors

> **Quiroga, Martha J.**, et al., "Ascorbate- and Zinc-Responsive Parkinsonism." *The Annals of Pharmacotherapy* 48, no. 11 (November 2014): 1515–20. doi:10.1177/1060028014545356. PMID: 25070397

➢ To report a case of Parkinsonism rapidly responsive to intravenous replacement of vitamin C and zinc. A 66-year-old man with Parkinsonism, pleural effusion, and bipolar disorder was found to have low serum vitamin C and zinc levels. Intravenous replacement of these micronutrients led to resolution of the movement disorder in less than 24 hours. Discussion: Parkinsonism has been associated with vitamin C deficiency, and recent cases of scurvy complicated by Parkinsonism have responded well to intravenous replacement of vitamin C. In this case, deficiency of zinc may have contributed to the development of a movement disorder. The likely pathophysiology of, and treatment recommendations for, Parkinsonism linked to deficiencies of vitamin C and zinc are reviewed. Conclusions: Whereas vitamin C has a strong link with Parkinsonism, the potential role of zinc has only been suspected. This case report highlights some of the potential links between zinc deficiency and Parkinsonism.

Vitamin E

Vitamin E Reduces Neuroleptic-induced Parkinsonism

Dorfman-Etrog, P., et al., "The Effect of Vitamin E Addition to Acute Neuroleptic Treatment on the Emergence of Extrapyramidal Side Effects in Schizophrenic Patients: An Open Label Study." *European Neuropsychopharmacology: The Journal of the European College of Neuropsychopharmacology* 9, no. 6 (December 1999): 475–77., Publisher: ELSEVIER BV PMID: 10625114

> ➤ "Addition of vitamin E to neuroleptics may reduce the severity of acute neuroleptic-induced Parkinsonism (NIP) in schizophrenic patients."

Prolactin Lowering Substances

Jasmine

Jasmin Flower Extract Has a Significant Drop in Serum Prolactin in Women on Antipsychotic Drugs

Finny, Philip, et al., "Jasmine Flower Extract Lowers Prolactin." *Tropical Doctor* 45, no. 2 (April 2015): 118–22. doi:10.1177/0049475514560212., PMID: 25505191

> ➤ Ten out of 35 women had a significant drop in the serum prolactin while on the JFE. The non-responders to JFE were on higher doses of antipsychotic drugs. The main side effect was a transient and mild burning sensation in the nose. A cost analysis favoured JFE over dopamine agonists. JFE contains a prolactin-lowering substance which needs further characterisation.

Wuji Powder

Wuji Powder and Abilify Both Lowered Prolactin in Schizophrenics with Amenorrhea

Xia, Shi-Yan, et al., "[Treatment of antipsychotic drug-induced phlegm dampness type amenorrhea by Wuji Powder and a small dose aripiprazole: a clinical study]." *Zhongguo Zhong Xi Yi Jie He Za Zhi Zhongguo Zhongxiyi Jiehe Zazhi = Chinese Journal of Integrated Traditional and Western Medicine / Zhongguo Zhong Xi Yi Jie He Xue Hui, Zhongguo Zhong Yi Yan Jiu Yuan Zhu Ban* 34, no. 12 (December 2014): 1440–43., PMID: 25632742

> ➤ Both WP and aripiprazole could lower high prolactin levels of schizophrenics with phlegm dampness type amenorrhea. They showed equivalent efficacy. But WP showed more obvious effect in reducing obesity indices.

CODEX ALTERNUS

Bradykinesia Side Effect Treatments

Nicotine Patches

Nicotine Patches Effectively Lowered Bradykinesia-rigidity in 30 Haldol Treated Patients

Yang, Yen Kuang, et al., "Nicotine Decreases Bradykinesia-Rigidity in Haloperidol-Treated Patients with Schizophrenia." *Neuropsychopharmacology: Official Publication of the American College of Neuropsychopharmacology* 27, no. 4 (October 2002): 684–86. doi:10.1016/S0893-133X(02)00325-1., PMID: 12377405

> ➢ We applied nicotine 21 mg and matching placebo transdermal patches to thirty haloperidol-treated patients with schizophrenia who smoked. Clinical assessments of bradykinesia-rigidity were lower during nicotine patch administration than during placebo patch administration.

Tardive Oculogric Spasm Side Effect Treatments

Vitamin E

Vitamin E is a Successful Treatment of Tardive Oculogric Spasms

Coupland, N., et al., "Successful Treatment of Tardive Oculogyric Spasms with Vitamin E." *Journal of Clinical Psychopharmacology* 15, no. 4 (August 1995): 285–86., Publisher: LIPPINCOTT WILLIAMS & WILKINS; PMID: 7593713

> ➢ "The baseline frequencies of episodes accorded with his history and their number fell substantially within a month on vitamin E, 1200 IU daily." "A trial of vitamin E seems merited in oculogric spasms that have not responded to standard approaches...."

Neuroleptic Malignant Syndrome Side Effect Treatment

Vitamin E and Vitamin B6

Vitamin E Plus Vitamin B6 for Supportive Management of Neuroleptic Malignant Syndrome

Dursun, S. M., et al., "High-Dose Vitamin E plus Vitamin B6 Treatment of Risperidone-Related Neuroleptic Malignant Syndrome." *Journal of Psychopharmacology (Oxford, England)* 12, no. 2 (1998): 220–21., Publisher: SAGE SCIENCE PRESS (UK); PMID: 9694035

> " This patient responded satisfactorily to the supportive management and vit E plus vit B6."

Catalepsy Side Effect Treatments

Bark Cloth Tree

Agbaje, Esther O., et al., "Antidepressant, Anxiolytic, and Anticataleptic Effects of Aqueous Leaf Extract of Antiaris Toxicaria Lesch. (Moraceae) in Mice: Possible Mechanisms of Actions." *Journal of Basic and Clinical Physiology and Pharmacology*, February 27, 2014. doi:10.1515/jbcpp-2013-0054.

> Haloperidol (1 mg/kg i.p.) induced cataleptic behavior in mice, which was reversed by A. toxicaria (300 mg/kg) (p<0.001) treatment. Conclusions: The results suggest that A. toxicaria possesses an antidepressant-like effect involving interaction with α1-adrenoceptor, D2 dopamine receptor, and nitrergic pathway; an anxiolytic-like effect linked to the benzodiazepine system; and a neuroprotective effect.

Bermuda Grass

Aqueous Extract of Bermuda Grass was found to Reduce Reserpine-Induced Catalepsy Significantly

Sharma, Neha, et al. "Effect of Aqueous Extract of Cynodon Dactylon on Reserpine Induced Catalepsy." *International Journal of Pharmacy and Pharmaceutical Sciences*, Vol.3, Issue 4, 2011

> "The extract was found to reduce catalepsy significantly (p<0.001) as compared to the reserpine treated mice showing greater effect at 300 mg/kg i.p. dose. Thus the present study reveals the anti-cataleptic activity of AECD."

Cannabidiol

Cannabidiol (CBD) Can Attenuate Catalepsy Induced by Pharmacological Mechanisms

Gomes, Felipe V., et al., "Cannabidiol Attenuates Catalepsy Induced by Distinct Pharmacological Mechanisms via 5-HT1A Receptor Activation in Mice." *Progress in Neuro-Psychopharmacology & Biological Psychiatry* 46 (October 1, 2013): 43–47. Publisher: ELSEVIER INC. doi:10.1016/j.pnpbp.2013.06.005., PMID: 23791616

> "These findings indicate that CBD can attenuate catalepsy caused by different mechanisms (D2 blockade, NOS inhibition and CB1 agonism) via 5-HT1A

receptor activation, suggesting that it could be useful in the treatment of striatal disorders."

Devil's Weed

Devil's Weed Can Prevent Catalepsy Induced By Haldol

Nishchal, B. S., et al., "Effect of Tribulus Terrestris on Haloperidol-Induced Catalepsy in Mice." *Indian Journal of Pharmaceutical Sciences* 76, no. 6 (December 2014): 564–67., PMID: 25593394

> ➤ The result of the present study demonstrates Tribulus terrestris has a protective effect against haloperidol-induced catalepsy, which is comparable to the standard drug used for the same purpose. Our study indicates Tribulus terrestris can be used to prevent haloperidol-induced extrapyramidal side effects.

Holy Basil

Holy Basil Protected Animals form Catalepsy Induced by Haldol as Effectively as Standard Drugs

Pemminati, S, et al., "Effect of Ethanolic Leaf Extract of Ocimum Sanctum on Haloperidol-Induced Catalepsy in Albino Mice." *Indian Journal of Pharmacology* 39, no. 2 (2007): 87. doi:10.4103/0253-7613.32526.

> ➤ In the present study, OS protected mice from catalepsy induced by haloperidol as effectively as the standard drugs, scopolamine and ondansetron. The protective effect of OS against HIC is consistent with our earlier report on anticataleptic effect of a polyherbal product, NR-ANX-C, in which OS is one of the components. Earlier behavioral studies in rodents have suggested that OS facilitates activation of dopaminergic neurons. Thus, the anticataleptic effect of OS might be due to both its dopamine facilitatory and antioxidant properties. The active principle of the ethanolic leaf extract of OS contains 2.7% ursolic acid, which has antioxidant properties and gives remarkable protection against lipid peroxidation. However, further studies are required to confirm the exact mechanism of action. Our results suggest that OS can be used as an alternative / adjuvant drug in preventing and treating the extrapyramidal side effects of antipsychotic agents in clinical practice.

NR-ANX-C

Polyherbal Formula NR-ANX-C has a Significant Reduction on Catalepsy

Nair, Vinod, et al., "Effect of NR-ANX-C (a Polyherbal Formulation) on Haloperidol Induced Catalepsy in Albino Mice." *The Indian Journal of Medical Research* 126, no. 5 (November 2007): 480–84., Publisher: INDIAN COUNCIL OF MEDICAL RESEARCH; PMID: 18160755

➢ In our study, maximum reduction in cataleptic score was observed in NR-ANX-C (25mg/kg) treated group. The maximum reduction in SOD activity was also observed in the same group. These findings suggest a possible involvement of the antioxidant potential of NRANX-C in alleviating haloperidol induced catalepsy.

Quercetin

Quercetin is a Potential Drug Candidate for the Treatment of Neuroleptic-induced Extrapyramidal Side Effects

Naidu, P. S., et al., "Quercetin, a Bioflavonoid, Reverses Haloperidol-Induced Catalepsy." *Methods and Findings in Experimental and Clinical Pharmacology* 26, no. 5 (June 2004): 323–26., Publisher: PROUS SCIENCE; PMID: 15319809

➢ "In conclusion, the findings of the present study strongly suggest that quercetin can be screened as a potential drug candidate or as an adjuvant for the treatment of neuroleptic-induced extrapyramidal side effects."

Shilajit

Shilajit Prevented Catalepsy Better than Scopolamine on Repeated Administration

Godpalakrishna, H.N., et al., "Role of Shilajit in Murine Model of Haloperidol Induced Catalepsy." *Drug Invention Today,* Jun 2010, Vol. 2, Issue 6, p300-302

➢ In the present study, pretreatment of aqueous extract of shilajit protected the mice better from catalepsy induced from haloperidol as effectively as the standard drug scolpolamine and in fact better than scopolamine on repeated administration. Out study suggests that shilajit can be explored as an adjuvant drug in preventing and treating the extrapyramidal side effects of antipsychotic agents in clinical practice.

Spikenard

Spikenard Has Potential in Reversing Haldol-induced Catalepsy

Rasheed, A. S., et al., "Evaluation of Toxicological and Antioxidant Potential of Nardostachys Jatamansi in Reversing Haloperidol-Induced Catalepsy in Rats." *International Journal of General Medicine* 3 (2010): 127–36., Publisher: Dove Medical Press; PMID: 20531975

> "Our findings of behavioral studies and biochemical estimations show that Nardostachys jatamansi reversed the haloperidol-induced catalepsy in rats."

Ursolic Acid

Ursolic Acid Has a Protective Effect Against Haldol-induced Catalepsy

Permminati, Sudhakar, et al., "Effect of Chronic Administration of Ursolic Acid on Haloperidol Induced Catalepsy in Albino Mice." *Drug Invention Today*, Jun 2011, Vol. 3, Issue 6, p83-85

> The results suggest that UA has a protective effect against haloperidol-induced catalepsy, which is comparable to the standard drug used for the same purpose. Our study indicates UA could be used to prevent neuroleptic drug-induced extrapyramidal side effects.

Tic Side Effect Treatments

Magnesium and Vitamin B6

Magnesium and Vitamin B6 are Effective in Reducing the Tic Score in Children with Tourette syndrome

Garcia-Lopez, Rafael, et al., "New Therapeutic Approach to Tourette Syndrome in Children Based on a Randomized Placebo-Controlled Double-Blind Phase IV Study of the Effectiveness and Safety of Magnesium and Vitamin B6." *Trials* 10 (2009): 16. Publisher: BIOMED CENTRAL LTD. doi:10.1186/1745-6215-10-16., PMID: 19284553

> "The total tic score decreased from 26.7 (t0) to 12.9 (t4) and the total effect on the YGTSS was a reduction from 58.1 to 18.8."

Glorybower Leaf

Glorybower Leaf Extract Dramatically Reduces Chronic Motor Tics

Fan, Pi-Chuan, et al., "Intractable Chronic Motor Tics Dramatically Respond to Clerodendrum Inerme (L) Gaertn." *Journal of Child Neurology* 24, no. 7 (July 2009): 887–90. Publisher: B.C./DECKER INC; doi:10.1177/0883073808331088., PMID: 19617461

> Tics are characterized by involuntary, sudden, rapid, repetitive, nonrhythmic, stereotyped movements or phonic productions. Those who suffer from either motor or phonic tics, but not both, for more than 1 year are diagnosed with chronic tic disorder. Several pharmacological interventions have been proposed for the treatment of tic disorder. Dopamine D2 receptor blockers and dopamine depletors are thought to be the most effective ones clinically. However, such treatments are suboptimal in terms of effectiveness and side effects, such as body weight gain and extrapyramidal symptoms. We report on a 13-year-old girl, with chronic motor tic disorder refractory to multiple anti-tic therapies, who showed dramatic improvement and remission after taking the crude leaf extract of Clerodendrum inerme (L) Gaertn. No side effects were observed during a follow-up of more than 2 years. To the best of our knowledge, this is the first report on the anti-tic effect of Clerodendrum inerme.

Akathisia Side Effect Treatments

Gluten-free Diet

Gluten-free Diet in People with Schizophrenia Leads to Improvement in Extrapyramidal Side Effects and Akathisia

Jackson, Jessica, et al., "A Gluten-Free Diet in People with Schizophrenia and Anti-Tissue Transglutaminase or Anti-Gliadin Antibodies." *Schizophrenia Research* 140, no. 1–3 (September 2012): 262–63. Publisher: ELSEVIER BV; doi:10.1016/j.schres.2012.06.011., PMID: 22771303

> Our results suggest that a GFD in people with antibodies to anti-tTG or AGA may lead to symptom improvements in schizophrenia as well as robust improvements in extrapyramidal side effects (EPS). Both participants saw notable improvements on the BPRS and SANS. Both participants also had improvements in akathisia and EPS with participant B having notable changes in both at the end of the trial. The data shows that a GFD can be maintained in individuals with schizophrenia with no negative effects on behavior or attitude and no need for medication changes. Overall the diet was easily maintained, however it is recognized that much education would be needed to help patients understand the importance of a GFD and the gluten content of food and snacks.

Iron

Minor Evidence that Iron Supplementation May aid in the Treatment of Akathisia

Gold, R., et al., "Is There a Rationale for Iron Supplementation in the Treatment of Akathisia? A Review of the Evidence." *The Journal of Clinical Psychiatry* 56, no. 10 (October 1995): 476–83., Publisher: PHYSICIANS POSTGRADUATE PRESS, INC. PMID: 7559375

> The rationale for iron supplementation in the treatment of akathisia is relatively weak, and there are potentially adverse long-term consequences as outlined in our review. More research is required to directly measure the level of iron in the brains of patients with akathisia…..before such therapeutic intervention can be recommended.

Improvement of Akathisia with Intravenous Iron in Iron Deficient Patient

Cotter, Paul E., et al., "Improvement in Neuroleptic-Induced Akathisia with Intravenous Iron Treatment in a Patient with Iron Deficiency." *Journal of Neurology, Neurosurgery, and Psychiatry* 78, no. 5 (May 2007): 548. Publisher: B M J PUBLISHING GROUP doi:10.1136/jnnp.2006.101014., PMID: 17435196

> "The close temporal relationship between administration of intravenous iron deficiency can contribute to the development or persistence of akathisia in some patients. Iron repletion may be valuable in such cases, although this requires further evaluation."

Neuroleptic Drugs May Chelate Iron and Cause Akathisia—Replenishment May Reverse This Mechanism

Chengappa, K. N., et al., "Iron for Chronic and Persistent Akathisia?" *The Journal of Clinical Psychiatry* 54, no. 8 (August 1993): 320–21., Publisher: PHYSICIANS POSTGRADUATE PRESS, INC. PMID: 7902835

> Thus, neuroleptic drugs, which are known to chealate iron, may strip iron from the D2 receptor, causing akathisia in humans. Oral replenishment of iron may reverse this mechanism, thereafter allowing homeostatic mechanisms to take over. There is evidence that serum iron and transferrin decrease significantly in patients receiving neuroleptic drugs who experience akathisia but not in nonakathisic patients.

L-tryptophan and Niacin

L-Tryptophan and Niacin May Reduce Akathisia

Kramer, M. S., et al., "L-Tryptophan in Neuroleptic-Induced Akathisia." *Biological Psychiatry* 27, no. 6 (March 15, 1990): 671–72., Publisher: ELSEVIER INC. PMID: 1969752

> Akathisia scores decreased an average of 39% of base line. Some patients and referring physicians felt that L-tryptophan was quite helpful and requested its continuation.. L-tryptophan, along with nicotinic acid appeared to reduce both objective and subjective components of akathisia in most patients.

N-acetylcysteine

N-Acetylcysteine has a Moderate Benefit in the Treatment of Akathisia

CODEX ALTERNUS

Berk, Michael, et al., "N-Acetyl Cysteine as a Glutathione Precursor for Schizophrenia--a Double-Blind, Randomized, Placebo-Controlled Trial." *Biological Psychiatry* 64, no. 5 (September 1, 2008): 361–68. Publisher: ELSEVIER INC. doi:10.1016/j.biopsych.2008.03.004., PMID: 18436195

➤ "A moderate benefit of NAC at end point for akathisia was also evident on the BAS, which approached significance."

Placebo

Placebo Approach to Tardive Akathisia Sometimes is of Value

Remington, G., et al., "Placebo Response in Refractory Tardive Akathisia." *Canadian Journal of Psychiatry. Revue Canadienne De Psychiatrie* 38, no. 4 (May 1993): 248–50., PMID: 8100184

➤ "A double-blind, crossover drug trial with a patient with treatment-resistant tardive akathisia is described. The finding of a placebo response was unexpected, but emphasizes the value of such an approach in refractory cases."

Relaxation

Structured Relaxation May Be a Promising Alternative to Traditional Treatment for Akathisia

---

Hansen, Lars K., et al., "Structured Relaxation in the Treatment of Akathisia: Case Series." *Neuropsychiatric Disease and Treatment* 6 (2010): 269–71, Publisher: DOVE MEDICAL PRESS LTD. PMID: 20520790

➤ "....the relaxation program appears to be a promising alternative to traditional treatment of akathisia. The patients appreciated the relaxation sessions but none of them managed to carry it out on their own without professional encouragement."

Vitamin B6

High Dose Vitamin B6 is an Available Treatment for Neuroleptic-induced Akathisia

---

Lerner, Vladimir, et al., "Vitamin B6 Treatment in Acute Neuroleptic-Induced Akathisia: A Randomized, Double-Blind, Placebo-Controlled Study." *The Journal of Clinical Psychiatry* 65, no. 11 (November 2004): 1550–54., Publisher: PHYSICIANS POSTGRADUATE PRESS, INC. PMID: 15554771

➤ The vitamin B6-treated patients in comparison with the placebo group showed a significant on the subjective-awareness of restlessness, subjective distress, and global subscales of BAS. Our preliminary results indicate that high doses of vitamin B6 may be useful additions to the available treatments for NIA....

Miodownik, Chanoch, et al., "Vitamin B6 versus Mianserin and Placebo in Acute Neuroleptic-Induced Akathisia: A Randomized, Double-Blind, Controlled Study." *Clinical Neuropharmacology* 29, no. 2 (April 2006): 68–72., Publisher: LIPPINCOTT WILLIAMS & WILKINS; PMID: 16614537

> ➤ "Our results indicate that high doses of B6 and low dose of mianserin may be a useful addition to current treatments of NIA."

Dopaminergic Supersensitivity Side Effect Treatments

Estradiol

Estradiol caused a 2.8-fold Reduction of Dopamine Receptor Affinity for a Typical Antipsychotic

Gattaz, W. F., et al., "[Estradiol inhibits dopamine mediated behavior in rats--an animal model of sex-specific differences in schizophrenia]." *Fortschritte Der Neurologie-Psychiatrie* 60, no. 1 (January 1992): 8–16. Publisher: Harofarma, S.A; doi:10.1055/s-2007-999120., PMID: 1312053

> ➤ "Since oestradiol caused a 2.8-fold reduction of dopamine receptor affinity for sulpiride, we assumed that the behavioural changes caused by oestradiol were accounted for by a down-regulation of the dopaminergic system."

Estradiol can Suppress Haldol-induced Supersensitivity

Bédard, P. J., et al., "Estradiol Can Suppress Haloperidol-Induced Supersensitivity in Dyskinetic Monkeys." *Neuroscience Letters* 64, no. 2 (February 28, 1986): 206–10., Publisher: ELSEVIER IRELAND LTD; PMID: 3960400

> ➤ We have studied a monkey model of lingual dyskinesia, due to midbrain lesion, which is markedly increased by apomorphine. In such animals a single large intramuscular dose of haloperidol (HAL), 1mg/kg, almost completely abolishes the apomorphine potentiation after 24 h, but 15 days later there is is a 5-fold increase in the response to aporphine which we attribute to supersenitivity. Estradiol benzoate (0.15mg/kg, subcutaneously) on days 3, 6, 9, and 12 after HAL completely suppresses the expected rebound supersensitivity to apomorphine. However, the suppression is not seen if the animals have received HAL and estradiol together in the initial treatment.

Estrogen

Estrogen May Down Regulate Brain Dopamine Receptors

CODEX ALTERNUS

Fields, J. Z., et al., "Estrogen Inhibits the Dopaminergic Supersensitivity Induced by Neuroleptics." *Life Sciences* 30, no. 3 (January 18, 1982): 229–34., Publisher: ELSEVIER INC. PMID: 7200183

> ➤ Administration of estrogen to rats during the period of withdrawal from chronic haloperidol attenuated the characteristic increase in apomorphine-induced stereotypy and the increase in (3H) spiroperidol binding. This apparent ability of estrogen to "down-regulate" brain dopamine receptors could lead to useful pharmacological treatments of tardive dyskinesia and possibly of other hyperdopaminergic states.

Estrogen May Attenuate the Development of Dopaminergic Supersensitivity

---

Gordon, J. H., et al., "Antagonism of Dopamine Supersensitivity by Estrogen: Neurochemical Studies in an Animal Model of Tardive Dyskinesia." *Biological Psychiatry* 16, no. 4 (April 1981): 365–71., Publisher: ELSEVIER INC. PMID: 7194695

> ➤ The administration of EB during the withdrawal from chronic haloperidol treatment or the continuous administration of EB decreases or prevents the proliferation of dopamine binding sites in the striatum that normally occur upon withdrawal of these two substances. These results indicate that exogenous estrogens may modulate the number of dopamine receptors in the central nervous system and, as such, may decrease the incidence and/or relieve the symptoms of tardive dyskinesia.

Gordon, J. H., et al., "Modulation of Dopamine Receptor Sensitivity by Estrogen." *Biological Psychiatry* 15, no. 3 (June 1980): 389–96., Publisher: ELSEVIER INC. PMID: 7189674

> ➤ Rats treated chronically with Haldol, and treated daily with EB following the Haldol treatment, showed an attenuation of drug-induced sterotypy. These preliminary data indicate that estrogen can attenuate the development or mask the display of the supersensitive dopamine receptor.

Insulin

Insulin May Attenuate Dopamine Receptor Supersensitivity

Lozovsky, D. B., et al., "Modulation of Dopamine Receptor Supersensitivity by Chronic Insulin: Implication in Schizophrenia." *Brain Research* 343, no. 1 (September 16, 1985): 190–93., Publisher: ELSEVIER BV; PMID: 3899277

> ➤ Haloperidol-induced increases in the number of dopamine receptors, as measured by [3H]spiperone binding to striatal membranes, do not occur in rats repeatedly treated with insulin in doses eliciting pronounced hypoglycemia. Given alone, however, insulin

has no effect on [3H]spiperone binding in normal rats. These findings demonstrate a modulating effect of insulin on brain dopamine receptor sensitization. This effect might be relevant to the mechanism of insulin coma therapy in schizophrenia and is consistent with and supports the dopaminergic hypothesis of this disorder.

Light

Continuous Exposure to Light Leads to Lower Dopaminergic Supersensitivity Function

Abílio, V. C., et al., "Effects of Continuous Exposure to Light on Behavioral Dopaminergic Supersensitivity." *Biological Psychiatry* 45, no. 12 (June 15, 1999): 1622–29., Publisher: ELSEVIER INC. PMID: 10376124

> The supersensitivity ratios were always lower for the animals kept under the LL cycle than those kept under the LD cycle regardless of the behavioral parameter used, suggesting that the development of the doperminergic supersensitvity was lower in animals continuously exposed to light. This effect could also be explained by increased endogenous dopamine availability, which would attenuate the postsynaptic dopaminergic blockade induced by haloperidol and, consequently, the compensatory dopaminergic supersensitivity.

L-Prolyl-L-Leucyl-Glycinamide

L-Prolyl-L-Leucyl-Glycinamide (PLG) Inhibits Haldol Dopamine Receptor Supersensitivity

Chiu, P., et al., "Mesolimbic and Striatal Dopamine Receptor Supersensitivity: Prophylactic and Reversal Effects of L-Prolyl-L-Leucyl-Glycinamide (PLG)." *Peptides* 6, no. 2 (April 1985): 179–83., Publisher: ELSEVIER INC. PMID: 2863809

> Functional supersensitivity of mesolimbic and striatal dopamine receptors has been suggested to contribute to the pathogenesis of schizophrenia and tardive dyskinesia. Using the rodent model of chronic administration of the neuroleptic haloperidol, we investigated the possible desensitizing effects of a tripeptide structurally unrelated to dopamine agonists, L-prolyl-L-leucyl-glycinamide (PLG) on mesolimbic and striatal dopaminergic receptor supersensitivity. Administration of PLG either prior to or after chronic haloperidol, inhibited the supersensitivity of dopamine receptors. The results have implications for pharmacological intervention in preventing tardive dyskinesia and relapse psychosis of schizophrenia.

Melatonin

Melatonin May Revert the Enhancement of Haldol-induced Dopaminergic Supersensitivity

CODEX ALTERNUS

Abílio, Vanessa C., et al., "Effects of Melatonin on Behavioral Dopaminergic Supersensitivity." *Life Sciences* 72, no. 26 (May 16, 2003): 3003–15., Publisher: ELSEVIER INC.; PMID: 12706487

> Acute treatment with melatonin reverted the enhancement of the haloperidol-induced doperminergic supersensitvity produced by concomitant long-term treatment with melatonin, as well as melatonin-induced dopaminergic supersensitvity per se. Our results support previous evidence of antidopaminergic effects of melatonin and demonstrate that repeated administration of this hormone modifies the plasticity of behaviors mediated by central dopaminergic systems.

Nicotine

Chronic Nicotine use Blocks Haldol-induced Increase in D2 Dopamine Receptor Density

Prasad, C., et al., "Chronic Nicotine Use Blocks Haloperidol-Induced Increase in Striatal D2-Dopamine Receptor Density." *Biochemical and Biophysical Research Communications* 159, no. 1 (February 28, 1989): 48–52., Publisher: ACADEMIC PRESS; PMID: 2522303

> Epidemiologic studies have suggested a positive association in man between nicotine use and the incidence of tardive dyskinesia, a disease characterized by dopaminergic supersensitivity after chronic neuroleptic therapy. In rats, repeated administration of neuroleptics results into dopaminerigic supersensitivity and increased density of striatal D2-dopamine receptors. We investigated the effects of 6-week continuous nicotine intake on the neuroleptic (haloperidol)-induced increase in murine striatal D2-dopamine receptor density. Contrary to expectations, our data show that nicotine blocked the increase in D2-dopamine receptor density after neuroleptic administration.

Vitamin E

Attenuation of Dopaminergic Supersensitivity with Vitamin E

Gattaz, W. F., et al., "Vitamin E Attenuates the Development of Haloperidol-Induced Dopaminergic Hypersensitivity in Rats: Possible Implications for Tardive Dyskinesia." *Journal of Neural Transmission. General Section* 92, no. 2–3 (1993): 197–201, Publisher: SPRINGER-VERLAG; PMID: 8369109

> "Within the context of the present experiment vitamin E attenuated the development of behavioral DA-supersensitvity after haloperidol treatment."

CODEX ALTERNUS™

SECTION FIVE

Electroconvulsive Therapy Side Effect Treatments

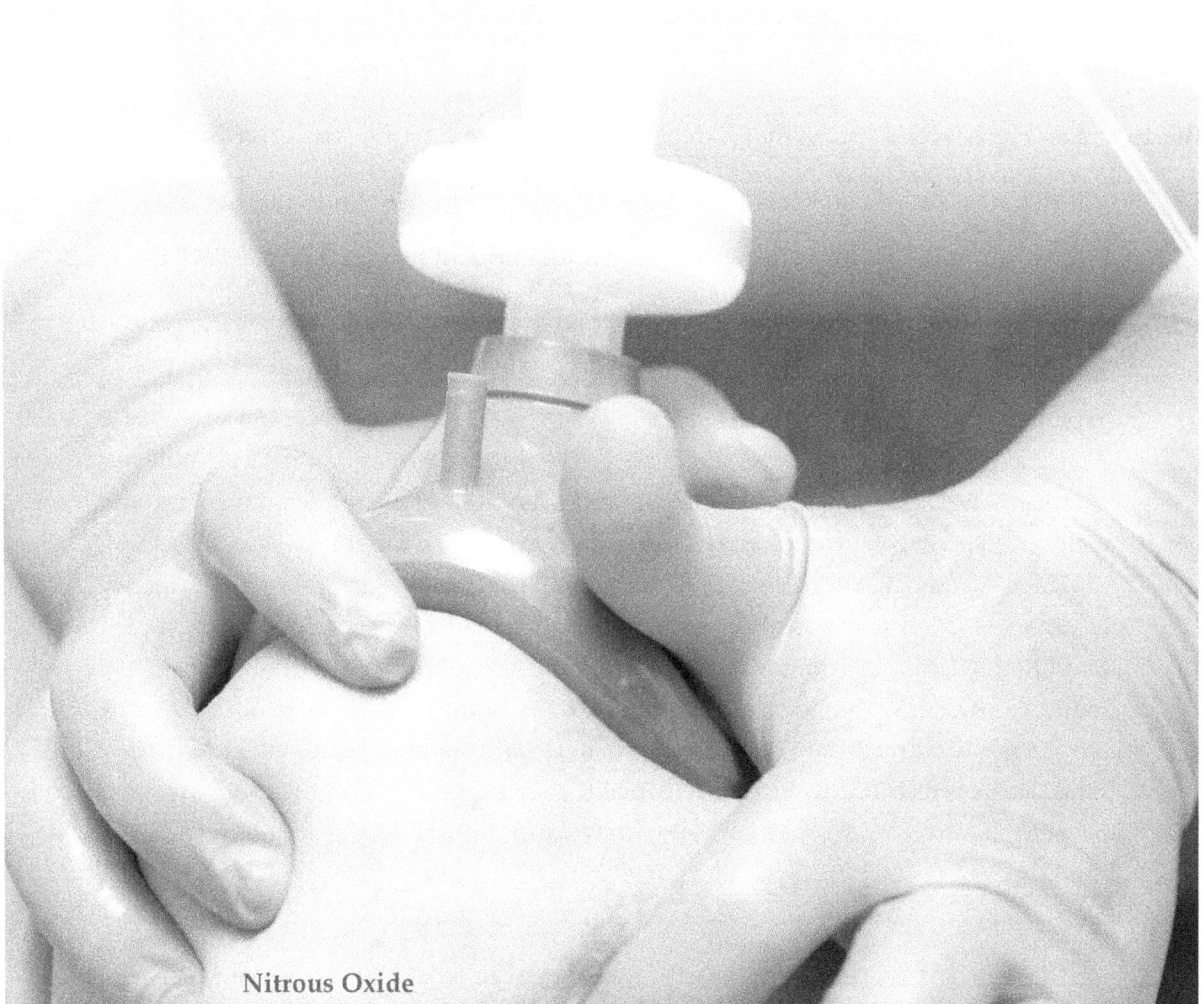

Nitrous Oxide

Brahmi and Mandookaparni

Brahmi and Mandookaparni Attenuate Effects of Electroconvulsive Shock

Andrade, Chittaranjan, et al., "Anti-Amnestic Properties of Brahmi and Mandookaparni in a Rat Model." *Indian Journal of Psychiatry* 48, no. 4 (October 2006): 232–37. Publisher: Indian Psychiatric Society; doi:10.4103/0019-5545.31554., PMID: 20703342

> ➤ Brahmi and Mandookparni do not in themselves improve learning; however, each attenuates the amnestic effects of ECS without showing synergism in this beneficial action. Exercises in research and development are indicated to further investigate the anti-amnestic properties of these herbs, and to identify the specific chemical constituents which have procognitive effects.

BR-16A

BR-16A is an Herbal Medication that Extends Protection against Electroconvulsive Shock Induced Anterograde Amnesia

Joseph, J., et al., "BR-16A Protects against ECS-Induced Anterograde Amnesia." *Biological Psychiatry* 36, no. 7 (October 1, 1994): 478–81., Publisher: ELSEVIER INC. PMID: 7811845

> ➤ BR-16A is an herbal (non allopathic) medication used in India to enhance cognition. In experiment 1, 28 Wistar rats received either BR-16A (200 mg/kg/day) or vehicle alone for 3 weeks. During the third week, the rats were tested for learning in the Hebb Williams complex maze. BR-16A-treated rats showed significantly better learning than did controls. Experiment 2 was conducted identically except that during the second week all of 32 rats additionally received six once-daily electroconvulsive shocks (ECS). An advantage for learning was again demonstrated for the BR-16A group. It is concluded that BR-16A facilitates learning, and that this effect extends to a protection against ECS-induced anterograde amnesia. Cognitive deficits induced by electroconvulsive therapy are a major disadvantage of the treatment and, to-date, no drug has been found to offer satisfactory protection against such deficits. It is suggested that BR-16A may hold promise in the containment of electroconvulsive therapy (ECT)-induced cognitive compromise.

Caffeine

Caffeine Pretreatment Enhances Clinical Efficacy and Reduces Cognitive Effects of ECT

> **Calev, Avraham,** et al., "Caffeine Pretreatment Enhances Clinical Efficacy and Reduces Cognitive Effects of Electroconvulsive Therapy." *Convulsive Therapy* 9, no. 2 (1993): 95–100., Publisher: RAVEN PRESS; PMID: 11941197

> ➢ In an open clinical trial, depressed patients received age-dosed, brief-pulse electroconvulsive therapy (ECT) either with or without 500 mg i.v. caffeine sodium benzoate before each treatment. Caffeine-pretreated patients required fewer ECT treatments, and after three to four treatments, their Hamilton Depression Scale (HDS) scores were significantly lower. At the end of the ECT course, both groups reached the same reduction in HDS scores. Of five memory tests, one showed better performance at the end of the ECT course for the caffeine-pretreated compared with the non-caffeine-pretreated patients. The results argue that caffeine-modified ECT differs from unmodified ECT in speed of response and the effects on cognitive tests.

Caffeine before ECT leads to Clinical Improvement in Patient who was Non-responsive to Treatment

> **Shapira, Baruch,** et al., "Potentiation of Seizure Length and Clinical Response to Electroconvulsive Therapy by Caffeine Pretreatment: A Case Report." *Convulsive Therapy* 1, no. 1 (1985): 58–60., Publisher: RAVEN PRESS; PMID: 11940806

> ➢ A patient with a history of nonresponse to electroconvulsive therapy (ECT) was treated with ECT modified by i.v. caffeine before electrical stimulation for some of the seizures. Seizures preceded by i.v. caffeine were longer, and led to marked clinical improvement. Caffeine pretreatment may be a method to enhance seizure length and efficacy in resistant patients.

Pretreatment with Caffeine Citrate Increases Seizure Duration during ECT

> **Pinkhasov, Aaron,** et al., "Pretreatment With Caffeine Citrate to Increase Seizure Duration During Electroconvulsive Therapy A Case Series." *Journal of Pharmacy Practice*, November 5, 2014, Publisher: SAGE SCIENCE PRESS (US) doi:10.1177/0897190014549838.

> ➢ Of the 12 ECT treatments utilizing caffeine citrate, 9 achieved at least 1 session lasting >30 seconds with an average seizure duration of 35 seconds. Increase in seizure duration ranged from −41% to 276% with an average increase of 48%. Only 3 treatment sessions utilizing caffeine citrate showed no increase in seizure duration. Doses ranged from 120 to 600 mg of both oral and parenteral caffeine citrate. Although increase in seizure duration was achieved for the majority of the ECT sessions, no dose–response correlation could be made. No significant adverse reactions were noted with the use of caffeine citrate during ECT.

Electric Acupuncture

Electric Acupuncture Convulsive Therapy is more efficient than Electroconvulsive Therapy

> **Chongcheng, Xue,** et al., "Electric Acupuncture Convulsive Therapy." *Convulsive Therapy* 1, no. 4 (1985): 242–51., Publisher: RAVEN PRESS; PMID: 11940829

> ➤ In 150 schizophrenic patients, a comparative investigation between electric acupuncture convulsive therapy (EACT) and electroconvulsive therapy (ECT) showed that the current used for eliciting a convulsion in EACT was only 3.6% of that for ECT when the electrodes were placed at acupoints Baihui and Renzhong. EACT is a modification of ECT in which stimulating currents are passed through acupuncture needle electrodes inserted in midline positions. In this study, the efficacy of EACT was better, the somatic and visceral reactions milder, and the incidence of spine fracture and changes in EEG and in memory were less than in ECT. The clinical efficacy of electroconvulsive therapy is seen to depend on changes in midline brain structures.

Galantamine

Galantamine May Be Protective Against Memory Impairment from ECT

> **Matthews, John D.,** et al., "A Double-Blind, Placebo-Controlled Study of the Impact of Galantamine on Anterograde Memory Impairment during Electroconvulsive Therapy." *The Journal of ECT* 29, no. 3 (September 2013): 170–78. Publisher: International Society for ECT and Neurostimulation; doi:10.1097/YCT.0b013e31828b3523., PMID: 23519225

> ➤ Galantamine may be protective against impairment in retention of new learning. Galantamine exhibited minimal adverse effects and was safe when administered during ECT. The present findings require replication by future researchers using larger samples before broad conclusions can be drawn.

Galantamine May Reduce Cognitive Impairment during ECT

> **Matthews, John D.,** et al., "The Impact of Galantamine on Cognition and Mood during Electroconvulsive Therapy: A Pilot Study." *Journal of Psychiatric Research* 42, no. 7 (June 2008): 526–31. Publisher: PERGAMON; doi:10.1016/j.jpsychires.2007.06.002., PMID: 17681545

> ➤ Our data support the hypothesis that galantamine may reduce cognitive impairment during ECT, especially with regards to new learning. In addition, galantamine may also enhance the antidepressant action of ECT. Galantamine was both safe and well tolerated during ECT.

Herbal Treatments

Herbal Medicine for Electroconvulsive Therapy

Andrade, C., et al., "Herbal Treatments for ECS-Induced Memory Deficits: A Review of Research and a Discussion on Animal Models." *The Journal of ECT* 16, no. 2 (June 2000): 144–56., Publisher: International Society for ECT and Neurostimulation; PMID: 10868324

> In this article, we have briefly introduced the practice of herbal medicine in India, summarized the studies that have examined the herbal attenuation of amnestic deficits induced by ECS, and discussed the application and limitations of animal models in the context of such research. We have primarily focused on our own work and insights, and have also examined practical issues that are involved in studies of this nature. For a comprehensive review of the effects of ECS on memory and cognition, the effects of pharmacological agents on ECS-induced memory deficits, and the effect of coadministered drugs on ECS seizure properties, the reader is referred to Krueger et al. (1992) and Fochtmann (1994).

Ice Pack Therapy

Ice Pack Therapy May Be Useful for the Treatment of ECT-Induced Headache

Drew, Brian I., et al.,"Cryotherapy for Treatment of ECT-Induced Headache." *Journal of Psychosocial Nursing and Mental Health Services* 43, no. 4 (April 2005): 32–39., Publisher: SLACK, INC. PMID: 15884476

> Because headache is a common side effect of electroconvulsive therapy (ECT), this study sought to determine the effectiveness of cryotherapy (i.e., a frozen gel band) in relieving pain in patients with post-ECT headaches, and whether headache intensity and physiological measurements could predict use of an alternative analgesic (rescue medication). We used a quasi-experimental, crossover design to collect data from 31 patients ages 24 to 85 who had been referred for ECT at two medical facilities in San Diego, California. Measurements of patients' pain intensity were made at three intervals: upon perceiving headache, and at 30 and 60 minutes following the cryotherapy or acetaminophen interventions, based on the order of the crossover design. Data were analyzed using Hotelling's T2 and logistic regression. No significant difference was found between cryotherapy and acetaminophen in relieving ECT-induced headaches ($p = .420$). There was no influence due to the crossover design ($p = .313$), nor where there significant changes in physiological measures from treatment ($p = .420$). Logistic regression showed that 50% of patients required rescue medication after 60 minutes for both treatments ($R2 = .498$, $p = .001$), and 66% required rescue medication based on pain level and physiological measures ($R2 = .662$, $p < .008$). Based on these results, cryotherapy is an alternative treatment that may be helpful to some patients with ECT-induced headaches.

Memoral Herbal

Memoral Herbal Showed Effective Prevention of ECT induced Cognitive Impairment

Mousavi, Seyed Ghafur, et al., "Efficacy of Memoral Herbal on Prevention of Electroconvulsive Therapy-Induced Memory Impairment in Mood Disorder Patients (isfahan - Iran 2011)." *International Journal of Preventive Medicine* 3, no. 7 (July 2012): 499–503., Publisher: Isfahan University of Medical Sciences; PMID: 22891152

➢ The Memoral herbal capsules, each contains 360 mg of Boswellia oleo-gum resin and 36 mg of Zimgiber rhizome. The most important constituent of Boswellia is gum resin 60%, mosilage 20-23% and essence 5-9%, which contains a-b-Thujon, p-cymen and linanol. Boswellia Serrata has Boswellic acid and acetyl- 11- keto-beta boswellic acid too, which are responsible for many therapeutic effect. The volatile oils in Boswellia dilate the vasculator of the brain thus can increase the blood passage through the brain. Boswellia extract has been demonstrated by a battery of rigorous tests to have anti-inflammatory effect. Boswellic acid has memory enhancing and anti-dementia properties. The mechanism by which Boswellia can improve memory is through its anti-inflammatory effect on the brain.

➢ Our work showed the effective prevention of ECT-induct cognitive impairment by using Memoral herbal. The cognitive status of patients not only declined, but also improved. The memory, attention and orientation, verbal fluency, and MMSE of patients showed improvement by Memoral use.

Nitrous Oxide

Nitrous Oxide Inhalation as an Alternative to Electroconvulsive Therapy

Milne, Brian, et al., "Nitrous Oxide (laughing Gas) Inhalation as an Alternative to Electroconvulsive Therapy." *Medical Hypotheses* 74, no. 5 (May 2010): 780–81. Publisher: CHURCHILL LIVINGSTONE; doi:10.1016/j.mehy.2009.11.021., PMID: 20006916

➢ Electroconvulsive therapy (ECT) is used widely in the treatment of psychiatric conditions; however, its use is not without controversy with some recommending a moratorium on its clinical use. Complications and side effects of ECT include memory loss, injury, problems originating from sympathetic stimulation such as arrhythmias and myocardial ischemia and the risk of general anesthesia. Nitrous oxide (laughing gas) could potentially substitute for ECT as it shares some similar effects, has potential beneficial properties for these psychiatric patients and is relatively safe and easy to administer. Nitrous oxide induces laughter which has been described as nature's epileptoid catharsis which one might surmise would be beneficial for depression. It also produces a central sympathetic stimulation similar to ECT and causes release of endogenous opioid peptides, which are potential candidates for the development of antidepressant drugs. Nitrous oxide is also associated with seizure like activity itself. Administration of nitrous oxide as a substitute for ECT is eminently feasible and could be given in a series of treatments similar to ECT therapy.

Percutaneous Electrical Nerve Stimulation

Percutaneous Electrical Nerve Stimulation (PENS) Proves Useful for Treating ECT-induced Headaches

> **Ghoname, E. A.,** et al., "Use of Percutaneous Electrical Nerve Stimulation (PENS) for Treating ECT-Induced Headaches." *Headache* 39, no. 7 (August 1999): 502–5., Publisher: BLACKWELL PUBLISHING, INC. PMID: 11279935

> ➢ Five patients who experienced migraine-like attacks associated with electroconvulsive therapy (ECT) were treated using a novel non-pharmacologic therapy known as percutaneous electrical nerve stimulation (PENS). In this sham-controlled preliminary evaluation, PENS therapy proved to be a useful alternative to opioid analgesics for the acute treatment and/or prevention of ECT-induced headache.

Phenylbutyric Acid

Phenylbutyric Acid Protects against Spatial Memory Deficits form ECT

> **Yao, Zhao-Hui,** et al., "Phenylbutyric Acid Protects against Spatial Memory Deficits in a Model of Repeated Electroconvulsive Therapy." *Current Neurovascular Research* 11, no. 2 (May 2014): 156–67., Publisher: BENTHAM SCIENCE PUBLISHERS LTD; PMID: 24712645

> ➢ Intraperitoneal injection of phenylbutyric acid (PBA), an aromatic short chain fatty acid acting as a molecule chaperon, could prevent rats from the rECS-induced memory deficits and synaptic potential enhancement by decreasing the levels of the abnormally increased memory-associated proteins and enhanced axon reorganization in hippocampus. Our data suggested that PBA might be potentially used to attenuate the rECS-induced memory impairment.

Transcutaneous Acupoint Electrical Stimulation

Transcutaneous Acupoint Electrical Stimulation Has a Good Response in Reliving Nausea and Vomiting in Patients Receiving Electroconvulsive Therapy

> **Kramer, Barry Alan,** et al., "Transcutaneous Acupoint Electrical Stimulation in Preventing and Treating Nausea and Vomiting in Patients Receiving Electroconvulsive Therapy." *The Journal of ECT* 19, no. 4 (December 2003): 194–96., Publisher: International Society for ECT and Neurostimulation; PMID: 14657771

> ➢ Transcutaneous acupoint electrical stimulation (TAES) is a nonpharmacologic method for preventing and treating nausea and vomiting. TAES can alleviate motion sickness, reduce the incidence of vomiting caused by chemotherapy, and treat pregnancy-induced nausea and vomiting. TAES has been shown to reduce the incidence of postoperative nausea after general anesthesia. This is the first report to review the effectiveness of

TAES in preventing and treating nausea and vomiting in 11 patients receiving ECT. Nine of these patients had a good response to TAES. One patient had a mixed response, and 1 did not respond to TAES.

T3 Thyroid

T3 Thyroid Hormone May Protect ECT Related Memory Impairment

Stern, R. A., et al., "Antidepressant and Memory Effects of Combined Thyroid Hormone Treatment and Electroconvulsive Therapy: Preliminary Findings." *Biological Psychiatry* 30, no. 6 (September 15, 1991): 623–27., Publisher: ELSEVIER INC. PMID: 1932410

> The most parsimonious explanation for possible °F~ protection against ECT-related memory impairment is that the T3 group received fewer ECT treatments. This would be consistent wit=h past observations that there is a direct relation- ship between number of ECT treatments and neurocognitive impairment (Daniel and Crovitz 1983). However, one additional explanation in- volves an alteration of available central thyroid hormone. It is known that diminished "1"4i n vitro markedly reduces neuronal actin polymerization and that replacement of "1"4 normalizes the actin cytoskeleton (Siegrist-Kaiser et al 1990). It is possible that temporary disorgization of the actin cytoskeleton in neurons located in the amygdala and hippocampus (structures that are highly susceptible to seizure and play important roles in learning and memory) may protect the cells from potential disruption by the seizure.

T3 Thyroid Hormone Accelerated the Antidepressant Effects and Diminished the Amnestic Effects of ECT

Stern, R. A., et al., "Influence of L-Triiodothyronine on Memory Following Repeated Electroconvulsive Shock in Rats: Implications for Human Electroconvulsive Therapy." *Biological Psychiatry* 37, no. 3 (February 1, 1995): 198–201. Publisher: ELSEVIER INC. doi:10.1016/0006-3223(94)00227-T., PMID: 7727629

> In tests of retrograde and anterograde amnesia, rats that received the thyroid hormone T3 in addition to ECS performed better than rats that received ECS with placebo. Stem and colleagues (1991) found that T3 administration in humans both accelerated the antidepressant effects and diminished the amnestic side effects of ECT; however, ECT in that study was discontinued as soon as clinical improvement was observed, which may have confounded the results. That is, the diminished amnesia may have been due to the reduced number of ECT exposures in the T3 group. In the present study, T3 diminished ECS-related amnesia in rats, when all groups received an equal number of ECS exposures. Other agents have been shown to diminish the amnestic side effects of ECS and ECT (Krueger et al 1992; Nobler and Sackeim 1993); however, the findings of the present animal study, along with those of our preliminary clinical report, suggest that T3 may be one of the first agents to reduce ECS/ECT-associated amnesia and also

414

improve the antidepressant efficacy of ECT. Replication of this animal study with a larger sample size, as well as additional clinical investigation with follow-up, is needed to support these promising results.

Wintergreen Oil

Topical Wintergreen Oil is Effective for Treatment of Post ECT Headache

Logan, Christopher J., et al., "Treatment of Post-Electroconvulsive Therapy Headache with Topical Methyl Salicylate." *The Journal of ECT* 28, no. 2 (June 2012): e17–18. Publisher: International Society for ECT and Neurostimulation doi:10.1097/YCT.0b013e318245c640., PMID: 22622298

> ➤ Headache after administration of electroconvulsive therapy (ECT) is common, affecting approximately half of patients treated. Post-ECT headache is typically treated with acetaminophen or nonsteroidal anti-inflammatory drugs but occasionally requires agents such as sumatriptan, opioids, or β-blockers. We report on a patient whose severe post-ECT headaches responded completely to methyl salicylate ointment, applied to the area of his temporalis and masseter muscles. Topical methyl salicylate is generally well tolerated and may be a viable option for some patients with post-ECT headache.

Vitamin B1

Vitamin B1 Helps Reduce Post-ECT Confusion

Linton, C. R., et al., "Using Thiamine to Reduce Post-ECT Confusion." *International Journal of Geriatric Psychiatry* 17, no. 2 (February 2002): 189–92., Publisher: JOHN/WILEY & SONS LTD. PMID: 11813284

> ➤ Cognitive side-effects are commonly seen following electroconvulsive therapy which convey no therapeutic benefit but are troublesome to both patient and clinician. Various efforts have been made in the past to minimize these symptoms. Although modification of technical parameters related to ECT administration has led to some limited improvement in this regard, attention is now being increasingly focused on pharmacological approaches. A number of agents have been explored in this context, however, as far as we are aware, the use of thiamine has not yet been investigated. We present three cases of elderly patients undergoing ECT for major depression in whom thiamine administration was associated with beneficial effects on post-ECT confusion. We review the evidence suggesting that thiamine deficiency may be implicated in the confusional state following ECT and recommend that consideration be given to its use in preventing and treating this problematic side-effect, especially in elderly patients.

Ogihara, T., et al., "Use of Thiamine in the Treatment of Post-Electroconvulsive Therapy Delirium." *Pharmacopsychiatry* 42, no. 1 (January 2009): 36–37. Publisher: GEORG/THIEME VERLAG; doi:10.1055/s-0028-1085440.

➢ In the present case, a series of ECT sessions led to the development of severe delirium, which was immediately resolved by thiamine administration. Additionally, further occurrence of post-ECT delirium was prevented. Unfortunately, we did not evaluate the blood thiamine levels prior to administration. However, the patient's response to thiamine indicates that the clinical manifestation of delirium is closely associated with thiamine deficiency.

➢ Both a decrease in thiamine supply and an increase in the need for thiamine promote a state of thiamine deficiency. Elderly patients with depression undergoing ECT are at a high risk of developing thiamine deficiency. This is because these patients often have an inadequate diet or suffer from anorexia. We speculate that thiamine deficiency caused by decreased dietary intake of thiamine and the effect of ECT procedures may together contribute to the development of post-ECT delirium. Linton et al. also suggested that thiamine deficiency arising from anorexia may mediate severe post-ECT delirium, and they reported that thiamine supplementation has a beneficial effect in treating post-ECT delirium. ECT-associated thiamine shortage may also be caused by another factor: neuronal discharges induced by ECT result in increased neuronal glucose metabolism, which in turn leads to thiamine consumption and hence results in relative thiamine deficiency. A previous study investigating the elevation levels of lactic acid and pyruvic acid in the rat brain following ECT seizure demonstrated that the rats treated with thiamine had significantly lower lactic acid level at 20 min following seizure, and suggested the possible advantages of thiamine use in human ECT To date, only a few studies, including this report, have suggested that thiamine supplementation has a beneficial effect in treating post-ECT delirium. Further clinical trials are required to clarify its efficacy in treating post-ECT delirium.

Miscellaneous Side Effect Treatments

Charcoal

Charcoal May Reduce Toxicity of Antidepressant Overdose and Put Mania in Remission

Jain, V., et al. "Charcoal Enhancement of Treatment for Tricyclic-Induced Mania." *Pharmacopsychiatry* 35, no. 5 (September 2002): 197–99. doi:10.1055/s-2002-34121., PMID: 12237792

➢ Induction of mania by tricyclic antidepressants (TCAs) is controversial, with indirect evidence for and against it. Unusual direct evidence of it was observed in a 77-year-old female patient having ingested an amitriptyline overdose. Mania developed while the TCA blood levels were high, and responded to a combination of charcoal and valproate. However, mania reappeared when charcoal was discontinued, and disappeared again when it was restarted. This time course suggests a therapeutic advantage for adding charcoal to valproate in treating tricyclic-induced mania. Presumably, charcoal might have removed a mania-inducing metabolite of amitriptyline. Moreover, repeated doses of oral activated charcoal accelerated the elimination of TCA from the blood stream to several times its original rate, which is consistent with interruption of the enterohepatic circulation. This enhanced elimination and improved outcome illustrate the value of repeated charcoal doses after TCA overdose, and suggest its use when mania develops in a patient who takes an antidepressant, at least amitriptyline or nortriptyline.

Melatonin

Melatonin is Useful for Inhibition of Antipsychotic-induced Side Effects

Anderson, George, et al., "Melatonin: An Overlooked Factor in Schizophrenia and in the Inhibition of Anti-Psychotic Side Effects." *Metabolic Brain Disease* 27, no. 2 (June 2012): 113–19. Publisher: SPRINGER NEW YORK LLC; doi:10.1007/s11011-012-9307-9., PMID: 22527998

> ➢ This paper reviews melatonin as an overlooked factor in the developmental etiology and maintenance of schizophrenia; the neuroimmune and oxidative pathophysiology of schizophrenia; specific symptoms in schizophrenia, including sleep disturbance; circadian rhythms; and side effects of antipsychotics, including tardive dyskinesia and metabolic syndrome. Electronic databases, i.e. PUBMED, Scopus and Google Scholar were used as sources for this review using keywords: schizophrenia, psychosis, tardive dyskinesia, antipsychotics, metabolic syndrome, drug side effects and melatonin. Articles were selected on the basis of relevance to the etiology, course and treatment of schizophrenia. Melatonin levels and melatonin circadian rhythm are significantly decreased in schizophrenic patients. The adjunctive use of melatonin in schizophrenia may augment the efficacy of antipsychotics through its anti-inflammatory and antioxidative effects. Further, melatonin would be expected to improve sleep disorders in schizophrenia and side effects of anti-psychotics, such as tardive dyskinesia, metaboilic syndrome and hypertension. It is proposed that melatonin also impacts on the tryptophan catabolic pathway via its effect on stress response and cortisol secretion, thereby impacting on cortex associated cognition, amygdala associated affect and striatal motivational processing. The secretion of melatonin is decreased in schizophrenia, contributing to its etiology, pathophysiology and management. Melatonin is likely to have impacts on the metabolic side effects of anti-psychotics that contribute to subsequent decreases in life-expectancy.

Milk Thistle

Milk Thistle is Effective in Preventing Psychotropic Drug-Induced Hepatic Damage

Palasciano G., et al., "The Effect of Silymarin on Plasma Levels of Malon-Dialdehyde in Patients Receiving Long-term Treatment with Psychotropic Drugs." *Current Therapeutic Research,* Vol 55(5), May 1994, 537-545, Publisher: EXCERPTA MEDICA, INC

> The data show that silymarin, when used at submaximal doses, reduces the lipoperoxidative hepatic damage that occurs during treatment with butyrophenones or phenothiazines. Results suggest that increased lipoperoxidation may contribute to PD-induced hepatotoxicity.

Vitamin C

Antipsychotic Drugs May Be Enhanced with Concurrent Administration of Vitamin C

De Angelis, L., et al., "Ascorbic Acid and Atypical Antipsychotic Drugs: Modulation of Amineptine-Induced Behavior in Mice." *Brain Research* 670, no. 2 (January 30, 1995): 303–7., Publisher: ELSEVIER BV; PMID: 7743194

> In conclusion, these data provide further in vivo support for the effect of ascorbic acid on dopaminergic system and demonstrate that the antidopaminergic effects of both typical and atypical antipsychotic drugs may be enhanced with concurrent administration of ascorbic acid.

Yi-gan san

Yi-gan san Add-on Treatment Improved Neuroleptic-induced Nocturnal Eating/Drinking Syndrome with Restless Legs Syndrome

Kawabe, Kentaro, et al., "Nocturnal Eating/drinking Syndrome with Restless Legs Syndrome Caused by Neuroleptics Improved by Yi-Gan San Add-on Treatment: A Case Report." *Clinical Neuropharmacology* 35, no. 6 (December 2012): 290–91. Publisher: LIPPINCOTT WILLIAMS & WILKINS; doi:10.1097/WNF.0b013e3182746a5b., PMID: 23151467

> "We report a middle-aged male patient with schizophrenia who had nocturnal eating/drinking syndrome with restless leg syndrome whose condition improved with the administration of the herbal medicine Yi-gan san (Yokukan-San in Japanese)."

Conclusion

<u>Discussion</u>

Putting it mildly, there has been significant research in the area of unconventional medicine for psychotic and affective disorders which is contrary to popular belief. From 1950 onward psychiatry has been researching numerous other alternative approaches for the treatment of psychotic and affective illnesses. In this book there are nearly 900 citations to treatments that are either well known, or have been experimented with for the treatment of these conditions. It has not been a lack of research that has slowed the acceptance of CAM therapies with traditional mental health professionals—it has been the overwhelming influence from the pharmaceutical companies promoting drugs as a primary treatment. Drugs are promoted in advertising campaigns on TV, magazine and in journals—pharmaceutical companies have market dominance and own a majority of the mental health education web sites. Further, promotion of pharmaceuticals to doctors by sales representivies, and pharmaceutical kickbacks to physicians which give them little incentive to prescribe anything but drugs. There is also the lack of training of mental health professionals in college about alternatives to pharmaceuticals, and the pharmaceutical companies' creation of false biological sciences (i.e. brain diseases (Zipursky, 2013), chemical imbalances (Lacasse & Leo, 2005; Whitaker & Cosgrove, 2015), mental illness pathophysiology (Cardinal & Bullmore, 2011; Whitaker & Cosgrove, 2015), etiology of mental illness (Whitaker & Cosgrove, 2015) which they promote to both mental health professionals and physicians and other medical students during medical school. These false sciences further the idealism that it takes psychopharmaceuticals to treat "broken brains". Chemical imbalances and the propagation of ideas of genetically predisposed people with an incurable sickness are also many of the pseudosciences which were promoted by the interests of the American Pyschiatric Association (APA) and pharmaceutical marketing campaigns for the sales of drugs (Whitaker & Cosgrove, 2015).

Drugs—though sometimes helpful for a small percentage of schizophrenics—are also leading patients onto a path of long-term illness (Whitaker, 2010). These antidepressant, anticonvulsant, and antipsychotic drugs cause more than just induction of mania, and dopamine supersenitivity psychosis; they induce progressive deterioration of the physical body in many different ways: obesity, sleep apnea, diabetes, brain damage, hyperdislipdemia, hypertension and cognitive decline. These natural complementary therapies are often a way to reduce the oxidative stress associated with antipsychotic monotherapy and psychotropic drug combination polytherapy. They also help treat cognitive decline associated with the drugs. They may be used to help treat many other side effects associated with psychotropic drugs use—including theoretically, possibly limiting the effects of dopaminergic supersenitvity psychosis.

Moreover, the use of integrative medicine is safer than the more toxic usage of monotherapy with psychotropics and it may be recommended by many physicians not to use psychotropics without nutraceuticals due to nutrient depletion caused by some drugs and the increased oxidative stress induced by many of these psychotropics. This oxidative stress caused by the drugs is most often the one of the primary causes of tardive dyskenisia in psychiatric patients and Codex Alternus has a plethora of antioxidants, vitamins and herbs that may help reduce oxidative stress associated with both the disease and the oxidative metabolites of the drugs.

In Codex Alternus there are a few therapies studied in drug-naïve patients, however they have shown superior efficacy over placebo or control group on psychotropic drugs. This may be an option for some patients. Below are some case examples:

Acupuncture Treatment of Schizophrenia Outcome

Three random controlled trials RCT's (two by Zhao YH, 2005, one by Wang L, 2006) compared the effects of manual acupuncture with antipsychotic drug therapies, while one RCT by Zhang LD, 1987, employed electroacupuncture (EA). The meta-analysis showed a significant effect of manual acupuncture for response rate compared with antipsychotic drugs (n = 360, RR: 1.18, 95% CI: 1.03– 1.34, p = 0.01; heterogeneity: s2 = 0.00, v2 = 2.98, p = .39, I2 = 0%). The RCT by Zhang LD, which employed EA, failed to show significant effects of EA on response rate compared with antipsychotic (Lee, 2009). Though the rate of recovery and the marked improvement in the four groups studied in this RCT was 46.5% for electric acupuncture (EA), 19.9% for herbal decoction: Dang Gui Cheng Qi Tang; 40.8% for electric acupuncture and herbal decoction combined and 37.8% for Chlorpromazine (Zhang, 1990). One RCT showed statistically significant effects of acupuncture on Brief Psychiatric Rating Scale (BPRS), Scale for the Assessment of Negative Symptoms (SANS) and Treatment Emergent Symptom Scale compared with drug therapy, but failed to show statistically significant effects of acupuncture on Scale for the Assessment of Positive Symptoms (Lee, 2009).

Omega-3 Fatty Acids for Pediatric Bipolar Mania Outcome

This is a drug-naïve study done in the European Neuropharmacology journal 2007. Study shows there was 8.9±7.8 point reduction in the YMRS at study endpoint (week 8 or LOCF). At study endpoint, 50% (n=10) of subjects had a 30% reduction in baseline YMRS scores and 35% (n =7) had a 50% reduction in baseline YMRS scores. The mean dose of omega-3 fatty acids at study endpoint was 2602.1±1013.5 mg/day. The range was 1290 mg–4300 mg per day or 3–10 Omegabrite capsules per day (Wozniak, 2007).

Sarcosine in Drug-naïve Schizophrenics

Lane et al. (2008) tested two dosages of sarcosine to treat drug-naïve acutely psychotic people with schizophrenia. Twenty individuals were randomly assigned for sarcosine at a dose of 2 grams or 1 gram for 6 weeks. Both positive and negative symptoms were decreased by an average of 20% for the antipsychotic naïve research participants (Lane, 2008; Litterell, 2015).

D-Serine Monotherapy in Treatment-Resistant Schizophrenia

An controlled pilot investigation compared the effectiveness of D-serine (DSR), (3 g/day) *versus* high dose olanzapine (30 mg/day) as antipsychotic monotherapy in 18 treatment resistant schizophrenic patients. The primary LOFC analysis indicated a lack of efficiency of DSR as compared to high dose olanzapine. However, DSR was not inferior to the prestudy antipsychotic drug treatment. Furthermore, among the patients who completed the nine study weeks, high dose olanzapine and DSR did not differ in their effectiveness, suggesting that a subgroup of patients may be successfully maintained on DSR (Durrant, 2014).

EPA Treatment of Schizophrenia Outcome

A study done by Malcolm Peet in 2001 Schizophrenia Research used 30 patients diagnosed with schizophrenia on no medication and a trial of 2 g a day EPA. Nine patients that were drug-naïve on entering the study, and the remainder had received no antipsychotic medication for at least two weeks. Four patients had no final PANSS rating completed (three on placebo, one on EPA); of these, three patients were lost to follow-up, and one died of accidental burns unrelated to the illness. In the placebo group, every patient required conventional antipsychotic medication by the end of the trial period. In contrast, six patients on EPA were not taking antipsychotic medication at the end of the study (Fisher's Exact test P < 0.02 vs. placebo). Of these six, four had gone through the entire treatment period without any antipsychotic medication (flupenthixol deconoate 25mg) at the start of the trial (regarded statistically as 14 days treatment). On average, EPA treated patients spent little more than a month on conventional treatment in contrast to more than 2 months for placebo group. Despite the substantial difference in the level of antipsychotic treatment, patients on EPA had significantly lower PANSS scores by the end of the study relative to the placebo treated group; this applied particularly to the positive symptom sub-scale. There was no obvious difference in outcomes between patients who had been medicated previously and those who were drug-naïve, but numbers were too small for statistical comparison. A responder analysis was also carried out, using 50% improvement in rating scale scores as criterion. On the positive PANSS rating, only two out of 12 patients on placebo showed more than 50% improvement, compared to 8 out of 14 patients on EPA (Fisher's Exact test, two-tail, P=0.05). No side effects were attributable to EPA (Peet, 2001).

Summary of Alternative Medicine Studies

As these studies show there is therapeutic efficacy in alternative medicine equal too, and above and beyond the therapeutic efficacy of psychotropic drugs. Some of these therapies such as Omega-3 fatty acids show modest effects and others such as acupuncture, sarcosine and D-serine have more proficient therapeutic benefits for psychosis. Theoretically, when these natural therapies are used in combinations as polytherapies with other alternatives such as exercises, dietary management, nutrition, etc. there is likely a significant synergistic therapeutic benefit psychotropics cannot compare too due to the fact there is little allostatic load with natural therapies. Allostatic load is created from the toxic metabolites of the drug that create a burden on the body, which cause the reactions of body to become overactive, underactive, or prolonged (Jackson, 2005). An example of combination polytherapy for schizophrenic psychosis with low allostatic load would be dietary management, exercise, use of vitamins and minerals, hormones such as DHEA, and testosterone, and sound therapy for hallucinations.

Codex Alternus Conclusion

Even though Codex Alternus is not a how to diagnose, and treat, type of book with dosages and product information, it is designed to give the reader a plethora of research on positive case reports, clinical trials and articles that support alternative and complementary medicine. Codex Alternus is a book full of scholarly, peer reviewed articles. Codex Alternus shows the reader there is ample scientific support for alternative and complementary medicine which it also inspires the reader to find suitable new therapies for any type of psychotic patient's condition or bipolar affective patient's condition. It sparks ideas, and is a reference guide for tough clinical situations that need a new approach. It can be concluded it is an alternative and complementary psychiatric research and clinical reference tool.

The author hopes that physicians overcome the stigma associated with prescribing natural substances to schizophrenic and bipolar patients and learn much of the cognitive defects and persistent relapse are often more associated with antipsychotic medications and polypharmacy with pharmaceuticals than "mental illness." Prescribing exercise, natural supplements and nutraceuticals with psychotropics only make more sense and reduces the side effects, decreases oxidative stress and increases clinical efficiency. Further, offering consulting and clinical experience to bipolar and schizophrenic patients who desire to use CAM therapies may offer new clients. A survey in 2015 on 23,393 US adults with neuropsychiatric symptoms were surveyed and 37% spent and estimated $14.8 billion dollars on out-of-the pocket CAM therapies (Purohit, 2015).

To sum the conclusion up; for decades pharmaceutical companies have dominated the marketplace leading many to believe there are few effective choices for treatment of psychotic and affective disorders. However not due to lack of research, but lack of physician's interest in prescribing alternative and complementary therapies the patient with serious mental illness has been "overdosed" with antipsychotic and other mood stabilizing drugs.

Psychotropic Drug-Nutrient-Herb Interactions

Introduction

In psychiatric patients with schizophrenia or bipolar disorder who are prescribed antidepressants, mood stabilizers, benzodiazepines, antipsychotics or hypnotics, you may find that some herbs, nutrients, amino acids, and other physiologics may cause an interaction. Often these add-on therapies work synergistically, enhancing the therapeutic efficiency of the psychiatric drug and in some cases the drugs may deplete specific nutrients. When there is polypharmacy involved with psychotropics and other drugs for physical problems, there may be a host of scenarios encountered (drug-supplement/herbal interactions, nutrient depletion, or synergistic enhancement) when utalizing nutrients, herbs and other supplements.

Interactions between psychotropic drugs and "natural" products such as nutrients and herbs is an area of immediate concern and growing awareness wherever patients are receiving psychiatric care. Many psychiatric patients naively assume that nutrient and herbal products are "natural" and that this somehow implies they are "safe." It is an acknowledged fact that psychiatric patients often withhold disclosure of nutrient and herbal intake from their conventional health care providers and psychiatrists. In fact only 48% of psychotic patients report their use of CAM therapies to their family physicians (Hazra, 2010). Accordingly, professional literature tends to assume that patients using nutrients and herbs (dietary supplements) are doing so without supervision of health care professionals trained and experienced in therapeutic application of nutritional and botanical therapies. Greater awareness, frank discussion, and informed decision making in these areas are necessary for effective clinical management as well as a patient's perception of respect for their choices. Similarly, in patients with complex and chronic conditions, the use of multiple providers from several different health care disciplines can increase clinical efficiency and patient safety though open dialogue and collegial (peer-to-peer) collaboration. However, without this open dialogue drug-nutrient herbal interactions are more likely if physicians are prescribing them. Often literature provided online and by physicians about any possible interactions, is prepared by health care professionals without training or experience in nutritional and botanical therapies. In addition, the interactions reference texts and guides developed for consumers are limited in depth, often avoid critical issues, and sometimes prey on readers' fears by exaggeration and headline hyperbole (Stargrove, Treasure, McKee 2008).

In this book we cite examples of drug-nutrient, herbal interactions on the charts below. They cover antidepressants, antipsychotics, mood stabilizers, and benzodiazepines. This book covers drug-nutrient interactions that are currently known and real examples of interactions between psychotropic drugs, nutrients and herbs commonly used in psychiatry.

Psychotropic Drug-Nutrient-Herb Interaction Charts

Antipsychotic Interactions

Antipsychotics have the least interactions with nutrients and herbs compared to mood stabilizers and antidepressants. Many of these natural supplements work synergistically with antipsychotics and several of these drugs deplete nutrients. The drugs listed here are both atypical and typical antipsychotics; Abilify (aripiprazole), Clozaril (clozapine), Haldol (haloperidol), Zyprexa (olanzapine), Seroquel (quetiapine), Risperdal (risperidone), Geodon (ziprasidone) and Phenothiazine class (Thorazine, Melaril, Prolixin). Many newer antipsychotics will not be represented due to the fact there is little data on nutrient interaction as of date.

Prescription Psychotropic Drug (Antipsychotics)	Vitamin B_{12} (Cobalamin)	Vitamin B_6 (Pyridoxine)	Vitamin B_3 (Niacin)	Folate or (Folic Acid)
Aripiprazole				
Clozapine				
Haloperidol		Reduction of adverse drug events		
Olanzapine	No interactions known		Synergistic effect	No interactions known
Phenothiazine		Enhancement of therapeutic outcome		
Quetiapine				
Risperidone				
Ziprasidone				

Antipsychotic Interactions

Prescription Psychotropic Drug (Antipsychotics)	Vitamin C	Vitamin E	Selenium	Iron
Aripiprazole	Reduces oxidative stress	No interactions known	No interactions known	N/A
Clozapine	Prevents agranulocytosis Reduce oxidative stress		Depletes Selenium	
Haloperidol	Potentiates Haldol/works synergistically	Depletes vitamin E		Reduces blood levels of iron
Olanzapine	Reduces Oxidative Stress	No interactions known	No interactions known	N/A
Phenothiazine	Beneficial Effect Anecdote to Amenorrhea			
Quetiapine	Reduces Oxidative Stress			
Risperidone				
Ziprasidone				

Antipsychotic Interactions

Prescription Psychotropic Drug (Antipsychotics)	5HTP	Omega-3'Fatty Acids	Melatonin	Chromium
Aripiprazole	Advisable to avoid due to interaction with serotonin	Clinical improvement added to atypical antipsychotics	Attenuates dopamine activity and counters side effects of antipsychotics	"Interaction between chromium and antipsychotics is theoretically plausible, but no substantive evidence from case reports or clinical trials has emerged to confirm or refute this occurrence."
Clozapine	N/A			
Haloperidol	N/A	Clinical improvement added to Haldol		
Olanzapine	Advisable to avoid due to interaction with serotonin	Clinical improvement added to atypical antipsychotics		
Phenothiazine	N/A	N/A		
Quetiapine	Advisable to avoid due to interaction with serotonin	Clinical improvement added to atypical antipsychotics		
Risperidone				
Ziprasidone				

Antipsychotic Interactions

Prescription Psychotropic Drug (Antipsychotics)	Potassium	Kava	Milk Thistle	CoQ10
Aripiprazole	N/A	Kava use for extrapyramidal symptoms may be appropriate therapy with professional management. (*Though there are small but finite case reports of Kava causing Parkinson-like or dystonic symptoms in some patients.*)	N/A	No Interactions Known
Clozapine	N/A		N/A	No Interactions Known
Haloperidol	Known to induce both hyperkalemia and hypokalemia		Coadministration of milk thistle extracts or silymarin with hepatotoxic drugs reduces biochemical and histopathological markers of drug-induced hepatocellular toxicity.	No Interactions Known
Olanzapine	N/A		N/A	No Interactions Known
Phenothiazine	Coadministration of potassium may reduce the incidence of ventricular arrhythmias associated with the use of Thioridazine in alcohol withdrawal.		Coadministration of milk thistle extracts or silymarin with hepototoxic drugs reduces biochemical and histopathological markers of drug-induced hepatocellular toxicity.	CoQ10 prevents and reverses impairment of myocardial respiration caused by phenothiazines
Quetiapine	N/A		N/A	No Interactions Known
Risperidone	N/A		Inhibits P-glycoprotein	No Interactions Known

Mood Stabilizer Interactions

Listed under prescription psychotropic drugs as "mood stabilizes" are several neurological drugs used in psychiatry. Apart from lithium carbonate these other drugs listed; carbamazepine (Tegratol), gabapentin (Neurotin), levetracetam (Keppra), oxcarbamazepine (Trileptal), topiramate (Topamax), valproic acid (Depakote), zonisamide (Zonegran) are antiepileptic drugs (AED's). Lamotrigine (Lamictal) wasn't used in this chart due to the fact there is little literature on interactions with herbs and nutrients. This does not exclude the drug from being neutral—it's just there is no current data on this drug.

Prescription Psychotropic Drug (Mood Stabilizer)	Vitamin B_{12} (Cobalamin)	Vitamin B_6 (Pyridoxine)	Vitamin B_3 (Niacin)	Folate or (Folic Acid)
Carbamazepine	Drug-induced nutrient depletion or deficiency	Pyridoxal 5'-phosphate (PLP) levels can be significantly decreased	Niacinamide may decrease clearance of AED's through inhibition of CYP450 and potentiate the anticonvulsant action of these drugs	Most AED's cause folate depletion by inhibiting nutrient absorption, inducing microsomal oxidase enzymes (cytochrome P450) increasing hepatic folate metabolism and impacting microbiota.
Gabapentin				
Levetracetam				
Oxcarbazepine				
Topiramate				
Valproic Acid				
Zonisamide				
Lithium	No interaction known	No interaction known	No interaction known	"folate at high concentrations enhances lithium prophylaxis"

Mood Stabilizer Interactions

Prescription Psychotropic Drug (Mood Stabilizer)	Vitamin B1 (Thiamine)	Vitamin B2 (Riboflavin)	Inositol	Vitamin D
Carbamazepine			Synergistic effect	
Gabapentin	Coadministration of 50-100mg of oral thiamine daily due to impaired uptake from AED's	AED's may alter riboflavin metabolism and deplete riboflavin	No interaction known	AED'st that induce CYP3A4 which degrades vitamin D AED's disturb vitamin D metabolism and may cause deficiency
Levetracetam				
Oxcarbazepine				
Topiramate				
Valproic Acid			Synergistic effect with VPA helps treat depressive phases	
Zonisamide			No interaction known	
Lithium	No Interaction known	No interaction known	Concomitant Inositol is beneficial for lithium-induced psoriasis	No interaction known

Mood Stabilizer Interactions

Prescription Psychotropic Drug (Mood Stabilizer)	Omega-3 Fatty Acids	Vitamin E	Vitamin C	Vitamin A
Carbamazepine	Synergistic effects (Recommended treatment)	Low plasma vitamin E levels associated with some AED's. Caution is advised for this class of drugs	Administration of vitamin C highly recommended to prevent DNA damage	AED's alter endogenous retinoid metabolism causing low blood levels of vitamin A
Gabapentin				
Levetracetam				
Oxcarbazepine				
Topiramate				
Valproic Acid				
Zonisamide				
Lithium	No interaction known	No interaction known	No interaction known	No interaction known

Mood Stabilizer Interactions

Prescription Psychotropic Drug (Mood Stabilizer)	Vitamin K	Potassium	Chromium	Selenium
Carbamazepine	Enzyme inducing AED's may increase the metabolic breakdown of vitamin K by inducing hepatic microsomal enzymes	N/A	No interaction known	No interaction known
Gabapentin				
Levetracetam				
Oxcarbazepine				
Topiramate		Due to possible potassium loss a diet of fresh fruits and vegetables is recommended		
Valproic Acid		N/A		Decreases plasma levels of selenium
Zonisamide	No interaction known	Due to possible potassium loss a diet of fresh fruits and vegetables is recommended	No interaction known	No interaction known
Lithium	No interaction known	N/A	Coadministration of chromium with lithium may decrease glucose levels and cause hypoglycemia in diabetics	No interaction known

Mood Stabilizer Interactions

Prescription Psychotropic Drug (Mood Stabilizer)	Magnesium	Zinc	Calcium	Copper
Carbamazepine	No interaction known	Reports have indicated zinc deficiency with AED's, especially combined with VPA	AED's may reduce serum calcium levels	No interaction known
Gabapentin				
Levetracetam				
Oxcarbazepine				
Topiramate				
Valproic Acid		VPA may alter zinc metabolism causing depletion especial when combine with other AED's		VPA may increase excretion of copper into bile causing abnormalities of serum copper concentrations
Zonisamide		Reports have indicated zinc deficiency with AED's, especially combined with VPA		No interaction known
Lithium	Lithium and magnesium interact. Monitor for high blood levels	No interaction known	No interaction known	No interaction known

Mood Stabilizers Interactions

Prescription Psychotropic Drug (Mood Stabilizer)	Carnitine	DHEA	5HTP	Milk Thistle
Carbamazepine	Many AED's depress acylcarnitine. Though loss is less than VPA, some could cause carnitine deficiency.	Enzyme inducing AED's of CYP3A4 may decrease circulating levels of DHEA and DHEA-S. Coadministration of DHEA may interfere with the action of AED's, however if patient has been safely using DHEA with medication cessation of DHEA may be deemed inappropriate. Monitor closely.	No interaction known	Coadministration of milk thistle extracts or silymarin with hepatotoxic drugs reduces biochemical and histopathological markers of drug-induced hepatocellular toxicity.
Gabapentin				
Levetracetam				
Oxcarbazepine				
Topiramate				
Valproic Acid	VPA depress renal absorption of both free carnitine and acylcarnitine causing carnitine depletion and VPA hepatotoxicity.			
Zonisamide	Same as most other AED's			
Lithium	No interaction known	No interaction known	5HTP may increase serotonin. Confirmed interactions are lacking. Clinical observations suggest 5HTP can be effective adjunctive to lithium.	No interaction known

Mood Stabilizer Interactions

Prescription Psychotropic Drug (Mood Stabilizer)	Tryptophan	Kava
Carbamazepine	No interaction known	Kava may potentiate side effects of AED's and have antiseizure effects
Gabapentin		
Levetracetam		
Oxcarbazepine		
Topiramate		
Valproic Acid		
Zonisamide		
Lithium	Theoretically lithium and tryptophan can increase serotonin and cortisol levels excessively. Confirmed interactions are lacking and clinical observations suggest tryptophan can be effective adjunctive to lithium.	No interaction known

Benzodiazepines Interactions

Commonly used benzodiazepines in psychiatry are Xanax (alprazolam), Klonopin (clonazepam), Valium (diazepam), and Ativan (lorazepam). Benzodiazepines are commonly prescribed for schizophrenic and bipolar patients for issues with anxiety, panic, and insomnia. They are almost always used as polypharmacy in combination with antipsychotics, antidepressants or mood stabilizers which excluding Klonopin, have few interactions with nutrients, however have a few herbal interactions.

*Note: Clonazepam (Klonopin) is considered an AED and though will be classified as a benzodiazepine in this section, but will have the same nutrient and herbal interactions as many AED's.

Prescription Psychotropic Drug (Benzodiazepines)	Vitamin B1	Vitamin B2	Vitamin B6	Vitamin B12
Alprazolam	No interaction known	No interaction known	No interaction known	No interaction known
Diazepam				
Lorazepam				
Clonazepam*	Coadministration of 50-100mg of oral thiamine daily due to impaired uptake from AED's	AED's may alter riboflavin metabolism and deplete riboflavin	Pyridoxal 5'-phosphate (PLP) levels can be significantly decreased	Drug-induced nutrient depletion or deficiency

Benzodiazepine interactions

Prescription Psychotropic Drug (Benzodiazepines)	Vitamin B3	Vitamin E	Vitamin C	Vitamin D
Alprazolam	Concomitant use of niacinamide and benzodiazepine could theoretically produce and additive effect of sedation hypnotic response. Evidence is lacking to confirm hypothetical interactions.	No interaction known	No interaction known	No interaction known
Diazepam				
Lorazepam				
Clonazepam		Low plasma vitamin E levels associated with some AED's though caution is advised for this class of drugs	Coadministration of vitamin C highly recommended to prevent DNA damage	AED'st that induce CYP3A4 which degrades vitamin D AED's disturb vitamin D metabolism and may cause deficiency

Prescription Psychotropic Drug (Benzodiazepines)	DHEA	Folic Acid	Vitamin K	Vitamin A
Alprazolam	DHEA inhibits CYP4A and CYP3A23 which may reduce the capacity for alprazolam and related medications. Thereafter leading to elevations of these medications.	N/A	No interaction known	No interaction known
Diazepam				
Lorazepam				
Clonazepam*		Most AED's cause folate depletion	Enzyme inducing AED's may increase the metabolic breakdown of vitamin K by inducing hepatic microsomal enzymes	AED's alter endogenous retinoid metabolism causing low blood levels of vitamin A

Benzodiazepine Interactions

Prescription Psychotropic Drug (Benzodiazepines)	Omega-3Fatty Acids	Zinc	Calcium	Melatonin
Alprazolam	N/A	No interaction known	No interaction known	Benzodiazepines deplete melatonin.
Diazepam				
Lorazepam				
Clonazepam*	Synergistic effects (Recommended treatment)	Reports have indicated zinc deficiency with AED's, especially combined with VPA	AED's may reduce serum calcium levels	Oral melatonin may reverse tolerance to benzodiazepine hypnotics

Prescription Psychotropic Drug (Benzodiazepines)	Kava	Valerian	Milk Thistle
Alprazolam	Kava has an additive pharmacodynamics action interaction between sedative and hypnotic effects with alprazolam.	Valerian reduces benzodiazepine withdrawal effects. It has GABAergic, antidepressant and antispasmotic activity which helps with withdrawal.	With polypharmacy of benzodiazepines with hepatotoxic drugs administration of milk thistle extracts or silymarin reduces biochemical and histopathological markers of drug-induced hepatocellular toxicity.
Diazepam			
Lorazepam			
Clonazepam*	Kava may potentiate side effects of AED's and have antiseizure effects		

Antidepressant Interactions

The antidepressant category has a diverse range of nutrient/herbal interaction which includes SSRI's, SNRI's, serotonin agonists, and tricyclic antidepressants. Drugs include Celexa (citalopram), Cymbalta (duloxetine), Effexor (venlafaxine), Lexapro (escitalopram), Luvox (fluvoxamine), Paxil (paroxetine), Prozac (fluoxetine), Serzone (nefazodone), Wellbutrin (bupropion) and Zoloft (sertiline).

Prescription Psychotropic Drug (Antidepressant)	Vitamin B1(Thiamine)	Vitamin B2 (Riboflavin)	Vitamin B3 (Niacin)	Vitamin B6 (Pyridoxine)
Citalopram				
Duloxetine				
Escitalopram			Vitamin B3 saturation might theoretically encourage diversion of tryptophan to serotonin synthesis and provoke excessive serotonin levels in individuals being treated with SSRI/SNRI's	Recommended coadministration of vitamin B6 or B-complex vitamins with SSRI/SNRI's to increase serotonin. Offers synergistic support.
Fluoxetine	No interaction known	No interaction known		
Fluvoxamine				
Nefazodone				
Paroxetine				
Sertiline				
Venlafaxine				
Tricyclic Antidepressants	Thiamine depletion and replacement has synergistic effects	TCA's can inhibit riboflavin absorption. Coadministration of riboflavin can augment the therapeutic activity of TCA's	Tryptophan supplementation can potentiate TCA's through serotonergic effects. Coadministration of niacinamide supports synergist action.	Vitamin B6 recommended with TCA's combined with B-complex nutrients and vitamin D though no known interaction

Antidepressant Interactions

Prescription Psychotropic Drug (Antidepressant)	Vitamin B12	Vitamin C	Folic Acid	Inositol
Citalopram	Enhances therapeutic response and decreases depressive symptoms	Enhances therapeutic response	Additive or synergistic effect when combined with antidepressants	Careful monitoring is advised for concurrent use or consecutive use of high-dose myo-inositol with SSRI's. However, no case reports have indicated an interaction of serotonin syndrome.
Duloxetine				
Escitalopram				
Fluoxetine				
Fluvoxamine		Helps reduce bleeding associated with Paxil And Luvox		
Paroxetine				
Sertiline		Enhances therapeutic response		
Venlafaxine				
Nefazodone	N/A	N/A	N/A	N/A
Tricyclic Antidepressants	Enhances therapeutic response and decreases depressive symptoms	N/A	N/A	N/A

Antidepressant Interactions

Prescription Psychotropic Drug (Antidepressant)	Omega-3 Fatty Acids	Chromium	Zinc	Melatonin
Bupropion	N/A	N/A	N/A	Monitor closely
Citalopram	Advised to co-administer fish oil with SSRI/SNRI's in patients who never eat fish or take OTC products containing fish oil	Physicians should consider prescribing 200 μg once to twice daily of chromium with SSRI medications especially in patients with a history of hypoglycemia, dysglycemia, insulin resistance or diabetes.	Pending essays of zinc depletion 25 to 40 mg of daily zinc should be administered to achieve therapeutic effect improving depression.	N/A
Duloxetine				
Escitalopram				
Fluoxetine				Prozac and Sarafem can reduce melatonin levels in humans . Not known whether supplementation helps.
Fluvoxamine				Luvox elevates melatonin levels. Monitor closely.
Paroxetine				N/A
Sertiline				
Venlafaxine				
Nefazodone	N/A	N/A	N/A	N/A
Tricyclic Antidepressants	N/A	N/A	Pending essays of zinc depletion 25 to 40 mg of daily zinc should be administered to achieve effect improving depression.	N/A

440

Antidepressant Interactions

Prescription Psychotropic Drug (Antidepressant)	CoQ10	Tyrosine	5HTP	Tryptophan
Citalopram	No interaction known	No interaction known	5HTP coadministration with SSRI/SNRI may cause serotonin syndrome.	Moderate risk of serotonin syndrome, however 2 to 4 grams daily may be used in conjunction with SSRI to enhance clinical effectiveness of medication
Duloxetine				
Escitalopram				
Fluoxetine				Tryptophan and fluoxetine can potentially cause serotonin syndrome
Fluvoxamine				Same as top box: risk of SS and enhance effectiveness of medications
Paroxetine				
Sertiline				
Venlafaxine				
Nefazodone				N/A
Tricyclic Antidepressants	TCA's may cause CoQ10 deficiency. Coadministration may prevent myocardial depression and other cardiac events associated with TCA's	Use of TCA's and tyrosine to restore depleted dopamine from cocaine abuse is helpful in the withdrawal process	N/A	N/A

Antidepressant Interactions

Prescription Psychotropic Drug (Antidepressant)	DHEA	SAMe	St. John's Wort	Ginkgo biloba
Citalopram	Speculative concerns that DHEA may induce mania combined with antidepressants	SAMe 400 to 800mg twice daily in graduated doses can be used adjunctively with SSRI/SNRI's to enhance clinical efficiency. Should not be used outside clinical management.	At a professional level SJW coadministered does not present significant problems, given appropriate monitoring. May also be used before starting drug therapy or assisting with SSRI antidepressant withdrawal.	Ginkgo leaf may be helpful in ameliorating sexual dysfuction from SSRI therapy
Duloxetine				
Escitalopram				
Fluoxetine	Potential supportive interaction reported between Prozac and DHEA			
Fluvoxamine	Speculative concerns that DHEA may induce mania combined with antidepressants			
Paroxetine				
Sertiline				
Venlafaxine				
Nefazodone		N/A		N/A
Tricyclic Antidepressants		N/A	N/A	N/A

All Drug-Nutrient-Herb Interaction Charts information came from the book:
Stargrove, Mitchell Bebel, Jonathan Treasure, and Dwight L. McKee. 2008. Herb, nutrient, and drug interactions clinical implications and therapeutic strategies. St. Louis (Mo.): Mosby/Elsevier.

Suppliers of High Quality Peptides, Nutraceuticals, Herbs and Chinese Traditional Medicines

Natural Product or Chemical Supplier	Type of Product Supplied	Description of Services
Sigma-Aldrich Corp. St. Louis, MO, USA Phone: 314-771-5765 Fax: 314-771-5757 E-mail: cssorders@sial.com Website: United States	Supplier of sarcosine, D-serine, D-alanine, sodium benzoate, caerulein diethylamine, gamma endorphin, guanosine, thymulin, secretin, leucine, genistein, sodium butyrate.	Sigma-Aldrich, a leading Life Science and High Technology company focused on enhancing human health and safety, manufactures and distributes more than 230,000 chemicals, biochemicals and other essential products to more than 1.4 million customers globally in research and applied labs as well as in industrial and commercial markets. The Company operates in 37 countries, has more than 9,000 employees worldwide and had sales of $2.7 billion in 2013.
PeptaNova GmbH Keplerstr. 26 69207 Sandhausen Germany Fon: +49 (0) 6224 - 9259777 Fax: +49 (0) 6224 - 9259800	Peptides of all sorts, Amylin peptide, gamma endorphins, CCK, Amino Acids and derivatives	With the special support of Peptide Institute, PeptaNova established a well sorted stock of biologically active peptides, enzyme - substrates, enzyme - inhibitors and peptide antisera, located in the heart of Europe.
KareBay Biochem, Inc. 11 Deer Park Drive, Suite 204 Monmouth Junction, NJ 08852 E-mail KareBay: product@karebaybio.com service@karebaybio.com support@karebaybio.com Telephone: 732-823-1545 Fax: 732-823-1349	Peptides of all sorts, Amylin, gamma endorphins, CCK, and Amino acid derivatives, etc.	KareBayTM Biochem's headquarters is located in New Jersey. It is a United States based, globally operated company dedicated to the innovation and manufacture of biochemical products and services.

PureFormulas Attn. Customer Happiness Team 11800 NW 102nd Road, Suite #2 Medley, FL 33178 E-mail: help@pureformulas.com Phone: 1.800.383.6008	Vitamins, minerals, fatty acids, amino acids and numerous other natural products	Sells natural health products from some the highest quality commercial suppliers in the vitamin, mineral, amino acid, fatty acid, supplement arena. Have at least 100 different companies' products to choose from.
Pacific Botanicals 4840 Fish Hatchery Road Grants Pass, OR 97527 Telephone: (541) 479-7777 Fax :(541) 479-7780	Carries organic herbs and spices, and fresh non-dried herbs.	Pacific Botanicals is a medicinal herb farm. The most experienced and diversified in North America. Carries organic herbs and spices, sea vegetables, super food powders, fresh non dried herbs, and bulk seeds.
MOUNTAIN ROSE HERBS PO Box 50220 Eugene OR 97405 (800) 879-3337 (541) 741-7307 support@mountainroseherbs.com	Carries organic dried herbs, spices, essential oils, extracts, herbal capsules, teas, etc.	Grows, markets and distributes herbs, spices, teas, aromatherapy, natural ingredients, bitters, elixirs, syrups, extracts, tinctures, herbal oils, salves and herbal capsules.
Ron Teegaurden's Dragon Herbs 5670 Wilshire Blvd., Suite #1500 Los Angeles, CA 90036 (310) 917-2288 info@dragonherbs.com	Carries herbal teas, Chinese herbal tonics, Chinese herbal formulations, herbal extracts, and super foods	Ron Teegaurden is a wild harvester and importer of the highest quality natural Chinese herbs available on the American market. He carries herbal teas, 350 herbal products, super foods, coffee, and books. He has several stores in California and does mail order.

Mr. Rahul Agarwal (Marketing Executive) Mother Herbs (P) Ltd C - 39, 2nd & 4th Floor, 13 - Street, Madhu Vihar, Patpadganj, Delhi - 110092, (India) Call Us : +(91)-8588810220 Fax: (+91)-(120)-3911010 E-mail : info@motherherbs.com	Manufactures a full range of Indian medicinal herbal products from antidepressant herbs, anxiety herbs, antioxidant herbs, sedative herbs, insomnia herbs and much more.	Mother Herbs is an organic grower and manufacturer of Indian herbal medicinal plants. They manufacture a diverse variety of herbs, herbal extracts, teas, essential oils, phytochemicals, oleoresins, on orders of the customer. They specialize in processing the natural plant product of whatever the client needs.
Blue Dragon Herbs Michael Sax, L.Ac. 855 1th Street, # 304 Santa Monica, CA 90403 Phone: (310)-393-6642 info@bluedragonherbs.com	Grows and manufactures organic, heavy metal free Chinese herbal formulas	The mission of Blue Dragon is to bring the healing power of Chinese herbs to the United States, in all their original potency, yet unadulterated by the toxins of herb farming in China. 88% of the herbs used in our formulas are either USDA or EU certified organically grown or certified organic wild-crafted. 28 of Blue Dragon's 66 formulas are comprised of 100% certified organically grown or wild-crafted herbs. 56 of our 66 formulas have 80% or higher certified organically grown or wild-crafted herbs.
Crazy Water 209 N.W. 6th Street Mineral Wells, Texas 76067 Tel: (940) 325-8870 http://drinkcrazywater.com/	Mineral Water with Lithium	Crazy Water comes in 4 different styles. Bulk home bottle use and 3 different strengths of bottled mineral water with lithium. No. 4 "The Craziest" has .17 mg/l of elemental lithium per bottle.

Himalaya Drug Company Makali, Bangalore, KA 562 162, India Phone: 1-800-425-1930 http://www.himalayawellness.com/	Makers of total rauwolfia serpentina alkaloid product Serpenia	60 strong product portfolio includes therapeutics, wellness products, prescription dermaceuticals and oral health products for men, women and children. Today, Himalaya is ranked thirty-one amongst 500 top pharmaceutical companies in India.
Orthomolecular Products 1991 Duncan Place Woodstock, IL 60098 Phone: (815)-337-0089 1-800-332-2351 Email: contact@ompimail.com http://www.orthomolecularproducts.com	Sells Lithium Orotate 10mg	Orthomolecular products offers a full line of supplements. Ortho Molecular Products is unique in that they operate their own 100,000-square-foot, cGMP, FDA-audited manufacturing facility that is based in Stevens Point, Wisconsin and staffed by highly trained personnel who share a passion for efficacy.
CannVest Phone: 855-PLUS-CBD (758-7223) Email: info@cannavest.com Web: http://cannavest.com/	Makers of Hemp CBD Products	CannaVest™ is in the business of developing, producing, marketing and selling raw oil and end-consumer products containing agricultural hemp-based compounds with a focus on cannabidiol (CBD). We are pioneering an emerging worldwide trend to re-energize the production of agricultural hemp and to foster its many uses for consumers. Our health and wellness raw agricultural and consumer products are produced with cannabidiol (CBD). We believe that we are the largest supplier of low-THC CBD oil in the world.

SOTERIX MEDICAL INC 160 Convent Ave New York, NY, 10031 contact@soterixmedical.com training@soterixmedical.com 1.888.990.TDCS (1.888.990.8327) Fax: 212-315-3232	Providers of tDCS and GVS devices for clinicians	Founded in 2008, SMI is the world leader in clinical trials for non-invasive neuromodulation working with over 150 medical centers in the US and worldwide. SMI has licensed and developed a comprehensive intellectual property portfolio that includes High-Definition transcranial Direct Current Stimulation (HD-tDCS), Limited Total Energy tDCS (LTE-tDCS), and Neurotargeting. From the most targeted non-invasive clinical systems to the most portable units, Soterix Medical provides clinicians and patients with unique and adaptable solutions.
Rogue Resolutions Ltd Sophia House 28 Cathedral Road Cardiff, Wales, UK CF11 9LJ Tel: +44 (0) 2920 660 198 Fax: +44 (0) 2920 660 199 Email: info@rogue-resolutions.com	Makers of Neuromodulation Equipment for clinical use and research: TMS, tRNS, tDCS and several more others.	Our portfolio of services and products includes a range of "best-in-class" devices in the fields of: Neuronavigation Neuroimaging Neuromodulation Neurosensory
VieLight Inc 346A Jarvis Street Toronto, Ontario M4Y 2G6 Canada. Tel: +1-855-875-6841 (Toll-free for US and Canada) or +1-416-316-6691 info@vielight.com	Makers of transcrainal-intranasal light therapy combination for patients with schizophrenia, depression, PTSD, Alzhiemer's and TBI	Lew Lim and his colleagues invented intranasal light therapy as a non-invasive method to introduce therapeutic light energy into the human body in California in 1995. The research and development continued under MedicLights Research Inc in the 2000's before Vielight Inc was founded to commercialize the invention.

Alternative Reading

Alternative Medicine

➤ Bragdon, Emma. *Resources for Extraordinary Healing: Schizophrenia, Bipolar and Other Serious Mental Illnesses*. [Woodstock, VT]: Lightening Up Press, 2012.

➤ Edelman, Eva. *Natural Healing for Bipolar Disorder: A Compendium of Nutritional Approaches*. Eugene, Or.: Borage Books, 2009.

➤ Edelman, Eva. *Natural Healing for Schizophrenia: And Other Common Mental Disorders*. Eugene, Or.: Borage Books, 2001.

➤ Flaws, Bob, and James Lake. *Chinese Medical Psychiatry: A Textbook & Clinical Manual : Including Indications for Referral to Western Medical Services*. Boulder, CO: Blue Poppy Press, 2001.

➤ Greek, Milt. *Schizophrenia: A Blueprint for Recovery*. Athens, Ohio: CreateSpace Independent Publishing Platform, 2012.

➤ Guyol, Gracelyn. *Healing Depression & Bipolar Disorder without Drugs: Inspiring Stories of Restoring Mental Health through Natural Therapies*. New York: Walker & Co., 2006.

➤ Hawkins, David R. *Orthomolecular Psychiatry: Treatment of Schizophrenia*. San Francisco: W H Freeman & Co, 1973.

➤ Hoffer, Abram. *Healing Schizophrenia: Complementary Vitamin and Drug Treatments*. Canada: CCNM Press, 2004.

➤ Hoffer, Abram. *Orthomolecular Treatment for Schizophrenia*. 1 edition. Los Angeles: McGraw-Hill, 1999.

➤ Lou, Baiceng, Thomas Dey, and Nigel Wiseman. *Soothing the troubled mind: acupuncture and moxibustion in the treatment of schizophrenia*. Brookline, Mass.: Paradigm Publications, 2000.

➤ M.D, Carl C. Pfeiffer Ph D. *Nutrition and Mental Illness: An Orthomolecular Approach to Balancing Body Chemistry*. Rochester, Vt: Healing Arts Press, 1988.

➤ Moyer, David. *10 Ways to Keep Your Brain from Screaming Ouch!* [S.l.]: Xlibris Corporation, 2014.

➤ Moyer, David. *Beyond Mental Illness Transform the Labels Transform a Life.* Xlibris Corp, 2014.

➤ Moyer, David. *Too Good to Be True?: Nutrients Quiet the Unquiet Brain : A Four Generation Bipolar Odyssey.* Penn Valley, CA: Nu-Tune Press, 2003.

➤ Sharma, Dr Krishna N. *Acupuncture for Schizophrenia Simplified: An Illustrated Guide.* Ill edition. CreateSpace Independent Publishing Platform, 2013.

➤ Wagner, Craig "*Choices in Recovery, Non-drug Approaches for Adult Mental Health - an Evidence-Based Guide.*" Create Space, 2015.

Psychotropic Drug Withdrawal

➤ Hall, Will. *Harm Reduction Guide to Coming Off Psychiatric Drugs.* 1 edition. Icarus Project, 2007.

➤ Harper, James. *How to Get Off Psychoactive Drugs Safely,* n.d.

➤ Lehmann, Peter, Loren R. Mosher, Judi Chamberlin, and Pirkko Lahti. *Coming off Psychiatric Drugs: Successful Withdrawal from Neuroleptics, Antidepressants, Mood Stabilizers, Ritalin and Tranquilizers.* Peter Lehmann Publishing, 2014.

➤ MD, Peter R. Breggin. *Psychiatric Drug Withdrawal: A Guide for Prescribers, Therapists, Patients and Their Families.* 1 edition. New York: Springer Publishing Company, 2012.

Iatrogenic Injury from Psychotropics and Conventional Mental Health Treatment

➤ Breggin, Peter R. *Toxic Psychiatry: Why Therapy, Empathy and Love Must Replace the Drugs, Electroshock, and Biochemical Theories of the "New Psychiatry."* 1 edition. New York: St. Martin's Griffin, 1994.

➤ Jackson, MD Grace E. *Drug-Induced Dementia: A Perfect Crime.* Bloomington, IN: AuthorHouse, 2009.

- Jackson, MD Grace E. *Rethinking Psychiatric Drugs: A Guide for Informed Consent.* Bloomington, Ind: AuthorHouse, 2005.

- Keshavan, Matcheri S. *Drug-Induced Dysfunction In Psychiatry.* 1 edition. New York: Taylor & Francis, 1991.

- Kirk, Stuart A., Tomi Gomory, and David Cohen. *Mad Science: Psychiatric Coercion, Diagnosis, and Drugs.* 1 edition. New Brunswick, N.J: Transaction Publishers, 2013.

- MD, Peter R. Breggin. *Brain Disabling Treatments in Psychiatry: Drugs, Electroshock, and the Psychopharmaceutical Complex.* 2 edition. New York: Springer Publishing Company, 2007.

- Moncrieff, Joanna. *The Bitterest Pills: The Troubling Story of Antipsychotic Drugs.* 1 edition. Houndmills, Basingstoke, Hampshire ; New York, NY: Palgrave Macmillan, 2013.

- Whitaker, Robert. *Anatomy of an Epidemic: Magic Bullets, Psychiatric Drugs, and the Astonishing Rise of Mental Illness in America.* 1 edition. New York: Crown, 2010.

- Whitaker, Robert, and Lisa Cosgrove. *Psychiatry Under the Influence: Institutional Corruption, Social Injury, and Prescriptions for Reform.* New York: Palgrave Macmillan, 2015.

Miscellaneous Books

- Stastny, Peter, and Peter Lehmann, eds. *Alternatives Beyond Psychiatry.* Berlin ; Eugene, Or: Peter Lehmann Publishing, 2007.

- Stradford, Dan, Garry Vickar, Christine Berger, and Hyla Cass. *The Flying Publisher Guide to Complementary and Alternative Medicine Treatments in Psychiatry.* Bernd Kamps Steinhäuser Verlag, 2012.

- Cardinal, Rudolf N., and Edward T. Bullmore. *The Diagnosis of Psychosis.* 1 edition. Cambridge, UK ; New York: Cambridge University Press, 2011.

- Sachdev, Perminder S., and Matcheri S. Keshavan, eds. *Secondary Schizophrenia.* 1 edition. Cambridge ; New York: Cambridge University Press, 2010.

Alternative Mental Health Practitioners Directories

There are a growing number of practitioners in the field of Integrative Psychiatry and alternative treatments for mental health, though the field has imprecise boundaries. Consider the following directories, clinics and practitioners when seeking integrative mental health care.

Directories of Integrative Psychiatrists
American Psychiatric Association directory
http://www.intpsychiatry.com/practitioner-directory.html (note: put this link in the Wayback Machine: https://archive.org/web/)

Integrative Medicine for Mental Health Referral
Registry http://www.integrativemedicineformentalhealth.com/registry.php

Directories of Naturopaths.
Find a Naturopath http://findanaturopath.com/

American Association of Naturopathic Physicians
directory http://www.naturopathic.org/AF_MemberDirectory.asp?version=1

Canadian Association of Naturopathic Doctors http://www.cand.ca/

Directories of Orthomolecular practitioners.

Orthomolecular.org worldwide practitioner directory
http://orthomolecular.org/resources/pract.shtml

Walsh Institute biochemical/nutrient therapy practitioner directory
http://www.walshinstitute.org/clinical-resources.html

Canadian Society of Orthomolecular Medicine practitioner directory
https://www.csom.ca/practitioner-list/

Directories of Alternative/Integrative Medicine practitioners.

AlternativeMentalHealth.com practitioner
directory http://www.alternativementalhealth.com/directory/search.asp

Directories of Alternative/Integrative Medicine practitioners.

American Board of Integrative Holistic Medicine physician directory
http://www.abihm.org/search-doctors

American College for Advancement in Medicine directory
of complementary and integrative medicine practitioners
http://acam.site-ym.com/search/custom.asp?id=1758

Food Matters directory of holistic healthcare practitioners
http://foodmatters.tv/resource/practitioner-directory

American Holistic Health Association practitioner directory
http://ahha.org/ahhasearch.asp

Hospitals with Integrative Psychiatry focus.
California: http://www.ucsfhealth.org/treatments/integrative_psychiatry/

Pennsylvania: http://www.upmc.com/Services/integrative-medicine/services/Pages/integrative-psychiatry.aspx

Ohio: http://www.uhhospitals.org/services/integrative-medicine/integrative-medicine/our-services/integrative-psychiatry

Minnesota: www.northmemorial.com/psychiatry#.VPM7ZvnF9qX
New
York: http://asp.cumc.columbia.edu/facdb/profile_list.asp?uni=rpb1&DepAffil=Psychiatry

Integrative Psychiatry clinics/practices.
Mensah Medical http://www.mensahmedical.com/_index.php

Orthomolecular clinics
http://www.nmrc.ca/

"Alternative Mental Health Practitioners Directory"
Information taken from Craig Wagner's *Beyond Psychotropics*, 2014

Web Resources for Persons with Serious Mental Illness

All Categories: Psychosocial, Alternative Medicine, Peer Support, Advocacy, Research

Safe Harbor, http://www.alternativementalhealth.com/
Tardive Dyskinesia Center, http://www.tardivedyskinesia.com/
International Society for Orthomolecular Medicine, http://www.orthomed.org/
National Empowerment Center, http://www.power2u.org/
Mad In America, http://www.madinamerica.com/
Will Hall, http://willhall.net/
The Icarus Project, http://www.theicarusproject.net/
Madness Radio, http://www.madnessradio.net/
Ron Unger LCSW, http://recoveryfromschizophrenia.org/about-ron-unger/
Jim Gottstein/PsychRights Law Project for Psychiatric Rights, http://psychrights.org/
International Society for Psychological and Social Approaches to Psychosis, http://www.isps-us.org/
Mindfreedom International, http://www.mindfreedom.org/
International Schizophrenia Foundation, http://www.orthomed.org/isf/isf.html

All Categories: Psychosocial, Alternative Medicine, Peer Support, Advocacy, Research

Walsh Research Institute, http://www.walshinstitute.org/
Hearing Voices Network USA, http://www.hearingvoicesusa.org/
Hearing Voices Network, http://www.hearing-voices.org/
Asylum Magazine, http://www.asylumonline.net/
Peter Breggin M.D., http://www.breggin.com/
Joanna Moncrief, http://joannamoncrieff.com/
David Moyer LCSW, http://www.bipolarodyssey.com http://beyondmentalillness.us/
Citizen Commission on Human Rights International, http://www.cchrint.org/
Craig Wagner www.OnwardMentalHealth.com
Citizens Commission on Human Rights International, http://www.cchr.org/
Monica Cassani http://beyondmeds.com/
Dr. Toby Watson http://www.drtobywatson.com/

Appendix A

The First Antipsychotic: Rauwolfia Serpentina and Alkaloid Drug Reserpine

History of Rauwofia Sepentina and Reserpine

The history of the therapeutic use of Rauwolfia serpentina goes back to the origins of ayurevedic medicine. Sarpagandha is the therapeutic properties of the plant are documented in the classical treatise Charaka Samhita (between 1000 and 2000 B.C.). It is referred to by such names as: in Sanskrit as Chandrika or Sarpangandha; in Hindi, as Chota-chand; in Bengali, as Chandra; in Tamil, as Chivin Melpodi; and in Patna, as Dhan Marua or Dhan Barua. A local definition of the plant is called "pagal-ka-dawa" and even means "herb against insanity (Kline, 1954; López-Muñoz, 2004)".

It has been variously used as a febrifuge, an emetic, and in the treatment of such conditions as hypertension, snake bite, insomnia, and insanity. The first reports on the tranquilizing and sedative effects of Rauwolfia serpentine occurred in India in the 1930's . In 1931, Gananath Sen and Kartick Chandra Bose reported on the use of an alkaloid extract from the Rauwolfia serpentina plant in the treatment of hypertension and "insanity with violent maniacal symptoms." They noted that dosages "of 20 to 30 grains of the powder twice daily produce not only a hypnotic effect but also a reduction of blood pressure and violent symptoms . . . within a week usually the patient's senses are restored, though he may show some mental aberrations." Outside of India, however, Sen and Bose's observations on the use of rauwolfia for psychotic disorders were generally ignored (Greenberg, 2006). Siddiqui and Siddiquil that same year also make mention of its general sedative action and its curative properties in certain kinds of insanity. These results did not reach Western medicine until 1949, when Indian cardiologist Rustom Jal Vakil published a study on the hypotensive effect of the root extracts in the *British Heart Journal* (Kline, 1954; López-Muñoz, 2004)

The pioneer for the use of reserpine in the treatment of psychosis was Nathan S. Kline from Rockland State Hospital of New York. In 1953, Kline read interesting news from Bombay in the New York Times. It read: "A special award was granted to Dr. R.A. Hakim (Ahmedabad) for the study titled 'Indigenous drugs in the treatment of mental disease'. Hakim studied "Siledin" which was a mixture of medicinal plants that contained Rauwolfia. His studies were a sample of 146 patients diagnosed with schizophrenia or manic depression which had a 51% positive response rate to Siledin. Combined therapy with Siledin and electroshock therapy was 80% positive. These results led Kline to think reserpine was a substance similar to chlorpromazine which was being published as treatment in France.

Kline designed a clinical study in which 411 patients (94.4% schizophrenics) were enrolled and the efficacy of reserpine was assessed. In this study, the sedative, anxiolytic and antiobsessive effect were verified. He also verified certain side effects (somnolence, nasal congestion or reduction of blood pressure) but Kline did not observe any substantial antipsychotic effects, possible due to the low dose of reserpine used (0.51 mg/day). This was reported to the New York Academy of Science on April 30, 1954 (López-Muñoz, 2004). This study was the first study to use 500mg of natural rauwolfia serpentine root extract daily on psychiatric inpatients showing it had a marked effect on reducing anxiety reactions (Kline, 1954). Later studies of the same research team, using larger dosage regimes (initial dose of 5mg intramuscular and 3 mg orally per day), verified the antipsychotic efficacy of reserpine in schizophrenic patients. Some 200 patients were treated for 9 months with improvements percentages of 86% and hospital discharge index of 22%.

On July 20, 1954, the second publication of reserpine use in psychiatry was published. This publication collected data obtained about the new alkaloid. Hospital Sainte-Anne de Paris, Y. Tardieu and Therese Lempérière are authors who studied the antipsychotic effects of reserpine comparing them with those of chlorpromazine, predicting that reserpine could have an efficacy greater than chlorpromazine in chronic schizophrenic patients.

In the latter half of the 50's , reserpine was used mostly for its two important pharmacological activities (antipsychotic and hypotensive) though in some places (University Psychiatric Clinic of Burghölzli, Zurich) it was used as a hypnotic agent to treat sleep disorders. However, the introduction of new, orally more effective hypotensive agents, reserpine's relationship with morality due to thrombosis and it's alleged association with breast cancer (later refuted, by controlled studies) and its drug-induced depressive states, with risk of suicide, considerably reduced its use (López-Muñoz, 2004). Though according to an article by David Healy, reserpine did not induce depression and was used to treat depression and had antidepressant effects. He indicated that in the 1955 when reserpine was being used that akathisia may have been the cause of suicides and psychiatrists and general physicians at that time were not familiar with akathisia as a side effect (Healy, 1998). Reserpine was also one of the drugs that played a role in the historical development of the monoamine hypothesis of depression which was later found to be untrue and now a myth (Baumeister, 2003). In 1991 a review still listed reserpine as 1 of 8 reasonable, evidence-based treatment options for persons affected with the refractory symptoms of schizophrenia (Christison, 1991).

Treatment of Psychotic Patients with Rauwolfia Total Alkaloid Product "Serpenia".

In an article wrote in (1958) *Journal of Neurolgical Neurosugical Psychiatry*, Dr. Homai M. Colabawalla did a study on the effects of rauwolfia serpentian alkaloid reserpine, total alkaloid product "serpenia" and placebo on 36 psychotic patients. The response and side effects were compared and the response to each drug was similar, but "serpina" was free from side effects.

Treatment response.—Two 4 mg tablets of "serpenia" were given thrice daily, and improvement began to be apparent after about three weeks. The unmanageable patients became manageable and all were employed –some without supervision. Most could sleep in unsupervised dormitories which had previously been impossible. Eighteen were able to shave themselves; none were wet and dirty, none had to be washed or dressed and a minimum of toilet supervision was needed. There were no impulsive outbursts; the destructive patient no longer tore his suits, and his table manners had improved so much that he could not eat with the other patients.

No patients could be discharged (often because they had been in-patients for years and no homes), but a few were well enough to be allowed out at week-ends for the first time.

Side Effects.--The response to "serpenia" and the absence of side effects were confirmed in a larger group treated for 22 weeks (Colabawalla, 1958).

More about Total Alkoloid Rauwolfia Products

Serpina is a single-ingredient formulation for the management of mild to moderate hypertension. The drug depletes peripheral catecholamine (noradrenaline) stores, which results in a reduction of blood pressure. Serpina decreases the adrenergic tone and controls anxiety, and is therefore beneficial in the treatment of anxiety disorders as well (Himalaya Drug Company, 2015).

According to the manufacturer of Serpenia (Himalaya Drug Company; http://www.himalayawellness.com/products/pharmaceuticals/serpina-tablet.htm), it does not have any side effects at the average fixed dosage for hypertension. However in other studies for hypertension "serpina" and other total alkaloid preparations may have some minor side effects. Side effects include; weight gain, nasal congestion, bradycardia, and sedation (reference needed). Other less common side effects include nausea and vomiting, diarrhea, lassitude, and anorexia (Vakil, 1949).

Weight gain with Serpina may be less than reserpine, which has been shown to cause an average weight gain of 2.2 kg (4.8lbs) in about 30 days for patients with hypertension (Melick, 1957). Total alkaloid rauwolfia serpetina products have extracts rauwolscine and yohimbine in them. These extracts are used in weight management and body building supplements (http://www.dexaprine.org/ingredients/rauwolfia-serpentina). This may keep the weight down when used as a psychotropic agent at doses of 4 grams a day or more as compared to reserpine.

The Serpenia drug can be purchased online at Himalaya Drug Company, or relatively cheap in bulk, at http://www.ebay.com/. It can cost as little as $10.00 to $20.00 US dollars on ebay.com for a 1 month to 3 month supply depending on dosage needed. It comes in 250 mg tablets, 100 and 300 tablet bottles. Dosage for chronic psychotic patients in current study was 4 mg, x thrice daily. For hypertension 1 to 4 tablets a day may be needed (http://www.himalayawellness.com/research/serpina.htm) or maintenance of psychiatric schizophrenia doses may be much lower than 4 mg x 3 daily. Speak to an experienced integrative psychiatrist, or doctor who specializes in Ayurvedic medicine for appropriate dosages.

If you use raw herbal root and other brands of rauwolfia serpentina it is not known of the side effects or efficiency. They may be generally safe however at high doses rauwolfia can cause parkinsonian tremors. It may also produce oxidative stress to the body like its alkaloid reserpine and it may be suggested to use antioxidants as adjunctive therapy. However, rauwolfia serpentina is a very effective and cost efficient medicine that has been used safely for thousands of years.

The History and Therapeutic Benefits of Lithium Mineral Water and Lithium Supplementation in the Treatment of Bipolar Manic Depression

History of Lithium Mineral Spring Water

The historical aspects of the use of lithium in psychiatry are quite interesting. As well are the reports of the therapeutic benefits of lithium mineral waters. Lithium salts may have inadvertently been used for the treatment of excitation in ancient and medieval times. Recommendations for drinking and bathing in alkaline mineral waters were made by Greek and Arabic physicians, including Avicenna, Galen, and Soranus (Baldessrini, 2013). The first therapeutic application of lithium in mania was prescribed in Rome in the second century AD by the Greek physician Seraus Ephesios (from Asian Minor) who, in his section on the treatment of mania, writes: *"Utendum quoque naturalibus aquis, ut sunt nitrosae....,"* which means: "use should also be made of natural waters, such as alkaline springs." The 5th century AD Roman physician Calelius Aurelianus recommended specific alkaline springs, many of which contained lithium, to treat certain physical and mental ailments. The tradition of natural spring water for the treatment of emotional illness was widely accepted throughout the centuries.

Around 1818, J.A. Arfwedson, working in the laboratory of Berzelius, discovered a silvery white substance which he called lithium, from the Greek *lithos*, which means stone. Arfwedson demonstrated that lithium resembled sodium and potassium in some reactions but not others. Robert Bunsen disclosed the presence of lithium in tobacco, sugar cane and seaweed which contradicted the exclusive occurrence of this element in minerals. Lithium's distribution in nature is extensive and diverse. It has been detected in trace amounts in plants, marine life, milk from several animals and various animal and human tissues, but not human bone (Georgotas, 1981).

The last half of the 19th century saw lithium grow in medicinal popularity and become a widely used proprietary drug. This was due, in part, to the writings of Alexander Haig which implicated uric acid as a factor in the causation of a myriad of diseases. These illnesses included headache, epilepsy, mental depression, melancholia, suicide, high blood pressure, angina, asthma, Raynaud's disease, gout, and rheumatism. Lithia tablets and litha spring waters "flooded" the market and were widely and vigorously extolled for their curative values in both lay and medical literature. A product called "Basic Litha Water" was advertised to be:

"Invaluable as a constant and exclusive drinking water, and in the prevention and cure of rheumatism, gout, malaria, typhoid fever and diseases of the kidney, liver, blood, and nerves."

Even respected medical journals touted the value of lithium waters for both bathing and drinking in search of cures. In response to this belief, for example, the Litha Springs Sanitarium was founded in Georgia in 1890 for the treatment of alcoholism, opioid dependence, and compulsive behaviors. Those who could not afford a holiday cure at a famous spa could at least buy bottled mineral water, such as the marketed Bear and Buffalo Lithia Waters from Virginia and District of Columbia, White Rock Spring water from upstate New York, and Lithia Beer from Wisconsin. In the early 1900's, over 40 products touting the presence of lithium salts made medicinal claims in the U.S. Some of them were eventually found to contain very little lithium.

Company after company glowingly proclaimed the therapeutic merits of mineral spring waters with lithium regularly touted as the critical component. When the lithium content in the waters was actually measured, however, it was generally found in negligible amounts and in certain samples was undetectable. The U.S. Bureau of Chemistry studied all of the most important lithia waters on the American market and found that nearly all of them contained only spectroscopic traces or less than one part per million of lithium. The contrast between claim and substance was noted by Harrington:

> This water claims to be a cure for almost all ills to which flesh is heir, and to contain over fourteen grains of lithium salts per gallon. It proves to be an exceedingly hard water, practically free from organic matter, absolutely free from lithia, but rich in undesirable lime salts. (Strobusch, 1980)

In the early 1900's the Supreme Court of District of Columbia declared that "in order to achieve a therapeutic dose of lithium by drinking Buffalo Lithia Water, a person should drink from 150,000 –225,000 gallons of water a day." And yet the public remained fond of lithium, despite its status as a form of medical quackery.

A lingering influence of the faddish use of mineral waters containing lithium is found in the popular non-alcoholic soft drink 7-Up, which was created by Charles Leiper Grigg two weeks before the crash of 1929. The lithium-laced drink was originally named "Lithiated Lemon Soda" before the name was changed to 7-UP. The soda was marketed as a hangover cure and general tonic that "neutralizes the acid blood…[and] soothes and smoothes the ragged nerves" It initially contained lithium until 1950 (Lewis, 2009).

Lithium in Drinking Water: Crime, Arrest Related Drug Addictions and Suicide Rates

A study published in the *British Journal of Psychiatry* (2009) was to examine lithium levels in tap water in 18 municiple cities of Oita prefecture in Japan in relation to the suicide standardized mortality ratio (SMR) in each municipality. They found that lithium levels were significantly and negatively associated with SMR averages for 2002–2006. The findings suggest that even very low levels of lithium in drinking water may play a role in reducing suicide risk within the general population. Their study concluded:

> These findings suggest that even very low lithium levels may reduce the risk of suicide and that within the levels there is a dose–response relationship. Although it seems unlikely that such low lithium levels can bring about mood-stabilizing effects and thereby reduce the risk of suicide, could the antisuicidal effect of lithium be unrelated to its prophylactic effect for mood disorders? Muller-Oerlinghausen et al. revealed that a significant reduction in suicide attempts occurred even in poor responders to lithium prophylaxis for mood disorders. Therefore, it seems probable that the antisuicidal effect of lithium may be unrelated to the mood-stabilising effects and that very low lithium levels may possess an antisuicidal effect. On the other hand, although lithium levels are extremely low in the drinking water, long-term exposure to lithium may be a factor which mitigates low absolute levels. It can be speculated that very low but very long lithium exposure can enhance neurotrophic factors, neuroprotective factors and/or neurogenesis, which may account for a reduced risk of suicide (Ohgami, 2009).

To evaluate the association between local lithium levels in drinking water and suicide mortality at district level in Austria, a study was published in the *British Journal of Psychiatry* (2011) that examined the association between lithium measurements with suicide rates per 100,000 population and suicide standardized mortality ratios across all 99 Austrian districts. Their findings were as follows:

> Owing to the sizeable magnitude of our finding, we provide conclusive evidence that lithium concentrations in drinking water are inversely correlated with suicide rates. Starting with anecdotic reports about the beneficial effects of lithium in drinking water on mental health in 1949 and earlier, there is increasing evidence from three independent countries and continents that lithium in drinking water is associated with reduced mortality from suicide (Kapusta, 2011).

In 1989, Gerhard Schrauzer et al. conducted a study that was published in *Biological Trace Element Research* that showed the relationship between lithium levels in drinking water and the rates of crime, suicides and arrests related to drug addiction. His study findings are as follows:

> Using data for 27 Texas counties from 1978-1987, it is shown that the incidence rates of suicide, homicide, and rape are significantly higher in counties whose drinking water supplies contain little or no lithium than in counties with water lithium levels ranging from 70- 170 I~g/L; the differences remain statistically significant ($p < 0.01$) after corrections for population density. The corresponding associations with the incidence

rates of robbery, burglary, and theft were statistically significant with $p < 0.05$. These results suggest that lithium has moderating effects on suicidal and violent criminal behavior at levels that may be encountered in municipal water supplies. Comparisons of drinking water lithium levels, in the respective Texas counties, with the incidences of arrests for possession of opium, cocaine, and their derivatives (morphine, heroin, and codeine) from 1981-1986 also produced statistically significant inverse associations, whereas no significant or consistent associations were observed with the reported arrest rates for possession of marijuana, driving under the influence of alcohol, and drunkenness. These results suggest that lithium at low dosage levels has a generally beneficial effect on human behavior, which may be associated with the functions of lithium as a nutritionally-essential trace element. Subject to confirmation by controlled experiments with high-risk populations, increasing the human lithium intakes by supplementation, or the lithiation of drinking water is suggested as a possible means of crime, suicide, and drug-dependency reduction at the individual and community level (Schrauzer, 1990).

Where Natural Lithium is Found

Lithium is found in trace amounts in all soils primarily in the clay fraction, and to a lesser extent in the organic soil fraction, in amounts ranging from 7 to 200 {g/g. It is present in surface water at levels between 1 and 10 {g/L, in sea water at 0.18 {g/L. The lithium concentrations in ground water may reach 500 {g/L, in river water of lithium-rich regions of northern Chile, 1508 and 5170 {g/L, respectively. In the latter regions, total Li intakes may reach 10 mg/day, without evidence of adverse effects to the local population. Still higher lithium levels, up to 100 mg/L are found in some natural mineral waters.

Everyone is exposed to small quantities of lithium. The U.S. Environmental Protection Agency (EPA) in 1985 estimated the daily Li intake of a 70 kg adult to range from 650 to 3100 mcgs (micrograms). Primary dietary sources of lithium are grains and vegetables, which may contribute from 66% to more than 90% of the total lithium intake; the remainder is from animal derived foods. In general, diets rich in grains and vegetables may be expected to provide more lithium than diets rich in animal proteins. However, due to the uneven distribution of lithium on the earth's crust, a predominantly vegetarian diet is not necessarily lithium rich. Common vegetables and spices as coriander seeds and leaves, nutmeg, cumin seeds, tomato and garlic, are rich in lithium. Millet and some variety of lentils, are also rich in lithium, though rice and wheat contain little. Some rock salts and crude sea salts, are rich in lithium, as are seafoods and sea vegetation. Seaweeds can be very rich in lithium. Accordingly, the estimated dietary lithium intakes in populations of different countries vary over a wide range and, as a rule, the standard deviations from the means are large. Tap water and beverages may contribute significantly to the total (Lewis, 2009; Schrauzer, 2002).

Lithium Deficiency in Humans

After many years of research, it appears that lithium is an essential nutrient. Lithium is normally present in all organs and tissues of both humans and animals. Lithium-deficient goats develop mammary cysts and inflammation, enlarged salivary glands, adrenal gland abnormalities, and ovarian cysts. One net effect of this deficiency state is to impair lactation and reproduction. Gerhard Schrauzer, one of the world's top lithium authorities, states:

> In studies conducted from the 1970s to the 1990s, rats and goats maintained on low-lithium rations were shown to exhibit higher mortalities as well as reproductive and behavioral abnormalities. In humans...lithium deficiency diseases have not been characterized, but low lithium intakes from water supplies were associated with increased rates of suicides, homicides and the arrest rates for drug use and other crimes. Lithium appears to play an especially important role during the early fetal development as evidenced by the high lithium contents of the embryo during the early gestational period (Lewis, 2009).

As Lithium deficiency in humans is unlikely ever to reach the degree of severity observed in experimental Li-depleted animals, any symptoms of lithium deficiency in humans, if at all observable, would be expected to be mild and manifest themselves primarily by behavioral rather than physiological abnormalities. Evidence linking low lithium intakes with altered behavior and aggressiveness in humans was reported by Dawson et al. These authors compared the regional mental hospital admission rates and homicide rates for 1967--1969 with the lithium concentrations in tap water samples and in urine samples obtained from 24 county sites in Texas. The highest significant inverse associations of water Li levels were observed with first mental hospital admissions for psychosis, neurosis and personality disorders. The decreasing order of magnitude of the associations was neurosis, schizophrenia, psychosis, first admission, all admissions, personality, homicide and secondary admissions. Urine lithium concentrations showed the statistically most significant inverse associations with the schizophrenic diagnosis, secondary with the first mental hospital admission for psychosis, neurosis and with homicide; associations with the suicide rates were inverse but not significant. Lithium deficiency may not only be caused by low dietary Li intakes but can also be secondary to certain diseases (Schrauzer, 2002).

Lithium Daily Requirements (RDA)

The minimum human adult (physiological) Li requirement was estimated to 100 {g/day, higher intakes are apparently needed to utilize "beneficial" effects of Li. Based on Li intake data in different countries, a provisional RDA of 1 mg Li/day for a 70 kg adult can be proposed, corresponding to 14.3 {g/kg BW, which can be reached by diet alone in Li-adequate regions. For subjects subsisting on special diets or for populations residing in naturally low Li areas, Li supplementation or other appropriate measures to meet this RDA would be required. Special attention should be accorded to the potentially higher relative Li needs of children, adolescents and lactating mothers. Lithium needs furthermore may be higher after physical exertion, in certain diseases and in dialysis patients. An adequate supply of Li should also be assured for subjects on formula diets and or on total or home parenteral nutrition (Schrauzer, 2002).

Low-Dose Lithium Supplementation

A study done by G.N. Schrauzer published in *Biological Trace Element Reseach* (1994) showed low-dose lithium was beneficial on mental well-being in former drug users. Here is a summary of the paraphrased abstract:

> A total of 24 subjects, 16 males and 8 females, average age 29.4 +/- 6.5 y, were randomly divided into two groups. The lithium group received 400 micrograms/d of lithium orally, in tablets composed of a naturally lithium-rich brewer's yeast, for 4 wk. All the subjects of the study were former drug users (mostly heroin and crystal methamphetamine). Some of the subjects were violent offenders or had a history of domestic violence. In the lithium group, positive mood test scores increased throughout the study, especially in the areas of "happiness", "friendliness" and "energy". Based on the results and the analysis of voluntary written comments of study participants, it is concluded that lithium at the dosages chosen had a mood-improving and -stabilizing effect (Schrauzer, 1994).

Lithium Orotate Supplementation

An article written by H.A. Nieper in the *Agressologie* journal (1973) on "The Clinical Applications of Lithium Orotate: A Two Years Study" made the following statement about lithium orotate supplementation:

> I cannot recall any medication which was able to achieve such remarkable results in so short a time as does lithium orotate. I have reason to believe that a number of patients, skeptical of low dosage, were taking lithium oratate capsules more frequently than necessary. This is, however, completely harmless in every respect (Nieper, 1973).

Many nutritionally oriented clinicians have found lithium orotate to be effective in patients seeking to improve mental health and well-being. Since lithium is a naturally occurring mineral, there is a growing opinion amongst physicians that lithium augmentation for nutrient deficient diets should be a consideration as clinically indicated.

How Lithium Orotate Works

The lithium salt of orotic acid (lithium orotate) increases the uptake of lithium and improves the specific effects of lithium many-fold. Based on intraperitoneal injections in a rat study, higher brain concentrations of lithium were obtained when lithium orotate was injected I.P. The study reported: "Furthermore, the 24-hour brain concentration of lithium after lithium orotate was approximately three times greater than that after lithium carbonate. These data suggest the possibility that lower doses of lithium orotate than lithium carbonate may achieve therapeutic brain lithium concentrations and relatively stable serum concentrations." Another study evaluated lithium orotate absorption in laboratory animals and showed the brain and blood serum concentrations of lithium orotate remained stable in the serum for up to 24 hours post-administration. Brain concentrations were also 3 times higher than found in the animals given lithium carbonate (CPMedical.net, 2011).

Lithium Orotate Compared to Other Lithium Salts

Lithium carbonate used in psychiatry, in the treatment of bipolar, has about 20% elemental lithium in it (the 80% is the "carbonate" part, not lithium). Hence, the typical dose of 900-1800 milligrams per day of lithium carbonate supplies about 180-360 milligrams of elemental lithium. This is the range that has potential long-term toxicity to the thyroid and other organs (Lewis, 2009).

Lithium is available in several forms; the most common are the lithium carbonate and lithium citrate forms. Because of the poor bioavailability of lithium carbonate and citrate, high dosages of these forms of lithium are normally required (2,400 mg-3,600 mg per day) to achieve the desired benefits. Research suggests the lithium salt of orotic acid (lithium orotate) may be more bioavailable than the carbonate and citrate forms. Because of this improved bioavailability, lower doses of lithium orotate than either lithium carbonate or lithium citrate may be used in the clinical setting to achieve beneficial concentrations and relatively stable serum concentrations. Standard lithium orotate 130 mg tablets provide only 4.8 mg of elemental lithium (CPMedical.net, 2011).

Because of the low dose of lithium orotate, none of the renal side effects, such as nephrogenic diabetes insipidus, partial distal renal tubular acidosis, interstitial nephritis, and reductions in glomerular filtration rate, are likely to develop by use of this compound. Moreover, mild renal insufficiency, which is common in patients with lithium intoxication, has not been reported with lithium orotate (Sartori, 1986).

Lithium Orotate vs. Lithium Aspartate

Lithium aspartate and lithium orotate are available over-the-counter and contain lower dosages of lithium than lithium carbonate, which must be prescribed by a doctor. Most proponents of low-dose lithium therapy such as Dr. Jonathan Wright recommend them equally. However, aspartate is thought to be an excitotoxin, a substance that binds to nerve cell receptors and may cause damaging over-stimulation. Marlina E. Borkwood, MSc states that excitotoxins can cause headaches, brain edema, eye inflammation, vascular system and central nervous system problems in sensitive individuals. Those who want to try low-dose lithium therapy and have experienced sensitivity to another excitotoxin, monosodium glutamate -- a food additive commonly known as MSG -- may wish to stick with lithium orotate (Jones, 2015).

Effects of Lithium Orotate: Physical, Mental and Side Effects

In a study done by H.E. Sartori published in the *Alcohol* journal (1986) found these effects of lithium orotate in alcoholic patients with mood disorders:

> All 42 patients received 150 mg lithium orotate in stomach acid resistant gelatin capsules every morning. Eight patients developed mild symptoms of muscle weakness, loss of appetite, mild apathy and listlessness after six to eight weeks. These symptoms disappeared promptly within a few hours after drinking one cup of bouillon with sodium glutamate. In these patients, lithium orotate dosage was reduced to 4 to 5 times weekly without development of major side effects. At the onset of the treatment most patients experienced a rapid excretion of fluids. Myopic or hyperopic patients showed changes in their vision because of dehydration of their eyes. Patients with migraine or with cluster headaches experienced a large reduction in severity and frequency of their attacks subsequent to lithium treatment. Ocular symptoms of migraine-like photopsia or teichopsia as well as flicker scotomata completely ceased after lithium orotate therapy. There was an improvement in the depressive mood of all patients. In addition, irritability, particularly in male patients prone to resort to violence, was improved markedly after a few weeks of the lithium orotate. The spouses reported that their husbands were less irritable and consequently were less violent in general. No recurrence of manic episodes was experienced during lithium orotate therapy by the three patients with major affective disorders and previous manic episodes.

> Chronic alcohol-induced depression of the majority of the patients showed favorable response to lithium orotate and the patients seemed cheerful and less tense. The three patients with manic depressive psychosis showed moderation of the depressive phase and the depression disappeared in one case. No manic episodes were evident in any of the three patients during the Li orotate treatment (Sartori, 2008)."

A study done by H.A. Nieper (1973) found that lithium orotate was effective for depressive moods:

> 12 patients were given lithium orotate to control depressive moods of larval endogenic depression, generally a maximum of five 150 mg capsules per week. 9 patients all reported an improved condition, of which 3, who also showed an accompanying hyperthyreosis and tendency towards migraine, noted an exceptional betterment (Neiper, 1973).

Conclusion

The historical aspects of lithium used in psychiatry are quite interesting and in ancient and medieval times, as well as in the 19th century, many have reported therapeutic benefits from lithium mineral waters. Lithium water became so popular that beers and sodas such as 7-Up became lithiated until 1950. Today we have beverages sold at Whole Foods that are lithated.

There are two brands of lithia water available on the internet, one is Crazy Water, and another is called Lithia Water.

Lithium has a proposed daily RDA of 1 mg per day and a minimum of 100 mcg a day before person reaches physical deficiency and manifests behavioral symptoms. Low dose lithium supplementation is proposed for these deficiency states. Lithium water, lithium orotate, or lithium aspartate can be used for low dose supplementation. Speak with your integrative physician. It can be concluded that low dose lithium is a safer way to balance moods in manic depressive patients than lithium carbonate, or lithium citrate. These OTC products are safe, and convenient and less toxic than prescription lithium.

Advanced Research Lithium Orotate Tablets designed by Dr. Hans Neiper are available online and at CVS Pharmacy, and Amazon.com. They are 120 mg tablets, in 200 count bottles for under $20.00 ea. Lower dosage 10 mg tablets are available by Orthomolecular Products—see Suppliers directory. Health product suppliers such as Pure Formulas have other lithium options such Li-Zyme a vegetable culture lithium product with 150 micrograms of naturally occurring lithium. Consult an integrative psychiatrist, or naturopathic doctor who is familiar with lithium supplements and find out what is right for you.

Appendix C

Unconventional Treatments in History that Outperformed Psychotropic Drugs of Today

Throughout the history of psychiatry there has been novel uses of unconventional medicine used to treat psychiatric in-patients. Many of these treatments were used before Thorazine came onto the market for the treatment of schizophrenia in the mid-1950's.

The mid-19th century was the beginning of homeopathic sanitariums in America. Some of the many homeopathic hospitals were New York State Homeopathic Asylum, Westborough Homeopathic State Hospital, and the Fergus Falls State Hospital. They most notably used hydrotherapy along with many other treatments including psychotherapy and materia medica. These institutions had high recovery rates for their patient populations. In 1866, the Battle Creek Sanitarium was built, it was better known as the Kellogg Sanitarium and they used over 200 kinds of hydrotherapy daily to treat their patients. The late 19th century also saw the use of organotherapy; the use of granular animal extracts for the treatment of mental illness. These were used in the Maudsley Hospital in London between 1923-1938 to treat psychiatric in-patients. These animal extracts were thyroid, testicular, pituitary, adrenal, brain, and ovary extracts (Evens, 2012, Borell, 1976). Some of these are still used today to treat endocrine diseases such as hypothyroid.

The early 20th century was the beginning of chiropractic and osteopathic sanitariums that specialized in the treatment of mental illness. They specialized in adjustments to the spine and cervical areas and used a host of other physical treatments, specialized diets, psychosocial therapies and recreational activities to achieve wellness with patients (Ching, 2015, Chiropractic Sanitarium News, 1926)[1]. Also in the early 1930's, there was a Spiritist hospital built in Brazil which reported a 41% recovery rate, and 16% improvement rate for mental patients using conventional treatments combined with prayer, laying of hands, and mediumistic séances (Silvia de Almeida, 2009). Today, there are 12,000 Spiritist Centers within Brazil and 160 Spiritist community centers in 34 countries outside of Brazil (including 70 in the USA). There are 50 Spiritist psychiatric hospitals in Brazil (Bragdon, 2015).

Expressive therapies such as art therapy, music therapy, poetry, letter writing, drama, dance, bibliography and photographic therapy were all used in the early mental asylums and are still used in state hospitals today. Chromology, better known as color therapy was used in the early institutions to aid in reliving depression or creating tranquility and is still used in interior

---

[1] Chiropractic Sanitarium News is a publication that came from Courtesy of Special Services, Palmer College of Chiropractic

design of some psychiatric hospitals mental wards (Young, 2015). Heliotherapy, and Phototherapy (light therapy) were used in some early psychiatric hospitals and sanitariums for the treatment of manic depression and schizophrenia (Jackson, 1927, Cormac, 1929).

Rauwolfia serpentina and it's alkaloid reserpine were used for a brief time during the early 1950's into the early 1960's for the treatment schizophrenia. It was the first antipsychotic used in America before Thorazine (Bhatara, 1997). Megavitamin treatment was born in the mid-1950's by Abram Hoffer and Humpry Osmond with the use of niacin trials on schizophrenic patients (Hoffer, 1974). Later, the term Orthomolecular Psychiatry was coined by two time Nobel prize winner Linus Pauling. Megavitamin therapy was used in some psychiatric hospitals and became a popular alternative treatment in America and Canada for the treatment of schizophrenia (Hawkins, 1970). In China in 1956, Hebei mental hospital used acupuncture and had an 84% recovery rate for patients with schizophrenia (Hiller, 2013). Allan Cott brought fasting to America in the early 1970's for the treatment of chronic schizophrenia. This practice was also popular in Russia at the Moscow Psychiatric Institute during the late 1960's and early 1970's (Cott, 1974). Usually one week after this treatment, Allan Cott would withdrawal the patients from their psychotropic drugs because they were well enough to endure without them (JOM, 2015). Controlled fasting had an average recovery rate of 70% in chronic schizophrenic patients, with results high as a 90% recovery rate (Cott, 1974, Boehme, 1977).

In retrospect, most of these unconventional therapies that were in use before the advent of Thorazine and other major tranquilizers were much more successful for treating chronic mental illness. According to the *Biennial Report of the Board of Trustees and Officers*, 1892, Fergus Falls Homeopathic State Hospital had nearly a 70% recovery rate for manic depressive patients (p. 166). Published in the *North American Journal of Homoeopathy*, 1907, Westborough Homeopathic State Hospital also had a high recovery rate for manic depressives—between 1903 and 1905, 159 cases were admitted and 80.71% recovered (p. 132). According to the *Journal of the American Institute of Homeopathy*, 1909, under the treatment of Dr. Henry Klopp at Westborough Hospital for the Insane, dementia praecox had a recovery rate 20.83% for hebephrenia, 42.3% for katatonia, and 25% for dementia paranoid. All totaled together there was a 29.36% average recovery rate for dementia praecox (p. 327). Also, in "An Osteopathic Study of 646 Cases of Mental Derangement" published in the *Journal of the American Osteopathic Association (December 1919)* found that paranoia had a 50% recovery rate at the Still-Hildreth Sanatorium(Gerdine, 1919).

In 1926 the Chiropractic Psychopathic Sanitarium better known as Forest Park Sanitarium, in Davenport, Iowa, had recovery rates of up to 81% for male patients and 71% for female patients. These figures included both full recovery and partial recovery (Chiropractic Sanitarium News, 1926)[2]. In 1952 the Clear View Sanitarium, also in Davenport, Iowa had published a recovery rate of 70% for schizophrenic patients and 33% for affective disorders

---

[2] Chiropractic Sanitarium News is a publication that came from Courtesy of Special Services, Palmer College of Chiropractic

(Quigley, 1973, p. 116)[3]. The osteopathic Still-Hildreth Sanatorium in 1933 had a 36% recovery rate for dementia praecox, and a 67% recovery rate for manic depressives (Ching, 2015).

Comparing these figures to modern figures on the recovery rates of patients on psychotropic drugs—in particular antipsychotics and mood stabilizers—they are much poorer. On July 31st 1900, in the *Biennial Report of the Board of Trustees and Officers*, 1898, Fergus Falls State Hospital for the Insane reported a recovery rate for manic depressives of 76 committed, 43 recovered, 14 improved. This is a functional recovery rate of 56.5% and a partial recovery rate of 18.4% (p. 177). The Westborough State Hospital for the Insane reported in the *Twenty-Seventh Annual Report of the Trustees of the Westborough State Hospital, November 30, 1911*, that a total of 70 patients committed, 43 recovered, 8 capable of self-support, 6 improved. This is a respective functional recovery rate of 61.42% and a total average partial recovery rate of 18.4% for manic depression (p. 39). Again printed in the *Annual Report of the Trustees of the Westborough State Hospital, November 30, 1927*, were reports for the Westborough State Hospital for the Insane. They had reported out of a total of 60 patients, 33 recovered and 20 improved (p. 29). This is a functional recovery rate of 55% and an average partial recovery rate of 33.3%.

Functional recovery rates for bipolar manic depression are lower today then before lithium carbonate and the use of other mood stabilizers and antipsychotics. According to a two year syndromal and functional recovery study in the *American Journal of Psychiatry* (2000)—functional recovery 2 years after hospitalization was 37.6% (Tohen, 2000). Another study done in the *American Journal of Psychiatry* (2003) by 2 years, patients achieved only 43% functional recovery after hospitalization (Tohen, 2003). A study in *European Neuropsychopharmacology* (2011) showed that at 2 years, patients achieved a 34% functional recovery rate (Haro, 2011).

Today, we have a recurrence rate of 1 year at 42.4% and 2 years at 61%, according to one study done on bipolar patients in the journal *Psychiatry Research* (2014). In this summary, the author has no data on the recurrence rate of mania, or depression in bipolar patients from historical data, however studies on hospital readmission rates may shed some light on today's environment compared to the past. A study done in the *Canadian Journal of Psychiatry* in 2013 reported that readmission after psychiatric hospitalization ranged from 39% to 89% (median 73%). In the *Annual Report of the Managers of the Middletown State Homeopathic Hospital at Middletown N.Y., to the State Commission of Lunacy*—readmission rates were reported as 66 patients readmitted, and there were 220 first admissions. Out of 66 patients being readmitted this would be a 30% readmission rate for the year 1926.

In 1927, the Westborough Hospital for the Insane reported functional recovery rates for dementia praecox at an average of 29.89%. They reported a total of 97 committed, 29 recovered, and 44 improved. Having an average total partial recovery rate of 45.36%--this was reported in the *Annual Report of the Trustees of the Westborough State Hospital, November 30, 1927 (p. 29)*. In 1933, Fred Still compared the results of patients treated with schizophrenia at Still-Hildreth

---

[3] Quigley, W.H., "Physiological Psychology of Chiropractic in Mental Disorders", Mental Health and Chiropractic, edited by Herman C. Schwartz, D.C. (New Hyde Park, N.Y., Sessions Publishers, 1973), p. 116 is Courtesy of Special Services, Palmer College of Chiropractic

Sanatorium with those at Colorado Psychopathic Hospital and reported 35% of patients with schizophrenia had total recovery (Ching, 2015). In the *Statistical Report of the Mental Patients Treated: March 1914 to March 1919 (p. 11)*, at the Still-Hilldreth Sanatorium it was reported that the recovery rate was 43% for dementia praecox (Hildreth, 1919). According to results from Fred Still in 1933, he said recovery rates were significantly better for dementia praecox during the first 6 months of treatment (68%) and duration of illness correlated to recovery rate. Resulting recovery rates at 6 months to 1 year were 48%, and from 1 to 2 years, at 29%. For duration over two years the recovery rate fell to 20% (Still, 1933).

According to a study published in *Schizophrenia Research* October, (2011), only 10% of patients had recovery at 6 months being treated with psychotropic drugs, and at 1 year recovery was at 1%, with a 22% symptom remission rate (Ventura, 2011). A study in the *American Journal of Psychiatry* (2004) claims the full recovery rate criteria at 2 years or longer for schizophrenics was only met in 13.7% of subjects in their study (Robinson, 2004). One study done in *Schizophrenia Research* (2011), shows that recovery rates adjusted at 15 years are 16.3% average for schizophrenia (Ventura, 2011). Another study done by Harrow in the *Journal of Nervous and Mental Disease* (2007) report a 5% recovery rate over 15 years and another done by Wunderink in *JAMA Psychiatry* (2013) report a 17.6% recovery rate for 7 year follow-up of first episode schizophrenics (Harrow, 2007, & Wunderink, 2013). This may not be a full review of all the studies done on the recovery rates of antipsychotic drugs; however these figures clearly show this paradigm of health care is not working and it's a myth that these drugs revolutionized modern treatment of mental illness. If anything we went backwards 70 plus years since the introduction of Thorazine.

References

Countercultural Healing: A Brief History of Alternative Medicine in America

1. James Whorton M.D., The Alternative Fix - Clash | FRONTLINE | PBS

Pbs.org,. 2015. 'The Alternative Fix - Clash | FRONTLINE | PBS'. Accessed April 30
2015. http://www.pbs.org/wgbh/pages/frontline/show

Prevalence and Most Common Types of CAM Medicine used in the Treatment of Serious Mental Illness

1. .Atmaca, Murad, Ertan Tezcan, Murat Kuloglu, Bilal Ustundag, and Ozlem Kirtas. "The Effect of Extract of Ginkgo Biloba Addition to Olanzapine on Therapeutic Effect and Antioxidant Enzyme Levels in Patients with Schizophrenia." Psychiatry and Clinical Neurosciences 59, no. 6 (December 2005): 652–56. doi:10.1111/j.1440-1819.2005.01432.x.

2. Babić, Dragan, and Romana Babić. "Complementary and Alternative Medicine in the Treatment of Schizophrenia." Psychiatria Danubina 21, no. 3 (September 2009): 376–81.

3. Behzadi, A. H., Z. Omrani, M. Chalian, S. Asadi, and M. Ghadiri. "Folic Acid Efficacy as an Alternative Drug Added to Sodium Valproate in the Treatment of Acute Phase of Mania in Bipolar Disorder: A Double-Blind Randomized Controlled Trial." Acta Psychiatrica Scandinavica 120, no. 6 (December 2009): 441–45. doi:10.1111/j.1600-0447.2009.01368.x.

4. Beitman, B. D., and D. L. Dunner. "L-Tryptophan in the Maintenance Treatment of Bipolar II Manic-Depressive Illness." The American Journal of Psychiatry 139, no. 11 (November 1982): 1498–99.

5. Berk, Michael, David Copolov, Olivia Dean, Kristy Lu, Sue Jeavons, Ian Schapkaitz, Murray Anderson-Hunt, et al. "N-Acetyl Cysteine as a Glutathione Precursor for Schizophrenia--a Double-Blind, Randomized, Placebo-Controlled Trial." Biological Psychiatry 64, no. 5 (September 1, 2008): 361–68. doi:10.1016/j.biopsych.2008.03.004.

6. Berk, Michael, Olivia Dean, Sue M. Cotton, Clarissa S. Gama, Flavio Kapczinski, Brisa S. Fernandes, Kristy Kohlmann, et al. "The Efficacy of N-Acetylcysteine as an Adjunctive Treatment in Bipolar Depression: An Open Label Trial." Journal of Affective Disorders 135, no. 1–3 (December 2011): 389–94. doi:10.1016/j.jad.2011.06.005.

7. Bhat, Amritha S., K. Srinivasan, Sunita Simon Kurpad, and Ravindra B. Galgali. "Psychiatric Presentations of Vitamin B 12 Deficiency." Journal of the Indian Medical Association 105, no. 7 (July 2007): 395–96.

8. Brewerton, T. D., and V. I. Reus. "Lithium Carbonate and L-Tryptophan in the Treatment of Bipolar and Schizoaffective Disorders." The American Journal of Psychiatry 140, no. 6 (June 1983): 757–60.

9. Brooks, S. C., L. D'Angelo, A. Chalmeta, G. Ahern, and J. H. Judson. "An Unusual Schizophrenic Illness Responsive to Pyridoxine HCl (B6) Subsequent to Phenothiazine and Butyrophenone Toxicities." Biological Psychiatry 18, no. 11 (November 1983): 1321–28.

10. Brown, C. H. Use Of Practitioner-Based Alternative Therapies By Psychiatric Outpatients: Psychiatric Services: Vol 56, No 11'. 2015. Psychiatric Services. http://ps.psychiatryonline.org/doi/full/10.1176/a

11. Bucci, L. "Pyridoxine and Schizophrenia." The British Journal of Psychiatry: The Journal of Mental Science 122, no. 567 (February 1973): 240.

12. Bulut, Mahmut, Haluk Asuman Savas, Abdurrahman Altindag, Osman Virit, and Alican Dalkilic. "Beneficial Effects of N-Acetylcysteine in Treatment Resistant Schizophrenia." The World Journal of Biological Psychiatry: The Official Journal of the World Federation of Societies of Biological Psychiatry 10, no. 4 Pt 2 (2009): 626–28. doi:10.1080/15622970903144004.

13. Cade, R., Privette, M., Fregly, M., Rowland, N., Sun, Z. J., Zele, V., ... & Edelstein, C. (2000). Autism and schizophrenia: intestinal disorders. Nutritional Neuroscience, 3(1), 57-72.

14. Chouinard, G., S. N. Young, and L. Annable. "A Controlled Clinical Trial of L-Tryptophan in Acute Mania." Biological Psychiatry 20, no. 5 (May 1985): 546–57.

15. Cohen, B. M., A. L. Miller, J. F. Lipinski, and H. G. Pope. "Lecithin in Mania: A Preliminary Report." The American Journal of Psychiatry 137, no. 2 (February 1980): 242–43.

16. Cohen, B. M., J. F. Lipinski, and R. I. Altesman. "Lecithin in the Treatment of Mania: Double-Blind, Placebo-Controlled Trials." The American Journal of Psychiatry 139, no. 9 (September 1982): 1162–64.

17. Cooke, Robert G., and Robert D. Levitan. "Tryptophan for Refractory Bipolar Spectrum Disorder and Sleep-Phase Delay." Journal of Psychiatry & Neuroscience: JPN 35, no. 2 (March 2010): 144.

18. Dohan, F. C., and J. C. Grasberger. "Relapsed Schizophrenics: Earlier Discharge from the Hospital after Cereal-Free, Milk-Free Diet." The American Journal of Psychiatry 130, no. 6 (June 1973): 685–88.

19. Dohan, F. C., J. C. Grasberger, F. M. Lowell, H. T. Johnston, and A. W. Arbegast. "Relapsed Schizophrenics: More Rapid Improvement on a Milk- and Cereal-Free Diet." The British Journal of Psychiatry: The Journal of Mental Science 115, no. 522 (May 1969): 595–96.

20. Doruk, Ali, Ozcan Uzun, and Aytekin Ozşahin. "A Placebo-Controlled Study of Extract of Ginkgo Biloba Added to Clozapine in Patients with Treatment-Resistant Schizophrenia." International Clinical Psychopharmacology 23, no. 4 (July 2008): 223–27. doi:10.1097/YIC.0b013e3282fcff2f.

21. Emsley, Robin, Piet Oosthuizen, and Susan J. van Rensburg. "Clinical Potential of Omega-3 Fatty Acids in the Treatment of Schizophrenia." CNS Drugs 17, no. 15 (2003): 1081–91.

22. Frazier, Elisabeth A., Barbara Gracious, L. Eugene Arnold, Mark Failla, Chureeporn Chitchumroonchokchai, Diane Habash, and Mary A. Fristad. "Nutritional and Safety Outcomes from an Open-Label Micronutrient Intervention for Pediatric Bipolar Spectrum Disorders." Journal of Child and Adolescent Psychopharmacology 23, no. 8 (October 2013): 558–67. doi:10.1089/cap.2012.0098.

23. Gately, Dermot, and Bonnie J. Kaplan. "Database Analysis of Adults with Bipolar Disorder Consuming a Micronutrient Formula." Clinical Medicine: Psychiatry 2 (2009).

24. Godfrey, P. S., B. K. Toone, M. W. Carney, T. G. Flynn, T. Bottiglieri, M. Laundy, I. Chanarin, and E. H. Reynolds. "Enhancement of Recovery from Psychiatric Illness by Methylfolate." Lancet 336, no. 8712 (August 18, 1990): 392–95.

25. Hazra, Monica "Complementary and Alternative Medicine in Psychotic Disorders : Journal of Complementary and Integrative Medicine." Accessed March 24, 2015. http://www.degruyter.com/view/j/jcim.2010.7.1/jcim.2010.7.1.1239/jcim.2010.7.1.1239.xml

26. Heresco-Levy, U., D. C. Javitt, M. Ermilov, C. Mordel, A. Horowitz, and D. Kelly. "Double-Blind, Placebo-Controlled, Crossover Trial of Glycine Adjuvant Therapy for Treatment-Resistant Schizophrenia." The British Journal of Psychiatry: The Journal of Mental Science 169, no. 5 (November 1996): 610–17.

27. Heresco-Levy, U., D. C. Javitt, M. Ermilov, C. Mordel, G. Silipo, and M. Lichtenstein. "Efficacy of High-Dose Glycine in the Treatment of Enduring Negative Symptoms of Schizophrenia." Archives of General Psychiatry 56, no. 1 (January 1999): 29–36.

28. Jackson, Jessica, William Eaton, Nicola Cascella, Alessio Fasano, Dale Warfel, Stephanie Feldman, Charles Richardson, et al. "A Gluten-Free Diet in People with Schizophrenia and Anti-Tissue Transglutaminase or Anti-Gliadin Antibodies." Schizophrenia Research 140, no. 1–3 (September 2012): 262–63. doi:10.1016/j.schres.2012.06.011.

29. Jamilian, Hamidreza, Hasan Solhi, and Mehri Jamilian. "Randomized, Placebo-Controlled Clinical Trial of Omega-3 as Supplemental Treatment in Schizophrenia." Global Journal of Health Science 6, no. 7 Spec No (2014): 103–8. doi:10.5539/gjhs.v6n7p103.

30. Javitt, D. C., I. Zylberman, S. R. Zukin, U. Heresco-Levy, and J. P. Lindenmayer. "Amelioration of Negative Symptoms in Schizophrenia by Glycine." The American Journal of Psychiatry 151, no. 8 (August 1994): 1234–36.

31. Kilbourne, Amy M., Laurel A. Copeland, John E. Zeber, Mark S. Bauer, Elaine Lasky, and Chester B. Good. "Determinants of Complementary and Alternative Medicine Use by Patients with Bipolar Disorder." Psychopharmacology Bulletin 40, no. 3 (2007): 104–15.

32. Kim, Tae Ho, and Seok Woo Moon. "Serum Homocysteine and Folate Levels in Korean Schizophrenic Patients." Psychiatry Investigation 8, no. 2 (June 2011): 134–40. doi:10.4306/pi.2011.8.2.134.

33. Knable, Michael B. "Extract of Ginkgo Biloba Added to Haloperidol Was Effective for Positive Symptoms in Refractory Schizophrenia." Evidence-Based Mental Health 5, no. 3 (August 2002): 90.

34. Kuo, Shin-Chang, Chin-Bin Yeh, Yi-Wei Yeh, and Nian-Sheng Tzeng. "Schizophrenia-like Psychotic Episode Precipitated by Cobalamin Deficiency." General Hospital Psychiatry 31, no. 6 (December 2009): 586–88. doi:10.1016/j.genhosppsych.2009.02.003.

35. Lee, Mei-Yi, Chun-Cheng Chiang, Hong-Yi Chiu, Ming-Huan Chan, and Hwei-Hsien Chen. "N-Acetylcysteine Modulates Hallucinogenic 5-HT(2A) Receptor Agonist-Mediated Responses: Behavioral, Molecular, and Electrophysiological Studies." Neuropharmacology 81 (June 2014): 215–23. doi:10.1016/j.neuropharm.2014.02.006.

36. Levkovitz, Yechiel, Orna Ophir-Shaham, Yuval Bloch, Ilan Treves, Shmuel Fennig, and Ettie Grauer. "Effect of L-Tryptophan on Memory in Patients with Schizophrenia." The Journal of Nervous and Mental Disease 191, no. 9 (September 2003): 568–73. doi:10.1097/01.nmd.0000087182.29781.e0.

37. Magalhães, P. V., O. M. Dean, A. I. Bush, D. L. Copolov, G. S. Malhi, K. Kohlmann, S. Jeavons, I. Schapkaitz, M. Anderson-Hunt, and M. Berk. "N-Acetyl Cysteine Add-on Treatment for Bipolar II Disorder: A Subgroup Analysis of a Randomized Placebo-Controlled Trial." Journal of Affective Disorders 129, no. 1–3 (March 2011): 317–20. doi:10.1016/j.jad.2010.08.001.

38. Masalha, R., B. Chudakov, M. Muhamad, I. Rudoy, I. Volkov, and I. Wirguin. "Cobalamin-Responsive Psychosis as the Sole Manifestation of Vitamin B12 Deficiency." The Israel Medical Association Journal: IMAJ 3, no. 9 (September 2001): 701–3.

39. Montgomery, P., and A. J. Richardson. "Omega-3 Fatty Acids for Bipolar Disorder." The Cochrane Database of Systematic Reviews, no. 2 (2008): CD005169. doi:10.1002/14651858.CD005169.pub2.

40. Morand, C., S. N. Young, and F. R. Ervin. "Clinical Response of Aggressive Schizophrenics to Oral Tryptophan." Biological Psychiatry 18, no. 5 (May 1983): 575–78.

41. Potkin, S. G., D. Weinberger, J. Kleinman, H. Nasrallah, D. Luchins, L. Bigelow, M. Linnoila, et al. "Wheat Gluten Challenge in Schizophrenic Patients." The American Journal of Psychiatry 138, no. 9 (September 1981): 1208–11.

42. Rajkumar, A. P., and P. Jebaraj. "Chronic Psychosis Associated with Vitamin B12 Deficiency." The Journal of the Association of Physicians of India 56 (February 2008): 115–16.

43. Reddy, R., S. Fleet-Michaliszyn, R. Condray, J. K. Yao, M. S. Keshavan, and R. Reddy. "Reduction in Perseverative Errors with Adjunctive Ethyl-Eicosapentaenoic Acid in Patients with Schizophrenia: Preliminary Study." Prostaglandins, Leukotrienes, and Essential Fatty Acids 84, no. 3–4 (April 2011): 79–83. doi:10.1016/j.plefa.2010.12.001.

44. Rice, J. R., C. H. Ham, and W. E. Gore. "Another Look at Gluten in Schizophrenia." The American Journal of Psychiatry 135, no. 11 (November 1978): 1417–18.

45. Richardson, A. J., T. Easton, J. H. Gruzelier, and B. K. Puri. "Laterality Changes Accompanying Symptom Remission in Schizophrenia Following Treatment with Eicosapentaenoic Acid." International Journal of Psychophysiology: Official Journal of the International Organization of Psychophysiology 34, no. 3 (December 1999): 333–39.

46. Robertson, J. M., and P. E. Tanguay. "Case Study: The Use of Melatonin in a Boy with Refractory Bipolar Disorder." Journal of the American Academy of Child and Adolescent Psychiatry 36, no. 6 (June 1997): 822–25. doi:10.1097/00004583-199706000-00020.

47. Rosenberg, G. S., and K. L. Davis. "The Use of Cholinergic Precursors in Neuropsychiatric Diseases." The American Journal of Clinical Nutrition 36, no. 4 (October 1, 1982): 709–20.

48. Rosse, R. B., S. K. Theut, M. Banay-Schwartz, M. Leighton, E. Scarcella, C. G. Cohen, and S. I. Deutsch. "Glycine Adjuvant Therapy to Conventional Neuroleptic Treatment in Schizophrenia: An Open-Label, Pilot Study." Clinical Neuropharmacology 12, no. 5 (October 1989): 416–24.

49. Ross-Smith, P., and F. A. Jenner. "Diet (gluten) and Schizophrenia." Journal of Human Nutrition 34, no. 2 (April 1980): 107–12.

50. Rucklidge, Julia J., and Rachel Harrison. "Successful Treatment of Bipolar Disorder II and ADHD with a Micronutrient Formula: A Case Study." CNS Spectrums 15, no. 5 (May 2010): 289–95.

51. Russinova, Zlatka, Nancy J. Wewiorski, and Dane Cash. "Use of Alternative Health Care Practices by Persons with Serious Mental Illness: Perceived Benefits." American Journal of Public Health 92, no. 10 (October 2002): 1600–1603.

52. Sagduyu, Kemal, Mehmet E. Dokucu, Bruce A. Eddy, Gerald Craigen, Claudia F. Baldassano, and Aysegül Yildiz. "Omega-3 Fatty Acids Decreased Irritability of Patients with Bipolar Disorder in an Add-On, Open Label Study." Nutrition Journal 4 (2005): 6. doi:10.1186/1475-2891-4-6.

53. Sarris, Jerome, David Mischoulon, and Isaac Schweitzer. "Omega-3 for Bipolar Disorder: Meta-Analyses of Use in Mania and Bipolar Depression." The Journal of Clinical Psychiatry 73, no. 1 (January 2012): 81–86. doi:10.4088/JCP.10r06710.

54. Schreier, H. A. "Mania Responsive to Lecithin in a 13-Year-Old Girl." The American Journal of Psychiatry 139, no. 1 (January 1982): 108–10.

55. Shamir, E., M. Laudon, Y. Barak, Y. Anis, V. Rotenberg, A. Elizur, and N. Zisapel. "Melatonin Improves Sleep Quality of Patients with Chronic Schizophrenia." The Journal of Clinical Psychiatry 61, no. 5 (May 2000): 373–77.

56. Shiloh, R., A. Weizman, N. Weizer, P. Dorfman-Etrog, and H. Munitz. "[Antidepressive effect of pyridoxine (vitamin B6) in neuroleptic-treated schizophrenic patients with co-morbid minor depression--preliminary open-label trial]." Harefuah 140, no. 5 (May 2001): 369–73, 456.

57. Singh, Vidhi, Surendra P. Singh, and Kelvin Chan. "Review and Meta-Analysis of Usage of Ginkgo as an Adjunct Therapy in Chronic Schizophrenia." The International Journal of Neuropsychopharmacology / Official Scientific Journal of the Collegium Internationale Neuropsychopharmacologicum (CINP) 13, no. 2 (March 2010): 257–71. doi:10.1017/S1461145709990654.

58. Strejilevich, S. A., M. J. Sarmiento, M. Scápola, L. Gil, D. J. Martino, J. F. Gil, and C. Gómez-Restrepo. "Complementary and Alternative Medicines Usage in Bipolar Patients from Argentina and Colombia: Associations with Satisfaction and Adherence to Treatment." Journal of Affective Disorders 149, no. 1–3 (July 2013): 393–97. doi:10.1016/j.jad.2012.08.029.

59. Strzelecki, Dominik, and Jolanta Rabe-Jabłońska. "[Changes in positive and negative symptoms, general psychopathology in schizophrenic patients during augmentation of antipsychotics with glycine: a preliminary 10-week open-label study]." Psychiatria Polska 45, no. 6 (December 2011): 825–37.

60. Strzelecki, Dominik, Paweł Kropiwnicki, and Jolanta Rabe-Jabłońska. "[Augmentation of antipsychotics with glycine may ameliorate depressive and extrapyramidal symptoms in schizophrenic patients--a preliminary 10-week open-label study]." Psychiatria Polska 47, no. 4 (August 2013): 609–20.

61. Suresh Kumar, P. N., Chittaranjan Andrade, Savita G. Bhakta, and Nagendra M. Singh. "Melatonin in Schizophrenic Outpatients with Insomnia: A Double-Blind, Placebo-Controlled Study." The Journal of Clinical Psychiatry 68, no. 2 (February 2007): 237–41.

62. Turnbull, Teresa, Mary Cullen-Drill, and Arlene Smaldone. "Efficacy of Omega-3 Fatty Acid Supplementation on Improvement of Bipolar Symptoms: A Systematic Review." Archives of Psychiatric Nursing 22, no. 5 (October 2008): 305–11. doi:10.1016/j.apnu.2008.02.011.

63. Waziri, R. "Glycine Therapy of Schizophrenia: Some Caveats." Biological Psychiatry 39, no. 3 (February 1, 1996): 155–56. doi:10.1016/0006-3223(95)00586-2.

64. Zhang, X. Y., D. F. Zhou, P. Y. Zhang, G. Y. Wu, J. M. Su, and L. Y. Cao. "A Double-Blind, Placebo-Controlled Trial of Extract of Ginkgo Biloba Added to Haloperidol in Treatment-Resistant Patients with Schizophrenia." The Journal of Clinical Psychiatry 62, no. 11 (November 2001): 878–83.

Evaluating Evidence-based Medicine: How to Appraise a Journal Article

1. Altman, D G. "Statistics and Ethics in Medical Research: III How Large a Sample?" British Medical Journal 281, no. 6251 (November 15, 1980): 1336–38.

2. Carta, Mauro Giovanni, Maria Carolina Hardoy, Bernardo Carpiniello, Andrea Murru, Anna Rita Marci, Fiora Carbone, Luca Deiana, Mariangela Cadeddu, and Stefano Mariotti. "A Case Control Study on Psychiatric Disorders in Hashimoto Disease and Euthyroid Goitre: Not Only Depressive but Also Anxiety Disorders Are Associated with Thyroid Autoimmunity." Clinical Practice and Epidemiology in Mental Health: CP & EMH 1 (November 10, 2005): 23. doi:10.1186/1745-0179-1-23.

3. Daly, L E. "Confidence Intervals and Sample Sizes: Don't Throw out All Your Old Sample Size Tables." BMJ : British Medical Journal 302, no. 6772 (February 9, 1991): 333–36.

4. Fowkes, F G, and P M Fulton. "Critical Appraisal of Published Research: Introductory Guidelines." BMJ : British Medical Journal 302, no. 6785 (May 11, 1991): 1136–40.

5. Greenhalgh, T. 2001, How to read a paper : the basics of evidence based medicine / Trisha Greenhalgh BMJ Books.

6. Huth, E. J. "Structured Abstracts for Papers Reporting Clinical Trials." Annals of Internal Medicine 106, no. 4 (April 1987): 626–27.

7. Lock, S. "Structured Abstracts." BMJ (Clinical Research Ed.) 297, no. 6642 (July 16, 1988): 156.

8. Patton, George C., Carolyn Coffey, John B. Carlin, Louisa Degenhardt, Michael Lynskey, and Wayne Hall. "Cannabis Use and Mental Health in Young People: Cohort Study." BMJ (Clinical Research Ed.) 325, no. 7374 (November 23, 2002): 1195–98.

9. UCL, "Critical appraisal of a journal article" Friends of the Children of Great Ormond Street Library, 2011

Cannabis for Treating Psychiatric Problems? A Clear Yes, Maybe.

---

1. Hall, Will. 2015. 'Cannabis For Treating Psychiatric Problems? A Clear Yes, Maybe. - Mad In America'. Mad In America. Accessed August 28 2015. http://www.madinamerica.com/2015/08/interest-in-marijuana-for-treating-psychiatric-problems-maybe/.

Conclusion

---

1. Cardinal, Rudolf N., and Edward T. Bullmore. The Diagnosis of Psychosis. 1 edition. Cambridge, UK ; New York: Cambridge University Press, 2011.

2. Durrant, Andrea R., Uriel Heresco-Levy, Andrea R. Durrant, and Uriel Heresco-Levy. "D-Serine in Neuropsychiatric Disorders: New Advances, D-Serine in Neuropsychiatric Disorders: New Advances." *Advances in Psychiatry, Advances in Psychiatry* 2014, 2014 (June 19, 2014): e859735. doi:10.1155/2014/859735, 10.1155/2014/859735.

3. Jackson, MD Grace E. *Rethinking Psychiatric Drugs: A Guide for Informed Consent*. Bloomington, Ind: AuthorHouse, 2005.

4. Lacasse, Jeffrey R, and Jonathan Leo. "Serotonin and Depression: A Disconnect between the Advertisements and the Scientific Literature." *PLoS Med* 2, no. 12 (November 8, 2005): e392. doi:10.1371/journal.pmed.0020392.

5. Lane, Hsien-Yuan, Yi-Ching Liu, Chieh-Liang Huang, Yue-Cune Chang, Chun-Hui Liau, Cheng-Hwang Perng, and Guochuan E. Tsai. "Sarcosine (N-Methylglycine) Treatment for Acute Schizophrenia: A Randomized, Double-Blind Study." *Biological Psychiatry* 63, no. 1 (January 1, 2008): 9–12. doi:10.1016/j.biopsych.2007.04.038.

6. LCSW, Jill Littrell PhD. *Neuroscience for Psychologists and Other Mental Health Professionals: Promoting Well-Being and Treating Mental Illness.* Springer Publishing Company, 2015.

7. Lee, M. S., B.-C. Shin, P. Ronan, and E. Ernst. "Acupuncture for Schizophrenia: A Systematic Review and Meta-Analysis." *International Journal of Clinical Practice* 63, no. 11 (November 2009): 1622–33. doi:10.1111/j.1742-1241.2009.02167.x.

8. Peet, M., J. Brind, C. N. Ramchand, S. Shah, and G. K. Vankar. "Two Double-Blind Placebo-Controlled Pilot Studies of Eicosapentaenoic Acid in the Treatment of Schizophrenia." *Schizophrenia Research* 49, no. 3 (April 30, 2001): 243–51.

9. Purohit, Maulik P., Ross D. Zafonte, Laura M. Sherman, Roger B. Davis, Michelle Y. Giwerc, Martha E. Shenton, and Gloria Y. Yeh. "Neuropsychiatric Symptoms and Expenditure on Complementary and Alternative Medicine." *The Journal of Clinical Psychiatry* 76, no. 7 (July 2015): e870–76. doi:10.4088/JCP.13m08682.

10. Whitaker, Robert, and Lisa Cosgrove. *Psychiatry Under the Influence: Institutional Corruption, Social Injury, and Prescriptions for Reform.* New York: Palgrave Macmillan, 2015.

11. Whitaker, Robert. *Anatomy of an Epidemic: Magic Bullets, Psychiatric Drugs, and the Astonishing Rise of Mental Illness in America.* 1 edition. New York: Crown, 2010.

12. Wozniak, Janet, Joseph Biederman, Eric Mick, James Waxmonsky, Liisa Hantsoo, Catherine Best, Joanne E. Cluette-Brown, and Michael Laposata. "Omega-3 Fatty Acid Monotherapy for Pediatric Bipolar Disorder: A Prospective Open-Label Trial." *European Neuropsychopharmacology: The Journal of the European College of Neuropsychopharmacology* 17, no. 6–7 (June 2007): 440–47. doi:10.1016/j.euroneuro.2006.11.006.

13. Zhang, L. D., Y. H. Tang, W. B. Zhu, and S. H. Xu. "Comparative Study of Schizophrenia Treatment with Electroacupuncture, Herbs and Chlorpromazine." *Chinese Medical Journal* 100, no. 2 (February 1987): 152–57.

14. Zipursky, Robert B., Thomas J. Reilly, and Robin M. Murray. "The Myth of Schizophrenia as a Progressive Brain Disease." *Schizophrenia Bulletin* 39, no. 6 (November 2013): 1363–72. doi:10.1093/schbul/sbs135.

1. Stargrove, Mitchell Bebel, Jonathan Treasure, and Dwight L. McKee. 2008. Herb, nutrient, and drug interactions clinical implications and therapeutic strategies. St. Louis (Mo.): Mosby/Elsevier.

2. Hazra, Monica "Complementary and Alternative Medicine in Psychotic Disorders : Journal of Complementary and Integrative Medicine." Accessed March 24, 2015. http://www.degruyter.com/view/j/jcim.2010.7.1/jcim.2010.7.1.1239/jcim.2010.7.1.1239.xml

Appendix A: The First Antipsychotic: Rauwolfia Serpentina and Alkaloid Reserpine

1. Baumeister, Alan A., Mike F. Hawkins, and Sarah M. Uzelac. "The Myth of Reserpine-Induced Depression: Role in the Historical Development of the Monoamine Hypothesis." Journal of the History of the Neurosciences 12, no. 2 (June 2003): 207–20. doi:10.1076/jhin.12.2.207.15535.

2. Christison, G. W., D. G. Kirch, and R. J. Wyatt. "When Symptoms Persist: Choosing among Alternative Somatic Treatments for Schizophrenia." Schizophrenia Bulletin 17, no. 2 (1991): 217–45.

3. Colabawalla, H. M. "A Preliminary Report on the Lack of Toxicity of a Preparation of Tatal Rauwolfia Alkaloids." Journal of Neurology, Neurosurgery, and Psychiatry 21, no. 3 (August 1958): 213–15.

4. Dexaprine.org,. 2015. '<? Single_Post_Title(); ?>'. Accessed August 29 2015. http://www.dexaprine.org/ingredients/rauwolfia-serpentina.

5. Greenberg, William M. "Treatment Resistance in Schizophrenia: The Role of Alternative Therapies | Psychiatric Times," October 30, 2006. http://www.psychiatrictimes.com/articles/treatment-resistance-schizophrenia-role-alternative-therapies.

6. Healy, David, "Reserpine exhumed" British Journal of Psychiatry (1998), 172, 376-378

7. Himalayawellness.com,. 2015. 'Serpina By Himalaya Herbal Healthcare'. Accessed August 29 2015. http://www.himalayawellness.com/products/pharmaceuticals/serpina-tablet.htm.

8. Kline, N. S. "Use of Rauwolfia Serpentina Benth. in Neuropsychiatric Conditions." Annals of the New York Academy of Sciences 59, no. 1 (April 30, 1 954): 107–32.

9. López-Muñoz, F., V. S. Bhatara, C. Alamo, and E. Cuenca. "[Historical approach to reserpine discovery and its introduction in psychiatry]." Actas Españolas De Psiquiatría 32, no. 6 (December 2004): 387–95.

10. Melick, R., and M. Mcgregor. "Reserpine and Extracellular-Fluid Volume." *The New England Journal of Medicine* 256, no. 21 (May 23, 1957): 1000–1002. doi:10.1056/NEJM195705232562107.

11. Vakil, Rustom Jal. "A CLINICAL TRIAL OF RAUWOLFIA SERPENTINA IN ESSENTIAL HYPERTENSION." *British Heart Journal* 11, no. 4 (October 1949): 350–55.

Appendix B: The History and Therapeutic Benefits of Lithium Mineral Water and Lithium Supplementation in the Treatment of Bipolar Manic Depression

1. Baldessarini, Ross J., and Leonardo Tondo. "Litio en Psiquiatría. / Lithium in Psychiatry." Revista de Neuro-Psiquiatria 76, no. 4 (February 24, 2014): 189.

2. Doongaji, D. R., V. S. Jathar, and R. S. Satoskar. "Manic Depressive Psychosis in India and the Possible Role of Lithium as a Natural Prophylactic. I--Hypothesis." Journal of Postgraduate Medicine 26, no. 1 (January 1980): 34–38.

3. Georgotas, A., and S. Gershon. "Historical Perspectives and Current Highlights on Lithium Treatment in Manic-Depressive Illness." Journal of Clinical Psychopharmacology 1, no. 1 (January 1981): 27–31.

4. Jathar, V. S., P. R. Pendharkar, V. K. Pandey, S. J. Raut, D. R. Doongaji, M. P. Bharucha, and R. S. Satoskar. "Manic Depressive Psychosis in India and the Possible Role of Lithium as a Natural Prophylactic. II--Lithium Content of Diet and Some Biological Fluids in Indian Subjects." Journal of Postgraduate Medicine 26, no. 1 (January 1980): 39–44.

5. Jones, Ann. 2015. 'Lithium Aspartate Vs. Lithium Orotate | LIVESTRONG.COM'. LIVESTRONG.COM. Accessed June 6 2015. http://www.livestrong.com/article/316987-lithium-aspartate-vs-lithium-orotate/.

6. Kapusta, Nestor D., and Daniel König. "Naturally Occurring Low-Dose Lithium in Drinking Water." The Journal of Clinical Psychiatry 76, no. 3 (March 2015): e373–74.

7. Kapusta, Nestor D., Nilufar Mossaheb, Elmar Etzersdorfer, Gerald Hlavin, Kenneth Thau, Matthäus Willeit, Nicole Praschak-Rieder, Gernot Sonneck, and Katharina Leithner-Dziubas. "Lithium in Drinking Water and Suicide Mortality." *The British Journal of Psychiatry: The Journal of Mental Science* 198, no. 5 (May 2011): 346–50. doi:10.1192/bjp.bp.110.091041.

8. Lewis, Alan E., Lithium: Under-Appreciated Brain Nutrient and Protector. Pacificbiologic.com,. 2015. Accessed May 30 2015. https://www.pacificbiologic.com/sites/default/files/Lithium%20article.pdf.

9. Lithium Orotate Technical Data, Cpmedical.net,. 2015. Accessed June 6 2015. http://www.cpmedical.net/pdf/TS_CP724

10. Nieper, H.A., "The clinical applications of lithium orotate: A two years study." *Agressologie* 1973, 14, 6: 407-411

11. Ohgami, Hirochika, Takeshi Terao, Ippei Shiotsuki, Nobuyoshi Ishii, and Noboru Iwata. "Lithium Levels in Drinking Water and Risk of Suicide." *The British Journal of Psychiatry: The Journal of Mental Science* 194, no. 5 (May 2009): 464–65; discussion 446. doi:10.1192/bjp.bp.108.055798.

12. Sartori, H. E. "Lithium Orotate in the Treatment of Alcoholism and Related Conditions." *Alcohol* (Fayetteville, N.Y.) 3, no. 2 (April 1986): 97–100.

13. Schrauzer, G. N., and E. de Vroey. "Effects of Nutritional Lithium Supplementation on Mood. A Placebo-Controlled Study with Former Drug Users." *Biological Trace Element Research* 40, no. 1 (January 1994): 89–101.

14. Schrauzer, G. N., and K. P. Shrestha. "Lithium in Drinking Water and the Incidences of Crimes, Suicides, and Arrests Related to Drug Addictions." *Biological Trace Element Research* 25, no. 2 (May 1990): 105–13.

15. Schrauzer, Gerhard N. "Lithium: Occurrence, Dietary Intakes, Nutritional Essentiality." *Journal of the American College of Nutrition* 21, no. 1 (February 2002): 14–21.

16. Strobusch, A. D., and J. W. Jefferson. "The Checkered History of Lithium in Medicine." Pharmacy in History 22, no. 2 (1980): 72–76.

Appendix C: Unconventional Treatments in History that Outperformed Psychotropic Drugs of Today

1. (N.Y.), Middletown State Homeopathic Hospital. Annual Report of the Managers of the Middletown State Homeopathic Hospital at Middletown, N.Y. to the State Commission in Lunacy ..., 1919.

2. .Annual Report of the Trustees of the Westborough State Hospital, November 30, 1927. Report, 1918-30. 2015. 'Report 1918-30.'. Hathitrust. Accessed June 5 2015. http://babel.hathitrust.org/cgi/pt?id=uc1.b3034483;view=1up;seq=441.

3. Bhatara, V. S., J. N. Sharma, S. Gupta, and Y. K. Gupta. "Images in Psychiatry. Rauwolfia Serpentina: The First Herbal Antipsychotic." The American Journal of Psychiatry 154, no. 7 (July 1997): 894.

4. Borell, M. "Brown-Séquard's Organotherapy and Its Appearance in America at the End of the Nineteenth Century." Bulletin of the History of Medicine 50, no. 3 (1976): 309–20.

5. Bragdon, Emma 2015, Mad In America, http://www.madinamerica.com/2015/04/spiritist-psychiatric-hospitals-brazil/

6. Ching, M Leslie., "The Still-Hildreth Sanatorium: A History and Chart Review." AO Journal - Winter 2014, Digital.turn-page.com,. 2015. 'AAO Journal - Winter 2014'. Accessed March 13 2015. http://digital.turn-page.com/i/448559/11.

7. Cott, Allan, "Controlled Fasting Treatment for Schizophrenia." Journal of Orthomolecular Psychiatry, (1974) Orthomolecular.org, http://www.orthomolecular.org/library/jom/1974/pdf/1974-v03n04-p301.pdf

8. Faedda, T. Suppes, P. Gebre-Medhin, and B. M. Cohen. "Two-Year Syndromal and Functional Recovery in 219 Cases of First-Episode Major Affective Disorder with Psychotic Features." The American Journal of Psychiatry 157, no. 2 (February 2000): 220–28.

9. Gerdine, L Van Horn "An Osteopathic Study of 646 Cases of Mental Derangement" Journal of the American Osteopathic Association (December 1919) 128-131

10. Haro, J. M., C. Reed, A. Gonzalez-Pinto, D. Novick, J. Bertsch, E. Vieta, and EMBLEM Advisory Board. "2-Year Course of Bipolar Disorder Type I Patients in Outpatient Care: Factors Associated with Remission and Functional Recovery." European Neuropsychopharmacology: The Journal of the European College of Neuropsychopharmacology 21, no. 4 (April 2011): 287–93. doi:10.1016/j.euroneuro.2010.08.001.

11. Harrow. M. (2007). Factors involved in outcome and recovery in schizophrenia patients not on antipsychotic medication. Journal of Nervous and Mental Disease. 195, 406-414.

12. Hawkins, D. R., A. W. Bortin, and R. P. Runyon. "Orthomolecular Psychiatry: Niacin and Megavitamin Therapy." Psychosomatics 11, no. 5 (October 1970): 517–21. doi:10.1016/S0033-3182(70)71622-8.

13. Hildreth, Arthur G "Statistical Report of the Mental Patients Treated: March 1914 to March 1919" Still-Hildreth Osteopathic Sanatorium (1919) 1-23

14. Hillier, S. M., and Tony Jewell. 2013. Health Care and Traditional Medicine in China 1800-1982. Hoboken: Taylor and Francis. http://public.eblib.com/choice/publicfullrecord.aspx?p=1539200.

15. Hoffer, John "The Controversy Over Orthomolecular Therapy," Journal of Orthomolecular Psychiatry, (1974) Orthomolecular.org, http://orthomolecular.org/library/jom/1974/pdf/1974-v03n03-p167.pdf.

16. JOM, Orthomolecular.org,. 2015. 'Orthomolecular.Org-History of Orthomolecular Medicine'. Accessed June 5 2015. http://orthomolecular.org/history/. "By the end of the first week, the medicines they had been on were usually discontinued."

17. Journal of the American Institute of Homeopathy. Board of Trustees of the American Institute of Homeopathy, 1909.

18. Minnesota Board of trustees for the hospitals and asylums for the insane, Biennial Report of the Board of Trustees and Officers, 1892.

19. Minnesota Board of trustees for the hospitals and asylums for the insane,. Biennial Report of the Board of Trustees and Officers, 1898.

20. North American Journal of Homoeopathy, 1907

21. Quigley, W.H., "Physiological Psychology of Chiropractic in Mental Disorders", Mental Health and Chiropractic, edited by Herman C. Schwartz, D.C. (New Hyde Park, N.Y., Sessions Publishers, 1973), p. 116

22. Robinson, Delbert G., Margaret G. Woerner, Marjorie McMeniman, Alan Mendelowitz, and Robert M. Bilder. "Symptomatic and Functional Recovery from a First Episode of Schizophrenia or Schizoaffective Disorder." The American Journal of Psychiatry 161, no. 3 (March 2004): 473–79.

23. Still, F. M. "Comparison of Osteopathic and Allopathic Results in Dementia Praecox. 1933." The Journal of the American Osteopathic Association 100, no. 8 (August 2000): 501–2.

24. Tohen, Mauricio, Carlos A. Zarate, John Hennen, Hari-Mandir Kaur Khalsa, Stephen M. Strakowski, Priscilla Gebre-Medhin, Paola Salvatore, and Ross J. Baldessarini. "The McLean-Harvard First-Episode Mania Study: Prediction of Recovery and First Recurrence." The American Journal of Psychiatry 160, no. 12 (December 2003): 2099–2107.

25. Twenty-seventh Annual Report of the Trustees of the Westborough State Hospital, November 30, 1911. Report, 1910/11-1914/15. 2015. 'Report 1910/11-1914/15.'. Hathitrust. Accessed June 5 2015. http://babel.hathitrust.org/cgi/pt?id=uc1.b3034482;view=1up;seq=1.

26. Ventura, Joseph, Kenneth L. Subotnik, Lisa H. Guzik, Gerhard S. Hellemann, Michael J. Gitlin, Rachel C. Wood, and Keith H. Nuechterlein. "Remission and Recovery during the First Outpatient Year of the Early Course of Schizophrenia." Schizophrenia Research 132, no. 1 (October 2011): 18–23. doi:10.1016/j.schres.2011.06.025.

27. .Wunderink, L, Nieboer, R., Wiersma, D., Sytema, S., Nienhius, J.F. (2013). Recovery in Remitted First-Episode Psychosis at 7 Years of Follow-up of an Early Dose Reduction/Discontinuation or Maintenance Treatment Strategy: Long-term Follow-up of a 2-Year Randomized Clinical Trial. JAMA Psychiatry. 70(9), 913-920. doi:10.1001/jamapsychiatry.2013.19.

28. Young, Mary De. Encyclopedia of Asylum Therapeutics, 1750-1950s. McFarland, 2015

Author Index/General Index

C

M

494

Q

R

T

U

V

W

X

Y

Z

www.ingramcontent.com/pod-product-compliance
Lightning Source LLC
Chambersburg PA
CBHW080122220326

41598CB00032B/4924